现代肛肠病小针刀综合疗法(汉英对照)

Application of Comprehensive Acupuncture Scalpel Therapy to Coloproctology(annotated bilingual edition)

(中西医结合的成果和 10 项专利,附临床光盘)

(Achievements and 10 Patents of Integrated Traditional Chinese and Western Medicine with DVD)

田淇第　著译

王西墨　主审

Chinese Author：Tian Qidi，M.D.

English Translator：Tian Qidi，M.D.

Peer Reviewer：Wang Ximo，M.D.

U0339046

天津出版传媒集团

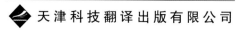

天津科技翻译出版有限公司

图书在版编目(CIP)数据

现代肛肠病小针刀综合疗法:汉英对照 / 田淇第著译. —天津:
天津科技翻译出版有限公司, 2013. 9
ISBN 978-7-5433-3281-2

Ⅰ.①现… Ⅱ.①田… Ⅲ.①肛门疾病—针刀疗法—汉、英
②直肠疾病—针刀疗法—汉、英 Ⅳ.① R245.31

中国版本图书馆 CIP 数据核字(2013)第 182354 号

出　　　版:天津科技翻译出版有限公司
出 版 人:刘 庆
地　　　址:天津市南开区白堤路 244 号
邮政编码:300192
电　　　话:022-87894896
传　　　真:022-87895650
网　　　址:www.tsttpc.com
印　　　刷:天津泰宇印务有限公司
发　　　行:全国新华书店
版本记录:787×1092　16 开本　21.5 印张　450 千字　彩插 1 印张
　　　　　2013 年 9 月第 1 版　2013 年 9 月第 1 次印刷
　　　　　定价:90.00 元

著 者 简 介

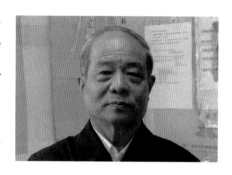

田淇第　男，汉族，1942 年 12 月出生于天津市，毕业于天津医学院和天津中医学院。天津市南开医院肛肠科主任，兼任北京中医药大学和北京高等中医学校教授、中国微型刀学会理事。从医 50 余年，在中医西结合治疗肛肠病方面取得突出成就，尤其是在微创小针刀综合疗法研究与应用技术方面获得 10 项专利，使肛肠病从以往的开放性大手术变为闭合性的微创手术。即采用小针刀专利技术挑、割、拨、刺、切方法，配合弯枪头负压、吸力套扎枪和外痔贴外敷纯中药治疗多种肛肠疾病，并获得国家级金奖、华佗杯一等奖、国外医学界的金奖等。发表论文 30 余篇，获发明专利 10 项。肛肠手术用多功能小针刀、肛肠激光小针刀、圆头缺口电池灯肛门镜、肛肠多功能手术治疗床等项技术是中西医结合的结晶，开创了中国特色微创肛肠外科的先例。

Tian Qidi, male, the Han nationality, born in Tianjin, in December, 1942, graduated from Tianjin Medical College and Tianjin Traditional Chinese Medical College, was a chief surgeon in Tianjin Nankai Hospital and a university professor in Beijing Traditional Chinese Medicine University and Beijing Higher Junior Traditional Chinese Medical College, a council in China Minimal Type Scalpel Association. He has been working as a doctor for 50 years, won out great achievement in coloproctology with the therapy of integrated traditional Chinese and Western medicine, especially got 10 patents for studying and applying comprehensive acupuncture scalpel therapy to minimally invasive surgical field. The diseases in anus, anal canal, rectum and colon are treated by the patent technique of acupuncture scalpel, such as puncturing, slicing, hooking, cutting and pricking at the same time combined angle head loop ligating gun with negative

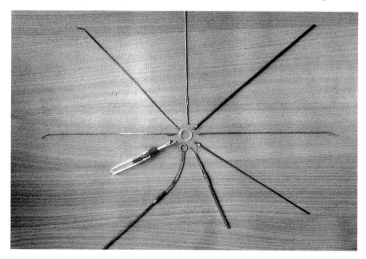

pressure –vacuum suction, herbs and laser. He has won a national gold medal, first prize of HuaTuo Cup and international gold prize. He has published 30 papers. These successful pioneering works are resplendent crystal of integrated traditional Chinese and Western medicine further to create a new epoch with Chinese characteristics in coloproctology.

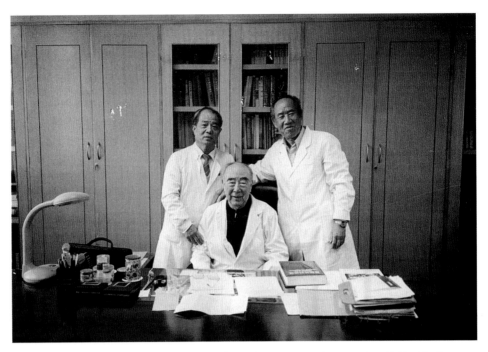

田淇第教授(左)、吴咸中院士(中)与专程学习小针刀疗法王名凡教授(美国)
Professor Tian Qidi (left), Academician Wu Xianzhong (middle) and Professor Wang Mingfan(right, special-purpose trip to study acupuncture scalpel therapy from U.S.A.)

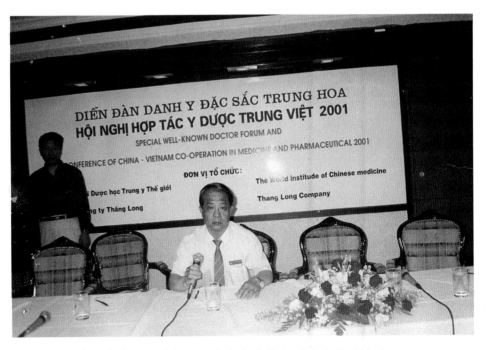

田淇第教授在越南中西医结合国际大会上宣讲肛肠病小针刀疗法
Professor Tian Qidi is giving lectures on applying Acupuncture Scalpel therapy to coloproctology in International Conference on Integrative Traditional Chinese and Western Medicine in Vietnam

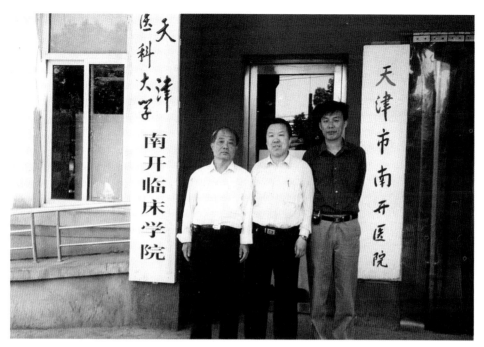

田淇第(左)、北京高等中医药学校校长刘长信(中)和针灸科主任吕福奎

Professor Tian Qidi （left）, President Liu Changxin of Beijing Higher Junior College of Traditional Chinese Medicine （middle）, and Dr. Lv Fukui, Department Chief of Acupuncture and Moxibustion （right）

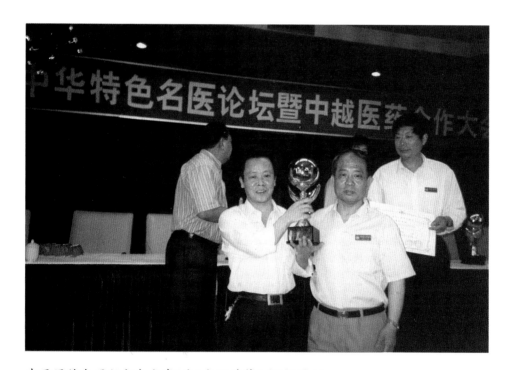

中西医结合国际大会主席(左)向田淇第(右)授奖杯

Professor Tian Qidi （right） won a laureate cup in the International Conference of Integrated Traditional Chinese and Western Medicine

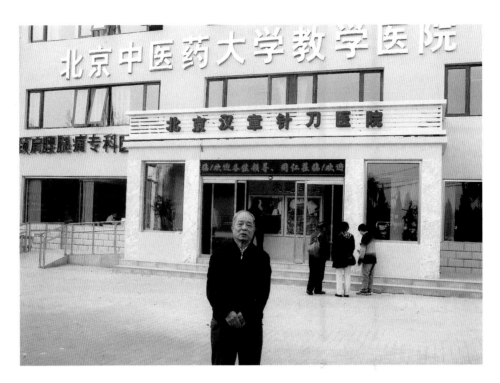

田淇第教授

Tian Qidi, M.D.

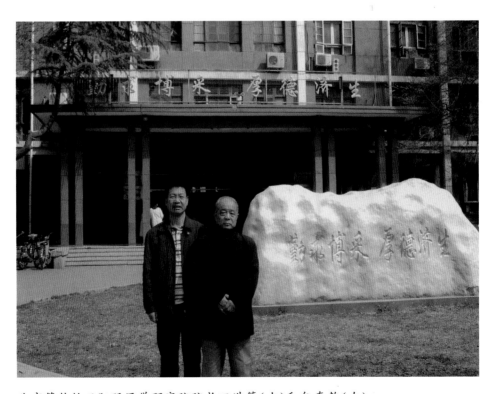

北京第乾针刀肛肠医学研究院院长田淇第(右)和包寿乾(左)

Tian Qidi (right), President of Beijing Diqian Acupuncture Scalpel of Coloproctology Research School, and Bao Shouqian(left)

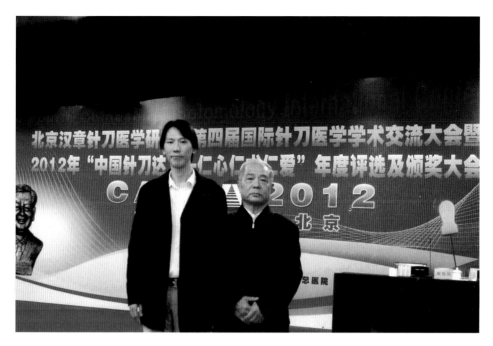

北京中医药大学教学医院院长、北京汉章针刀医院院长朱秀峰(左)和田淇第教授(右)

Zhu Xiufeng (left), President of Teaching Hospital of Beijing University of Chinese Medicine, and President of Beijing Hanzhang Acupuncture Scalpel Hospital, and Professor Tian Qidi(right)

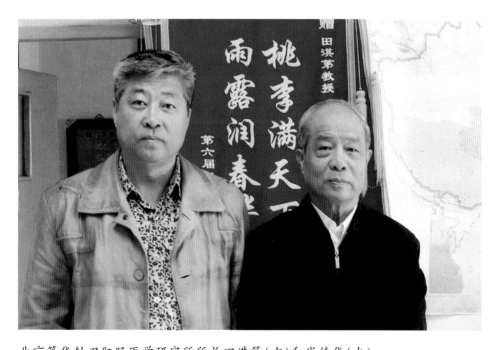

北京第华针刀肛肠医学研究所所长田淇第(右)和肖德华(左)

Tian Qidi (right), President of Beijing Dihua Acupuncture Scalpel of Coloproctology Research School, and Xiao Dehua(left)

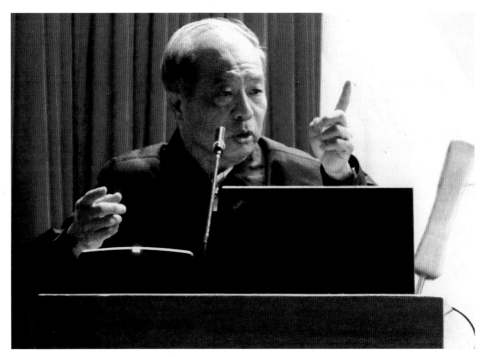

田淇第教授在中国北京国际论坛宣讲肛肠病小针刀疗法

Professor Tian Qidi gave a lecture on acupuncture scalpel therapy to coloproctology in International Forum of Beijing, China

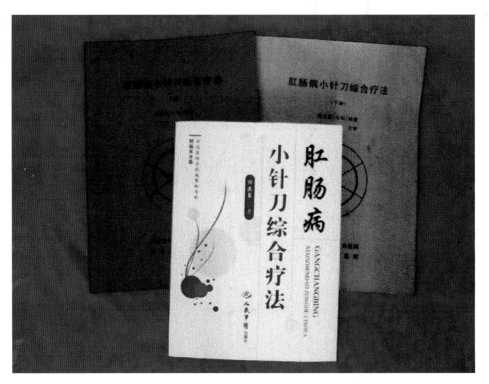

田淇第所著 3 种"肛肠病小针刀疗法"专著

Three kinds of monographs on acupuncture scalpel therapy to coloproctology by Tian Qidi

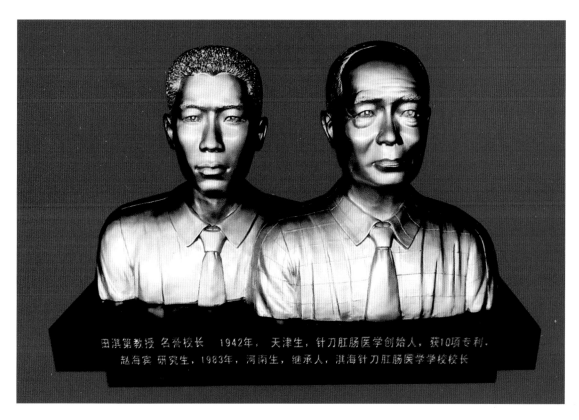

田淇第教授铜像(右),针刀肛肠医学创始人,淇海针刀肛肠医学学校名誉校长

Professor Tian Qidi bronze statue(right),the founder of Acupuncture Scalpel Therapy to Coloproctology,and the Chancellor of Qi Hai Acupuncture Scalpel Therapy to Coloproctology Medical College

赵海宾铜像(左),针刀肛肠医学继承人,淇海针刀肛肠医学学校校长

Zhao Haibin bronze statue (left),the successor of Acupuncture Scalpel Therapy to Coloproctology,and the President of Qi Hai Acupuncture Scalpel Therapy to Coloproctology Medical College

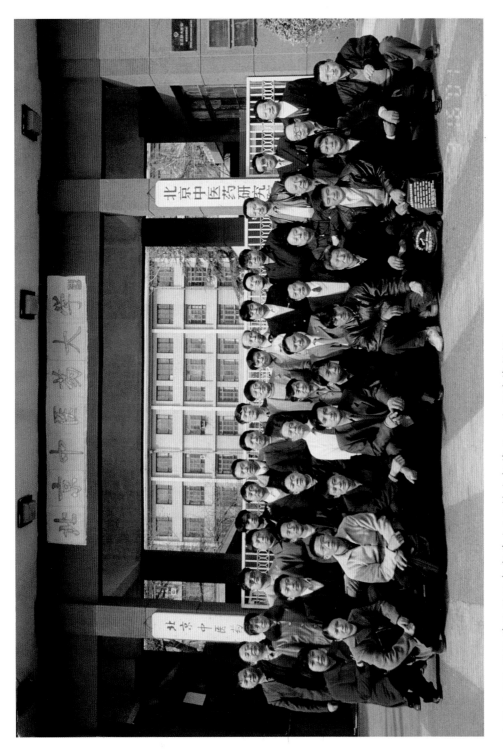

全国针刀肛肠医学培训班在京举办（二排左起第五人为田淇第教授）

National Training Class of Acupuncture Scalpel Therapy to Coloproctology was held in Beijing (Professor Tian Qidi was in the fifth of the second row from the left)

吴咸中院士题词

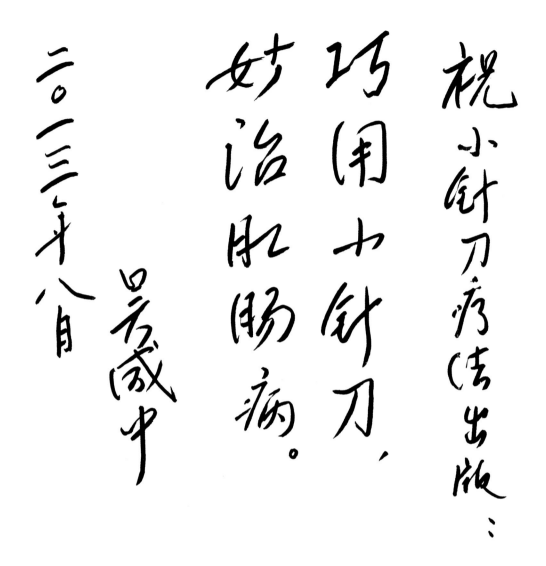

祝小针刀疗法出版；

巧用小针刀，

妙治肛肠病。

二〇一三年八月　吴咸中

Congratulations on publishing *The application of comprehensive acupuncture scalpel therapy to coloproctology*. The book shows that the author is an ingenious and intelligent coloproctology doctor.

Wu Xianzhong
August 2013

内 容 简 介

本书作者总结自己 50 余年的实践经验和多次开办培训班的讲稿,详细阐述了肛肠病小针刀综合疗法的基本知识、基础理论和操作技术。内容包括肛门、直肠解剖生理,肛肠科检查方法,中医对肛肠疾病的认识及非手术治疗,小针刀疗法的原理、临床应用和操作要点,痔、肛瘘、肛门狭窄、盆底松弛、肛肠肿瘤等各种肛肠疾病的诊断要点和小针刀综合治疗方法,以及肛肠科常用方药、专用器材等,并附有典型病例、作者的 10 项发明专利证书和 1 张约 2 小时 10 分钟的专利工具使用、小针刀肛肠疾病手术多媒体光盘。

本书将基础与临床、中医与西医、图书与光盘紧密结合,内容独具特色,操作方法具体,指导性、实用性强,适于肛肠科医师、基层医务人员和肛肠病患者阅读参考。

Abstract

The author sums up 50-years' clinical experience and prolonged training text of speech by himself, and states basic knowledge, theory and technique of "the application of comprehensive acupuncture scalpel therapy to coloproctology" in detail, such as anorectal anatomy, physiology, pathology, physical examination, the cognition of traditional Chinese medicine of anorectal diseases, operations, nonoperative therapies, etc. He introduces the diagnosis and treatment in coloproctology, including hemorrhoids, anal fistula, and specific equipments, demonstrated with classical clinical cases, ten patents and a DVD.

The book contributes a tight integration of basic theory and clinical practices, traditional Chinese medicine and Western medicine, text and disk. The work has great originality, specific technique. It's a guidance which owns infinitely practical charm suiting for coloproctology surgery, for both primary doctor and patients.

序

《现代肛肠病小针刀综合疗法(汉英对照)》一书,是集中医针与西医刀的优势为一体的中西医结合的结晶。这一疗法属中西医结合微创外科范畴。肛肠病小针刀综合疗法的发明人是我院肛肠科田淇第主任,他从事中西医结合肛肠科工作50年,在针刀技术治疗肛肠病领域有很深的造诣。田淇第教授虽年逾花甲,但仍工作在临床一线。他执著追求,不辍努力,且颇有心得而著书立说。我欣然接受田淇第教授的邀请,愿为此书作序并主审。

天津市　南开医院院长

天津市大肠肛门病研究所所长

王西墨

2013 年 8 月 8 日

Foreword

The book *Application of Comprehensive Acupuncture Scalpel Therapy to Coloproctology (annotated bilingual edition)* is a crystal of integrated traditional Chinese and Western medicine to combine the superiorities of the needle of traditional Chinese medicine and of the knife of Western medicine, in the minimal invasive surgical fields of integrated traditional Chinese and Western medicine. The patent inventor who applies acupuncture scalpel therapy to coloproctology is a chief surgeon in Tianjin NanKai Hospital, has been going for coloproctology of traditional Chinese and Western medicine for 50 years, and has owned masterly skill in applying acupuncture scalpel therapy to coloproctology. Although he is over 60 years old, he still works hard in first clinical line. The book gaining in depth comprehension results from persistent pursuing and unremitting effort for career. I am glad to accept the Professor's invitation to become his main peer reviewer meanwhile I prefer to write the preface for his book.

President, Tianjin Nankai Hospital

Director, Tianjin institue of coloproctology

Peer Reviewer: Wang Ximo, M.D.

August 8, 2013

前　言

　　肛肠病为常见病、多发病,且患者常因病情缠绵而苦不堪言。仅就痔疮而言,即有"十人九痔"之说,足见其发病之广;而"如坐针毡"之痛,则非病者难有此切肤之感。但肛肠科在浩大的医学领域中仅有一隅之地,执业者少而患者多,需求高而地位低。有志于肛肠专业的医务工作者们怀着高度的责任心,在不断追踪现代医学发展的同时,也努力挖掘中医学宝库的精华,以提高肛肠专业的学术地位和技术水平。

　　诚如太史公司马迁在《扁鹊传》中所言:"人之所病,病疾多;而医之所病,病道少。"肛肠专业的专家们在探究治疗常见肛肠病的方法中,一直把"简、便、验、廉"作为重要的追求目标,而中西医结合的小针刀综合疗法便成为实现这种目标的捷径之一。

　　《现代肛肠病小针刀综合疗法(汉英对照)》是中西医结合的结晶,并获中国专利。全书共15章,其中插图170余幅。其治疗方法获专利10项。希望此书能成为渴望掌握小针刀治疗技术同道的良师益友,同时企盼更多的有丰富实践经验的专家不遗余力,整理经验,以期集腋成裘,宏扬瑰宝,造福人类。

田淇第

2013 年 8 月 8 日

Preface

　　The diseases of colon and rectum are common and frequent pathological changes, so the effective handling of the diseases constitutes our most urgent problem, for example, the hemorrhoids is one of these diseases. An old maxim in China showed "If there are ten persons, there may be nine patients with hemorrhoid among them." So this kind of disease is universal in human being's. The doctor should have high responsibility whacever subject they are in, whatever they do. Just like a celebrity said: these are all to the good career and no inferior job can come of them. The doctors not only pursue frequently modern medicine, but also excavate hard traditional Chinese medicine for improving academic status and technical level in coloproctology.

　　A great man in ancient China ever said that common people woried about suffering from diseases easily while the doctors' anxiety was to treat them difficultly.

　　The works *Application of Comprehensive Acupuncture Scalpel Therapy to Coloproctology (annotated bilingual edition)* being a crystal of integrated traditional Chinese and Western medicine, got the Chinese patents. The book includes 15 chapters and about 170 figures. The methods of treatment won 10 patents. I expect that the book is a good teacher and helpful friend of doctors. I am sure the wide awake people of this occupation will bring great height of development to the medicine and unique benefit to the mankind.

Tian Qidi

August 8, 2013

目　录
CONTENTS

第1章 肛肠解剖基础
Chapter 1 Basic Anatomy of Anorectum

一、会 阴
I. The Perineum

1.范围 会阴包括盆膈以下的全部软组织皮肤与骨盆出口的菱形区域。

1.Space Total soft tissues inferior to pelvic diaphragm, diamond shape of pelvic outlet.

2.结构 会阴由皮肤、皮下组织、会阴浅部、深部筋膜及会阴部肌肉构成。

2.Frame Skin, hypodermis, shallow perineal space, perineal fascia and muscles.

3.器官 肛门三角和尿生殖三角,以两侧的坐骨结节连线划分。后方止点,尾骨尖,为肛门三角;前方止点,耻骨联合低点的会阴,为尿生殖三角。

3.Organ Anal and urogenital triangles by an interischial line between ischial tuberosities, tip of coccyx and two ischial tuberosities making up of posterior triangle-anal triangle, inferior margin of pubic symphysis and two ischial tuberosities making up of anterior triangle-urogenital triangle.

（1）男性尿生殖三角、器官、尿道、前列腺、阴囊见图1-1。

（1）Male urogenital triangle ,organ, urethra, prostate,scrotum, see Fig. 1-1.

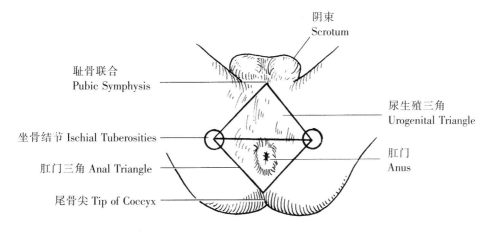

图1-1 男性会阴

Figure 1-1 Perineum in male

(2)女性尿生殖三角、器官、阴道、尿道、阴阜见图1-2。

(2)Female urogenital triangle, organs, vagina,urethra ,mons pubis , see Fig. 1-2.

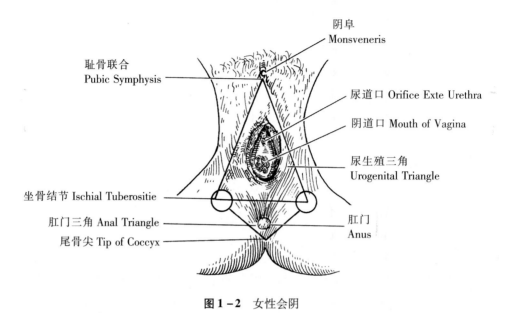

图1-2 女性会阴

Figure 1-2 Perineum in female

4.功能

4. Function

(1)肛门三角与尿生殖三角解剖相邻,相互影响。

(1)The anal triangle and the urogenital triangle are contiguous, so they may influence each other.

(2)肛门三角结构或功能紊乱,会造成排粪便困难或失控。

(2)The anal triangle dysfunction or disorders may cause difficult defecation or encopresis.

(3)尿生殖三角结构或功能紊乱会造成排尿或生殖异常。

(3)The urogenital triangle dysfimction or disorders may cause urinary or genital diseases.

二、盆 底

II. The Pelvic Floor

盆底又称为盆膈,起封闭骨盆出口作用。

The pelvic floor or pelvic diaphragm is the closure of pelvic outlet.

1. 范围 由耻骨联合下缘起,延两侧耻骨支、坐骨支、坐骨结节,止于骶尾骨。

1. **Space**　Pubic branches, ischium branches and ischial tuberosities on the sides and lower edge of pubic symphysis in front, and sacrum and coccyx behind.

2. **结构**　盆底,后侧边缘是骶尾骨与其骶结节韧带相连。盆底两侧是提肛肌与后侧尾前肌合成盆膈,并和盆筋膜共同悬吊盆底。

2. **Frame**　The pelvic floor is composed of muscle fibers of the levator ani, the coccygeus, and associated connective tissue spanning the area underneath the pelvis. The pelvic diaphragm is a muscular partition formed by the levatores ani and coccygei, with which may be included the parietal pelvic fascia on their upper and lower aspects.

3. 器官
3. Organ

(1)男性盆底纵向前侧有膀胱、前列腺和尿道;后侧有直肠、肛管(图 1 - 3)。

(1)The male pelvic floor from vertical plane, urinary bladder, prostate gland and urethral canal in front, and rectum and anal canal behind(Fig. 1 - 3).

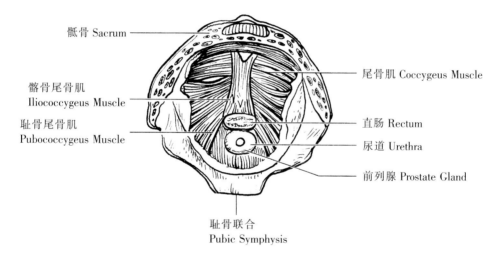

图 1 - 3　男性盆底(平面)

Figure 1 - 3　Pelvic floor of males (horizontal plane)

(2)女性盆底纵向前侧有膀胱、尿道、中间有子宫、阴道,后侧有直肠、肛管(图1 -4)。

(2)The female pelvic floor from vertical plane, urinary bladder and urethral canal in front, rectum and anal canal behind, and uterus and vagina in the middle of them (Fig. 1 -4).

4. 功能
4. Function

(1)承托盆腔和腹腔的脏器。

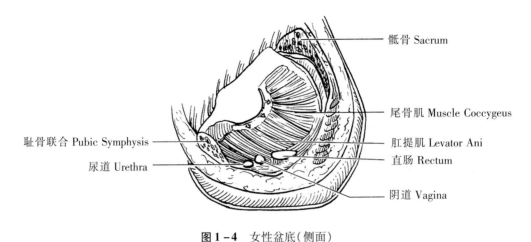

图 1 - 4　女性盆底(侧面)

Figure 1 - 4　Pelvic floor of females (lateral plane)

(1) To hold and sustain pelvic and abdominal organs.

(2) 调节排粪便的自控作用。

(2) To control defecation by self-regulation.

(3) 盆底结构或功能紊乱会造成排粪便困难,或失控,或引起排尿、生殖异常。

(3) The pelvic floor dysfunction or disorders may cause difficult defecation or encopresis, or urinary and genital diseases.

三、肛　门

III. The Anus

中医学称肛门为魄门。肛门是结肠与体外连通的出口,前面是会阴,后面是尾骨。在肛门与尾骨之间有一明显的沟,称为肛尾门沟。沟里面有肛尾韧带。平时肛门皱缩像收紧的袋口一样,排便时括约肌松弛,张开呈圆形洞口,肛门口周围的皮肤内有毛囊、汗腺及皮脂腺。肛门常因肌肉收缩,形成许多放射状皱襞。

The anus which is called corporeal soul gate in traditional Chinese medicine is outlet of large intestinal tract, whose front is the perineum, and behind, the coccyx. Between anus and coccyx there is a suleus of muscular and fibrous tissue, the anococcygeal ligament. The anus shrinks like the fastened mouth of a bag as usual while it opens like round hole as defecating. Around the anus there are folliculus pili, sweat glands amd sebaceous glands in subcutaneous fissue, forming many radial plicae during muscle contraction.

四、肛　管

IV. The Anal Canal

1.**肛管**　是从肛门口到齿线的一段,全长 2～3cm,是直肠末端(直肠之下),始于提肛门肌的止点。男性与前列腺尖端齐高;女性与会阴体齐高。肛管没有腹膜遮盖,周围肌肉有内外括约肌及肛提肌围绕着,平时为纵裂状,排便时呈管形。肛管两侧有坐骨直肠窝。男性肛管前部有尿道及前列腺,女性有阴道及子宫颈;肛管后部是尾骨。肛管上部被覆移行上皮,下部为鳞状上皮(图 1-5)。

1. **The Anal Canal**　It is the terminal portion of the rectum, 2～3 cm in length, from anus to dentate line. It begins at the end of levator ani muscle. The anal canal is as high as the level of the apex of the prostate gland in the male, and as that of the perineal body in the female. There is no peritoneal covering, but it is surrounded by sphincter ani internus, sphincter ani externus and levator ani muscles. In the empty condition it presents the appearance of an antero-posterior longitudinal slit while in the defecating an dition it shows tubiform. The two sides of it show fossae ischiorectalis. In front of it, in the male, there are urethra and prostate; and in the female, vagina and cervix uterus; behind the anal canal part is the coccyx. The upper part of the anal canal is covered by transitional epithelium, and the lower is squamous epithelium(Fig. 1-5).

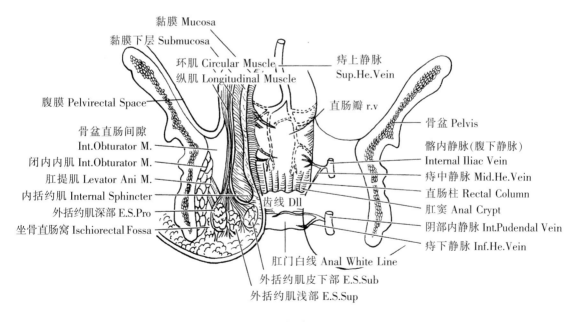

图 1-5　肛门直肠纵切面

Figure 1-5　Coronal section of anus and rectum

2.**肛门白线**　又称为括约肌线,在内、外括约肌交界处(距肛门缘约 1.5cm),如将食指插入肛管,可以摸到一沟,即为肛门白线(图 1-6),因该处血管少,颜色淡而叫白线。

2. **The Anal White Line**   The intermuscular sulcus (about 1.5cm from the anal orifice) is the space between the internal sphincter muscle and external sphincter muscle. When a finger is inserted into the anal canal a depression will be formed by retraction of the skin of the canal (Fig. 1 –6). It is called the white line because of a few vessels and light color here.

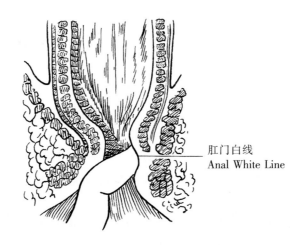

肛门白线
Anal White Line

图 1 – 6   手指在肛管内摸到肛门白线

Figure 1 – 6   The finger touchs the anal white line in the anal canal

3. **栉膜带**   肛门白线上齿线之下为宽 0.8 ~ 1.2cm 的灰白色环形带,被覆移行上皮,与下面的组织紧密粘连,并不受神经支配,没有弹力,经常保持收缩状态,故妨碍括约肌松弛。肛裂即因此种收缩状态影响而不易愈合(图 1 – 7)。

3. **The Pecten Band**   It is a gray white round band between the dentate line above and white line below, about in 0.8 ~ 1.2cm in width. It's covered with transitional epithelium, and connected closely to deep tissues. This area is not controlled nerves, and with no stretch, but often keeping constriction, to interfere with relaxation of sphincter muscles. That's why the anal fissure is not easily healed(Fig. 1 –7).

4. **肛瓣**   是肛管上端的黏膜,边缘不整齐,与直肠柱底相连,每两个直肠柱底之间有一个半月形皱襞,即肛瓣(图 1 – 8)。

4. **The Anal Valves**   The so-called anal valves are semilunar folds bridging adjacent top of anal canal with untidy edges between ends of rectal columns(Fig. 1 – 8).

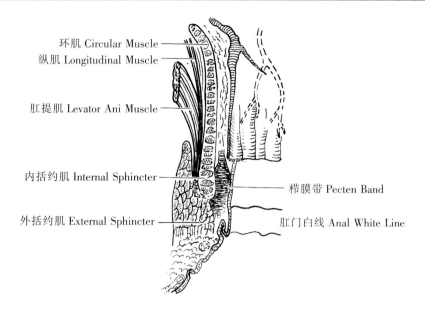

图 1 - 7　栉腹带的位置

Figure 1 - 7　Position of pecten band

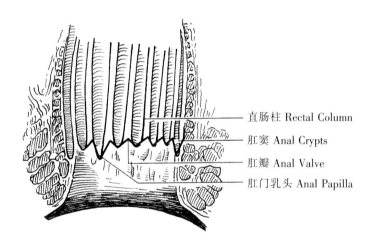

图 1 - 8　肛瓣、肛窦、肛门乳头、直肠柱位置

Figure 1 - 8　Position of anal valves，crypts，papillae and rectal columns

　　5. 肛窦　在肛瓣与直肠柱之间有许多凹陷的小窝，即肛窦(图 1 - 8)。肛窦口朝上,底向下,深约 0.3cm。肛窦基底有肛腺,平时分泌黏液,排便时受压迫流出,以滑润肛管,减少摩擦。

　　5. The Anal Crypts　They are between anal valves and rectal columns(Fig. 1 - 8), and are vertical with upward mouths and downward bases, and about 0.3cm long from mouth to bottom. Normally there are anal glands in the circumference of the anus. Each gland has a duct and discharges into an anal crypt, with secreting mucus. The mucus is discharged by pressure of defecating stool, to lubricate anal canal and to reduce friction.

6. **肛门乳头** 肛管与直肠连接处(齿线附近)有 2～6 个三角形略呈黄白色的乳头状突起,即肛乳头(图 1－8)。有时因受大便摩擦发炎而肥大,排便时脱出肛外,如锥体形小瘤,即为乳头瘤。

6. **The Anal Papillae** There are 2～6 triangular, yellow white papillary projections at the juncture between anal canal and rectum (near dentate line) (Fig. 1－8). Sometimes infection originates friction of defecating stool causing hypertrophy of anal papillae, while the anal papillae with hypertrophy frequently project toward the outside of anus, like a cone tumor called papilloma.

五、齿　线
V. The Dentate Line

齿线,也叫梳状线,因为它像锯齿或梳子;又因位于肛管和直肠交界处,所以又叫肛门直肠线。距肛门约 3cm,是胚胎时内胚叶与外胚叶的交界处。它在解剖学上十分重要,其上、下组织显著不同。

The dentate line, or pectinate line (like the sawtooth or comb) also known as anal rectum line is at the juncture of anal canal and rectum, 3cm from the anal verge. It's also the juncture of endoderm and ectoderm in embryo, and it's an important landmark in anatomy because of remarkable differences between dentate line above and below.

齿线以上的血管为痔上血管,其静脉属门静脉系统,血流入门静脉后再入肝脏;齿线以下的血管是痔下血管,其静脉属下腔静脉系统,血流入下腔静脉。

The blood vessels above this line are superior hemorrhoidal vessels, and the veins link to portal system, then into the liver; the blood vessels below this line are inferior hemorrhoidal vessels, and the veins link to inferior vena cava, then into systemic circulation.

齿线以上的神经属自主神经系统(没有痛感的神经);齿线以下的神经属脊髓神经系统(对疼痛敏锐)。

The epithelium above this line is supplied by sensory fibers from the autonomic nervous system and therefore is insensitive to painful stimuli; the epithelium below this line is innervated by spinal nerves and with somatic sensation.

齿线以上的淋巴液流入主动脉旁淋巴结,齿线以下的淋巴液则入腹股沟淋巴结(图 1－9)。

The lymph from the upper part of dentate line can be drained to the paraaortic lymph nodes while the below one, to the inguinal lymph nodes (Fig. 1－9).

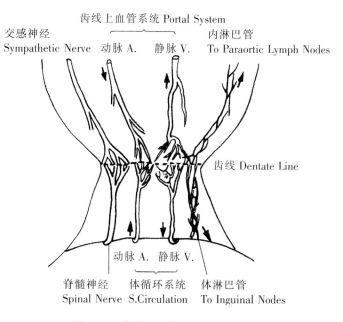

图 1 - 9 齿线上下神经血管淋巴分布

Figure 1 - 9 Distribution of nerves, arteries, veins and lymph above and below dentate line

六、肛　垫
VI. The Anal Cushions

肛垫,位于齿线上方,宽 1.5~2.6cm,由直肠黏膜层、黏膜下层、直肠柱区组织构成。1975 年,美国学者 Thomson 提出肛门衬垫概念,并发现健康人右前、右后及左侧排列着 3 个垫状组织,以 Y 形沟分为 3 块。

The anal cushions are above the dentate line, 1.5~2.6cm in width, in the anal canal lumen. They consist of mucosa, submucosa and rectal columns. There are three discrete and separated elastic tissues like cushion shape – right anterior, right posterior and left lateral forming Y-type stem, lying in constant sites. The term anal cushions was named by Thomson, an American scholar in 1975.

肛垫被黏膜下肌肉和弹性纤维组织贴固在括约肌上。肛垫内动脉和静脉相互构成血管网,血液充盈时可维持肛门闭合。肛垫内有神经末梢,其中的感觉神经构成肛门内感受器,参与控制排便的功能(图 1 - 10)。

The anal cushions are stuck and fixed on the sphincter by muscularis mucosa and fibroelastic tissue. They contain arteries and veins ramifying in a supportive syncytial network, and aid in anal continence, and they become engorged with blood during the act of defecation. There are terminal nerve fibers, and the sensory nerve endings constitute receptors within the anus, and participate in controlling the act of defecation(Fig. 1 – 10).

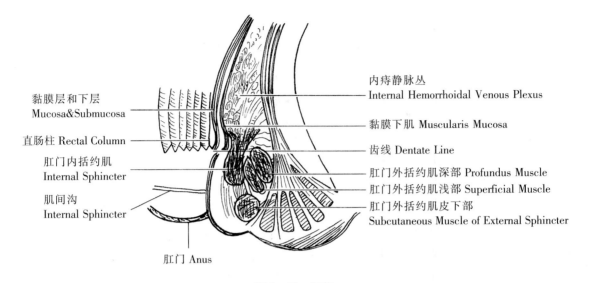

图 1 – 10　肛垫
Figure 1 – 10　The anal cushions

七、直　肠
VII. The Rectum

　　直肠上端与第三骶椎齐高，上段连接盆结肠，下段连接肛管，长约 12.5cm。在直肠和盆结肠连接处内径狭窄；向下的中段较大处为直肠壶腹；下段与肛管连接处又变狭窄。直肠行径弯曲，上部弯向后、向右，下部弯向前、向左。直肠上 1/3 的前面及其两侧有腹膜覆盖，中 1/3 处仅前面有腹膜，并形成反折回。腹膜反折与肛门距离约 7.5cm，女性则小于 7.5cm。直肠后面距肛门 12.5cm 处没有腹膜覆盖。

　　The rectum, measuring 12.5cm, is the distal portion of the large intestine, beginning at the sigmoid colon, the level of the third sacral vertebra, and ending at the anal canal. The level corresponds to the site of the rectal narrowing to join the sigmoid; the middle rectal lumen is inflated, being called rectal ampulla; the lower rectum is narrow again to join the anal canal. The rectum presents lateral curvatures and antero-posterior curves:an upper, with its convexity right and backward, and a lower, with its convexity left and forward. The upper one-third of the rectum is covered by peritoneum anteriorly and laterally; the middle one-third is covered anteriorly only, and the peritoneum forms its reflection. The peritoneal reflection in the male is 7.5cm from the anal verge, while in females it is lower than 7.5cm. The posterior peritoneal reflection is 12.5cm from the anal verge.

　　1. 直肠壁　分为内、中、外三层，内层为黏膜，中层是肌层，外层是浆膜。直肠黏膜较厚,血管较多,黏膜下层组织比较松弛,容易与肌层分离,如内痔经常脱出即因为反复被粪便推动,使黏膜与肌层分离之故。

1. The Rectal Coat　The adult rectum has three coats:the inner layer is mucous, the middle, muscular and the outer, serous. The mucosa of the rectum is thick and highly vascularized; the submucosa is slack ramifying and considerably mobile, and it separates easily from the muscular coat. So in hemorrhoids, the inner layer of rectal coat is strained during defecation, with repeated straining, the mucosa tends to be separated from the muscularis, forming the exclusion of the hemorrhoid.

2. 直肠肌肉　属于不随意肌(即不能任意收缩或松弛),其内层为环状肌,外层为纵状肌(图 1-11)。纵肌在直肠前后比两侧稍厚,上连盆结肠纵肌,下与肛提肌及内外括约肌相连。环肌在直肠上部,肌纤维较少,下部比较发达,到肛管处形成内括约肌。直肠由于有环、纵两层肌肉,所以比较坚固,不易破裂。

2. The Musculature of the Rectum　It belongs to involuntary muscle (not to constrict and relax voluntarily). The rectum, like the colon, has inner circular and outer longitudinal layers of muscle (Fig. 1-11). The longitudinal fibers at the front and back wall of the rectum are thicker than those at the lateral walls. The outer longitudinal muscle of the rectum is formed by an expansion of the colonic longitudinal muscle at the termination of the sigmoid colon. The expansion of the longitudinal muscle continues down on the rectum, at the levator-rectal junction. The circular fibers are thicker at the lower part of the rectum, and form internal sphincter at the anal canal. The Rectum has both circular and Longitudinallayers, so it is very strong and not easily broken.

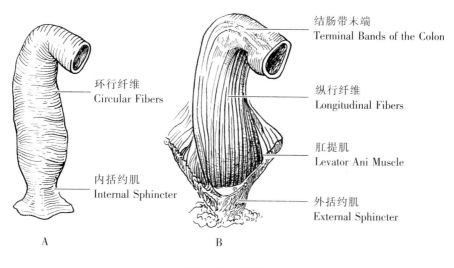

图 1-11　直肠肌

A. 内层环肌;B. 外层纵肌

Figure 1-11　The rectal muscle

A. The inner circular muscular layers;B. The outer longitudinal muscular layers

3. **直肠神经** 直肠由交感神经及副交感神经支配。

3. **The Rectal Nerve** The rectum is subject to sympathetic and parasympathetic nervous system.

4. **直肠柱** 也叫肛柱,在直肠下部。因受肛门括约肌收缩勒紧的影响,在黏膜上形成许多圆柱形皱襞(像一个扎紧口的口袋),突出在齿线上的直肠腔内,长1~2cm,共约10个。当直肠扩张或排便时,因括约肌松弛,皱襞消失(图1-8)。痔内静脉丛就包括在这里,也是内痔发生的部位。

4. **Rectal Columns** Another name is anal columns. These are a number of mucosal longitudinal folds formed in the lumen of the lower rectum above dentate line by fastening contractions of anal sphincter (like a bag fastened), 1~2cm length. There are about 10 columns. The folds disappear while the sphincters relax associated with dilations of the rectum or acts of defecation (Fig. 1-8). The hemorrhoidal veniplex is here, so inner hemorrhoids occur in this position.

5. **直肠瓣** 直肠全部黏膜有上、中、下3个皱襞,襞内有环肌纤维,好像把直肠分成三部分,即直肠瓣。直肠充满粪便时皱襞回缩,其主要作用是防止排便时粪便逆行(图1-12)。

5. **Rectal Valves** Usually there are three folds of mucosa, inferior, middle and superior, including the circular muscle coat of the rectal wall. They are formed to serve as steps or spiral supports to modify the flow of the feces as they descend into the lower rectum. When the rectum is full of feces, the rectal valves shrink trying to prevent feces upwards during defecation(Fig. 1-12).

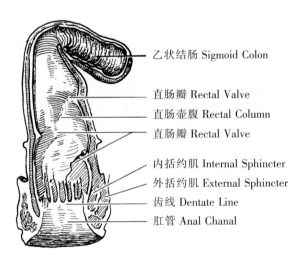

图1-12 直肠(纵切面图)

Figure 1-12 Rectum(vertical section)

八、肛门直肠肌肉

VIII. Muscles of the Anus and Rectum

1. **肛门外括约肌**　属于随意肌(可以随意收缩和松弛),有环形肌束及椭圆形肌束。后自尾骨起,向前下行到肛管后方分为两部分,沿两侧围绕肛管下部,至肛门前方,又会合为一,终止于会阴。外括约肌可分为三部分。

1. **Anal External Sphincter**　It belongs to voluntary muscle (voluntary contraction and relaxation). The circular and ellipse fascicles from the tip of the coccyx pass anteriorly and inferiorly inserting into the posterior part of anal canal, and then being divided into two parts, loop around the lower part of the anal canal on both sides, finally arriving at the anterior part of the anus to form the sphincter. It has three components.

(1)外括约肌皮下部:是环形肌束,只围绕于肛管下部,不附于尾骨,在肛门皮下可以摸到像索条状,与肛门内括约肌在同一平面上,肛门白线即位于两肌之间。这部分括约肌即为外括约肌,皮下部手术时切断它不会有大便失禁的危险。

(1)The Subcutaneous Muscle:It is situated below the transitional anal skin, and forms the lower wall of the anal canal. The bulk of the muscle is annular and disposed on the same plane with the internal sphincter. This forms the anal white line. The subcutaneous muscle lies in a septal network formed by the fibro-elastic muscle, and interweaves with the subcutaneous, presenting support. These terminal extensions into the skin form the corrugator cuis ani.

(2)外括约肌浅部:是椭圆形肌束,在皮下部与深部中间,有直肠纵肌纤维使其分开。

(2)The Superficial Muscle:This is an elliptical band of muscle fibers. It is the largest, longest and strongest portion. Arising from the sides of the coccyx and forming the important muscular component of the anococcygeal body, its diverging halves surround the mid-portion of the anal canal.

(3)外括约肌深部:也是环行肌束,在浅部之上。外括约肌深、浅两部分围绕直肠纵肌及肛门内括约肌,并连接肛提肌的耻骨直肠部,构成一个环形,即肛门直肠环(图 1 – 13)。此肌环有括约肛门作用,如手术不慎或其他原因被全部切断或损坏,会引起大便失禁。

(3)The Profundus Muscle:It is situated above the superficial muscle. Anteriorly, the profundus forms the upper margin of the anorectal muscle ring, but posteriorly the puborectalis muscle forms the upper margin of this ring(Fig. 1 – 13).

2. **肛门内括约肌**　是直肠环肌纤维下段较厚的部分(图 1 – 13)。它围绕肛管上部,属于不随意肌,宽约3cm,其下部有2cm,由外括约肌所包绕。单独的内括约肌没有括约肛门的功能。

2. Anal internal sphincter The terminal portion of the circular muscle coat of the rectum gradually thickens to become the component of the internal sphincter(Fig. 1 – 13). This muscle is surrounded by the superficial portion of the external sphincter.

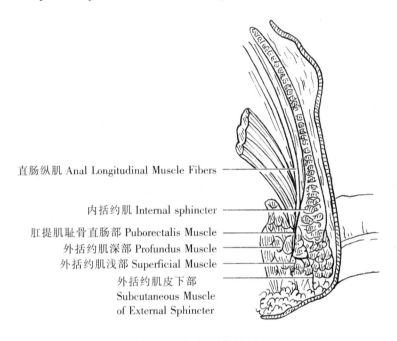

直肠纵肌 Anal Longitudinal Muscle Fibers

内括约肌 Internal sphincter

肛提肌耻骨直肠部 Puborectalis Muscle
外括约肌深部 Profundus Muscle
外括约肌浅部 Superficial Muscle
外括约肌皮下部
Subcutaneous Muscle
of External Sphincter

图 1 – 13 肛门直肠环

Figure 1 – 13 The anorectal muscle ring

3. 肛提肌 在肛管左右侧各一,联合成盆膈膜,可分为三部分。

3. The Levator Ani Muscle The levator ani muscle with external and internal sphincters, ischiococcygeus make up the pelvic diaphragm. Some principal paired muscles forming the levator are described as follows.

(1)前部:起于耻骨支后面,行向下后,有的纤维止于会阴;大部分纤维在内外括约肌之间,止于肛管,并与直肠外纵层肌纤维会合,故又称耻骨直肠肌。

(1) The anterior puborectalis muscle arises practically in common with the pubococcygeus, but on a slightly lower plane, the posterior surface of the pubic arch. It is a large part of the levator ani muscle between the internal and external sphincters, and the fibers continue until it begins to swing on the posterior side of the rectum, to encircle the rectum and become part of the anorectal muscle ring.

(2)中部:起于耻骨联合与闭孔肌膜,向后与对侧肌联合,附着于直肠下部的两侧,有的纤维与外括约肌相连,最终止于尾骨前面,故也称耻骨尾骨肌。

（2）The middle pubococcygeus muscle has a common origin with the puborectalis, its main portion continues posteriorly along with the puborectalis and is interlaced to a point of being insepararable, until it passes around the rectum and continues to insert into the anococcygeal body and the coccyx. Some fibers of pubococcygeus conjoined with the fibroelastic extensions of the external sphinefer.

（3）后部：起于坐骨棘内面，斜向下后内与对侧联合，附着于肛门尾骨之间，故又称髂骨尾骨肌（图 1 – 14）。

（3）The posterior：iliococcygeus muscle arises from the fascial covering of the obturator internus muscle and is directed posteriorly and medially, and they conjointly insert into the coccyx and lower sacrum. This muscle supports the anorectal shelf in the act of defecation（Fig. 1 – 14）.

肛提肌是一种阔而薄的肌膜，主要作用是使直肠下部和肛管收缩，向上提能帮助排便，并能使肛门闭合。如肛管黏膜和直肠脱出，可能因肛提肌松弛而失去作用所致。

The levator ani muscle is a kind of wide and thin muscular membrane. Its main affection is to make anal canal and inferior rectum contract, and it lifts anus upwards to help defecation and then to close anus, so that muscular relaxation or even loss of action can lead to prolapse of anal canal mucosa and the rectum.

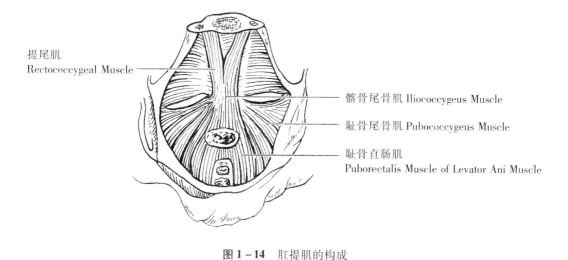

提尾肌 Rectococcygeal Muscle

髂骨尾骨肌 Iliococcygeus Muscle

耻骨尾骨肌 Pubococcygeus Muscle

耻骨直肠肌 Puborectalis Muscle of Levator Ani Muscle

图 1 – 14 肛提肌的构成

Figure 1 – 14 The structure of the levator ani muscle

4. **直肠尾骨肌** 起于尾骨前韧带，向前与直肠下部纵肌联合，主要作用是排便时使直肠下端固定不动。

4. **Rectococcygeal Muscles** It is a firm composite musculo-fascial structure arising from the second and third coccygeal vertebr, and passes downwards and forwards to blend with the longitudinal muscular fibers on the posterior wall of the anal canal, which supports the rectal ampulla.

九、肛门直肠血管

IX. The Blood Supply to the Anorectal Region

1. 动脉部分 肛门直肠有以下几条主要动脉(图 1 – 15)。

1. The Arterial Supply The arterial supply to the anorectal region shows somewhat distinct from that to the rectum(Fig. 1 – 15).

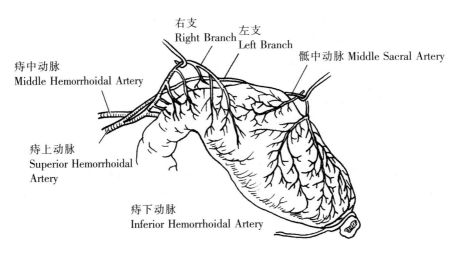

图 1 – 15 肛门直肠动脉分布

Figure 1 – 15 Arterial supply of the anal canal and rectum

(1)痔上动脉:在肠系膜下动脉的末端。在直肠上端后面分为左、右两支,沿着直肠两侧下行,穿过肌层抵达黏膜下层,在直肠柱内下行至齿线。在齿线上部分出许多小支,与痔中动脉、痔下动脉吻合。此动脉主要供给齿线以上直肠部分的血液。

(1) The superior rectal(hemorrhoidal)artery:It is the continuation of the terminal inferior mesenteric artery and descends posteriorly to the upper of the rectum, where it supplies above dentate line of the rectum, and divides into right and left main branches, which run down either side of the rectum, and pierce the muscular coat to reach the submucosa. After its main division, the right and left branches give off several smaller secondary branches above the anorectal line ,as far as the sphincter ani internus, where they anastomose with the other hemorrhoidal arteries and form a series of loops around the anus.

(2)痔中动脉:由腹下动脉(髂内动脉)分出,但也有与膀胱中动脉及阴道、前列腺或阴部外动脉合为一干者。此动脉在骨盆直肠间隙内,分布于直肠下部,在黏膜下层与痔上、痔下动脉吻合供给直肠下部的血液。

(2)The middle rectal(hemorrhoidal)arteries:They arise from the internal iliac artery on each side, coursing down the medial aspect of the sacrum behind the deep fascia, and enter the lower portion of the rectum. These arteries anastomose with the branches of the superior hemorrhoidal artery and the inferior hemorrhoidal arteries in the submucosa layer, where they supply the inferior rectum.

（3）痔下动脉：由阴部内动脉发出，经过坐骨直肠窝后，又分几个小支到达肛门内外括约肌和肛管末端，直到肛门外口，与痔上、痔中动脉吻合，供给肛管部分血液。

（3）The inferior rectal（hemorrhoidal）artery：It arises on each side from the internal pudendal arrery, a branch of the internal iliac artery, and traverses the ischiorectal fossa on each side, and then commonly divides into some large or small branches, entering the anal internal and external sphincter to supply terminal anal canal. There is no evidence of anastomosis between the superior and inferior hemorrhoidal arteries till the outside of the anus.

（4）骶中动脉：由腹主动脉发出，向下至直肠，与其他动脉吻合。

（4）The middle sacral artery：It arises posteriorly, just above the bifurcation of the aorta, descends to the rectum, where it provides an insignificant amount of blood supply to the rectum, and anastomoses with other arteries.

2.静脉部分
2. Venous Parts

（1）痔内静脉丛（痔上静脉）：由数个血管汇集而成，穿过肌层形成痔上静脉，再向上经肠系膜下静脉流入门静脉系统。痔内静脉丛在齿线上部的直肠黏膜下层内，尤其是在以下 3 个区域内比较显著：一支在右侧前方，一支在右侧后方，一支在左侧。它们是容易发生内痔（母痔）的部位。另外，还有 3～4 小支分布在左后和前、后方，是续发内痔（子痔）的部位（图 1－16，图 1－17）。

（1）The internal hemorrhoidal venous plexus（the superior hemorrhoidalvein）：The several branches pierce musculature, reach the submucosa where they are free to anastamose, and then drain the rectum and upper part of the anal canal into the portal system via the inferior mesenteric vein. The primary internal hemorrhoidal venous plexus forms in the submucosa above dentate line. Well-developed internal hemorrhoids are then situated usually in the right anterior, right posterior and left lateral areas. In addition, several smaller secondary branches reach the mid-lateral aspect and the posterior midline of the annulus hemorrhoidalis（Fig. 1－16, Fig. 1－17）.

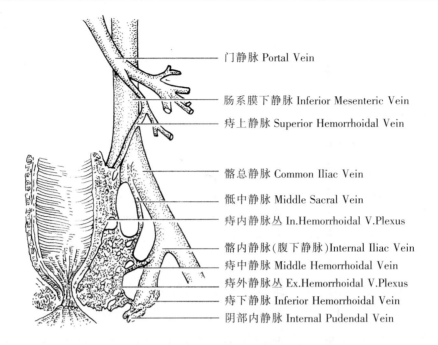

图 1 - 16　肛门直肠静脉分布

Figure 1 - 16　Venous drainage of the anal canal and rectum

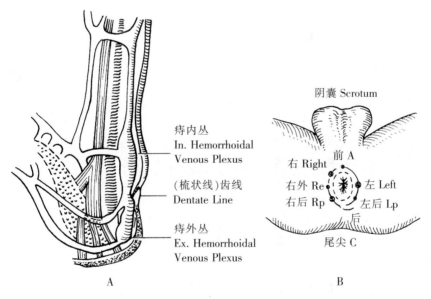

A:Anterior; Re:Right Exterior; Rp:Right Posterior; Lp:Left Posterior;C:Tip of Coccyx

图 1 - 17　易发生内痔的静脉分支及其位置

A. 痔内外静脉丛位置；B. 痔的位置

Figure 1 - 17　Venous drainage and positions of hemorrhoids

A. The position of internal and external hemorrhoidalvenous plexus；

B. The position of hemorrhoids

（2）痔外静脉丛（痔中、下静脉）：由肛管内静脉、直肠肌层外部静脉和皮下静脉联合形成痔外静脉丛。下部经过痔下静脉流入阴部内静脉；中部经痔中静脉流入腹下静脉，再流入髂总静脉。痔外静脉丛在齿线下部肌层外，分布于肛管、肛门边缘部分，是容易发生外痔的部位。

（2）The external hemorrhoidal venous plexus（the middle and inferior hemorrhoidalveins）: The middle hemorrhoidal veins drain the lower part of the rectum and the upper part of the anal canal and terminate in the internal iliac veins. The inferior hemorrhoidal veins drain the lower part of the anal canal via the internal pudendal veins, which empty into the internal iliac veins. At the anal verge, the inferior hemorrhoidal veins are prominent and form the indefinite plexiform arrangement, which is commonly referred to as the external hemorrhoidal plexus.

以上静脉内没有瓣膜（如同没有闸门），只借肌肉和肠的蠕动向上回流。因此，如上端压力增大，就容易发生静脉循环障碍，引起瘀滞，使静脉内压增高而扩张。

There are no valves in the lumen of hemorrhoidal venous plexus. Only by relying on muscular contraction and intestinal peristalses can the veins drain upwards, so that if the upper pressure increases, the obstacles of venous circulation will occur easily, leading to blood stasis, internal high pressure and distension in the venous lumen.

十、肛门直肠淋巴组织
X. Lymphatic Drainage of the Anal Canal and Rectum

1. **上组淋巴组织**　在齿线以上，包括直肠黏膜下层、肌层、浆膜下及肠壁外淋巴网。从肠壁外淋巴网，淋巴液循以下三个方向回收。

1. **Superior Lymphatic Tissues**　Around the rectum and anal canal are several spaces filled with connective tissue or fat, which may become sites of abscesses, fissures and fistulae and hemorrhoids.

（1）向上至直肠后骶骨前淋巴结，再至乙状结肠系膜根部淋巴结，最后至主动脉周围淋巴结。

（1）Perianal Group（Inferior）: This group drains the superficial and deep layers of the perineal skin, and terminates in the inferolateral group of inguinal nodes.

（2）向侧方至肛提肌上淋巴结，再至闭孔淋巴结，最后至髂内淋巴结。

（2）Anorectal Group（anal and rectal portions）: They are the mucosal, submucosal and intermuscular. The mucosal and submucosal sets anastamose with the perineal plexus, draining into the inguinal nodes. The rectal portion of the anorectal group is similar to that of the sigmoid with the same division of plexuses. The rectum and the submucous plexus bear relation to the pelvic superficial fascia in the supralevator and retrorectal spaces.

（3）向下至坐骨直肠窝淋巴结,然后到髂内淋巴结。

（3）Extrarectal Group:The downward zone arises in the anal canal and rectum, and extending lateralward and downward, may involve the anal sphincters or tissues of the ischiorectal fossae. The perianal skin may also be considered an important location in the lower zone.

2. 下组淋巴组织　包括外括约肌、肛管及肛门处皮下组织的淋巴网,经会阴流至腹股沟淋巴结(图1-18)。

2. **Inferior Lymphatic Tissues**　The upward zone of the retrorectal space extends to those of the mesorectum and sigmoid, and drains into the intercolated nodes and those of the obturator, paracolic, iliac, and aortic groups. Inferior zone drains into inguinal nodes(Fig. 1-18).

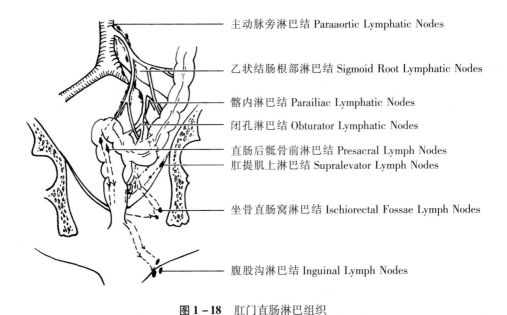

主动脉旁淋巴结 Paraaortic Lymphatic Nodes

乙状结肠根部淋巴结 Sigmoid Root Lymphatic Nodes

髂内淋巴结 Parailiac Lymphatic Nodes

闭孔淋巴结 Obturator Lymphatic Nodes

直肠后骶骨前淋巴结 Presacral Lymph Nodes
肛提肌上淋巴结 Supralevator Lymph Nodes

坐骨直肠窝淋巴结 Ischiorectal Fossae Lymph Nodes

腹股沟淋巴结 Inguinal Lymph Nodes

图1-18　肛门直肠淋巴组织

Figure 1-18　Lymphatic drainage of the anal canal and rectum

十一、肛门直肠神经

XI. Nerve Supply to the Anorectal Region

1. 交感神经　由肠系膜下丛及腹下丛组成,分布于直肠黏膜、直肠肌层及内括约肌间,在直肠附近形成痔上交感神经丛;兴奋时可抑制直肠运动,增加内括约肌张力。

1. **Sympathetic Fibers**　Sympathetic fibers from the inferior mesenteric plexus are distributed in the mucosa, submucosal and intermuscular layer of the rectum, in which the terminal distribution

of the sympathetics consists of the hemorrhoidal sympathetic plexus. It causes contraction of the sphincters, and inhibition to rectal peristalsis.

2. **副交感神经**　由第 2～4 骶神经组成,分布到直肠环行肌,有运动及抑制作用;兴奋时与交感神经作用相反。

2. **Parasympathetic Fibers**　Parasympathetic fibers reach their pelvic destination via the second, third, and fourth sacral spinal nerves. The sacral outflow of the parasympathetics supplies motor fibers to the circular musculature of the rectum, and inhibitory fibers to the internal anal sphincter.

3. **脊髓神经**　由第 4 骶神经组成阴部内神经的痔下支,经过坐骨直肠窝,分布到肛门外括约肌、肛管及肛门皮肤部分。

3. **Spinal Nerve**　It is the perineal branch from the fourth sacral spinal nerve which innervates inferior hemorrhoidal nerves of the pudendal. They supply the three divisions of the external sphincter and the terminal filaments in the skin, or continue to the anorectal junction.

齿线上都为无痛觉神经。齿线以下为脊髓神经,它感觉非常灵敏。肛门部感觉神经与膀胱颈部神经都来自第 4 骶神经。因此,肛门部病变常发生尿闭(有尿不能排出),或排尿困难;膀胱颈病变常有里急后重或均为神经反射所致。肛门部神经与会阴、臀部及股部神经也互有关联。因此,肛门疼痛常波及会阴、臀部及两侧股部。

No-sensory nerves are above the dental line, while below the dental line the spinal nerves are very sensitive. The anal and bladdery sensory nerves come from the fourth sacral nerve, so anal diseases often accompany urinary block and difficult urination, vice versa. Bladder lesions with tenesmus belong to nervous reflex act. The anal nerves are connected with the perineum, two sides of hip and thigh, so that anal pain often affects them.

十二、肛门直肠周围间隙
XII. Perianal and Perirectal Spaces

1. **肛门周围间隙**　也叫皮下间隙,在肛管下段的周围,内有外括约肌皮下部,是容易患外痔和发生皮下脓肿的部位。

1. **The Perianal Space**　This space surrounds the anus and the lower third of the anal canal, and the extensions continue downward into the perianal skin. The inner and outer extensions contain the subcutaneous muscle of external sphincter and the external hemorrhoidal plexus of veins. The space is the most common site of abscess in this region.

2. **黏膜下间隙**　在肛管上 2/3 部分及直肠下部,位于黏膜及内括约肌之间,内有痔内静脉丛和淋巴管,与内痔的发生有关,也可能因感染形成黏膜下脓肿。

2. **The Submucosal Space**　It lies between the submucosal and perianal spaces, above the

anorectal line, which occupies the submucosa. It contains the internal hemorrhoidal plexus of veins, lymphatics, and arterial and venous capillaries. This space is particularly important in formation of hemorrhoids.

3. **坐骨直肠间隙**　在坐骨结节和直肠之间,呈锥形,内有大量脂肪组织,富有弹性。有时坐骨直肠窝内发炎感染也可形成脓肿,如溃破即形成肛瘘。

3. **The Ischiorectal Space**　The conformation of the ischiorectal fossae depends upon the disposition of the levator ani muscle, which forms the inner wall and roof of the ischiorectal fossa between the coccyx and the ischium. It is smaller, narrower and deeper from 6 ~ 8cm anteroposteriorly, 2 ~ 4cm in width, and 6 ~ 8 cm in depth. The space is filled completely with fat and contains blood vessels and lymphatics, and an infection can lead to a horseshoe abscess or fistula.

4. **骨盆直肠间隙**　位于提肛肌与盆肌膜之间,是疏松结缔组织,为骨盆直肠窝脓肿的易发部位(图1 – 19)。

4. **The Pelvirectal Space**　It is situated on each side of the rectum above the levator ani. The presacral fascia, which covers the sacrum and coccyx, runs forward and downward and attaches to the posterior wall of the rectum. Infections vary according to the conformation of the spaces (Fig. 1 – 19).

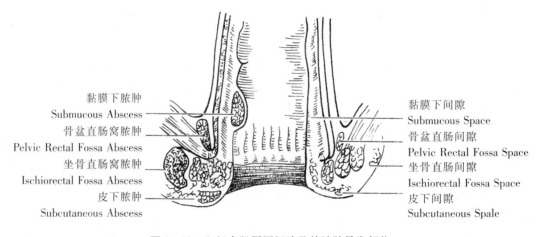

黏膜下脓肿　Submucous Abscess
骨盆直肠窝脓肿　Pelvic Rectal Fossa Abscess
坐骨直肠窝脓肿　Ischiorectal Fossa Abscess
皮下脓肿　Subcutaneous Abscess

黏膜下间隙　Submucous Space
骨盆直肠间隙　Pelvic Rectal Fossa Space
坐骨直肠间隙　Ischiorectal Fossa Space
皮下间隙　Subcutaneous Spale

图 1 – 19　肛门直肠周围间隙及其脓肿易发部位

Figure 1 – 19　The perianal and perirectal spaces, and the common site of abscess

十三、肛门直肠与周围组织的关系
XIII. Relations of the Rectum

男性直肠前方有前列腺、精囊、输精管及膀胱,直肠与膀胱之间有直肠膀胱陷凹;女性直肠前方有子宫颈及阴道,直肠与子宫之间有直肠子宫陷凹。直肠后部有骶骨、尾骨及提肛门肌,两侧有输尿管。直肠借其纤维鞘附着于盆腔筋膜,并有侧韧带及肛门尾骨韧带固定直肠。

The upper part of the rectum is separated in front and above, in the male, from the fundus of the bladder; in the female, from the intestinal surface of the uterus and its appendages, and in either sex, by some convolutions of the small intestine, and frequently by the sigmoid colon. Behind the lower part of the rectum there are the sacrum, coccyx, and levator ani, a dense fascia alone intervening; below it is in relation in the male with the triangular portion of the fundus of the bladder, the vesiculae seminales, and ductus deferentes, and more anteriorly with the posterior surface of the prostate, and the rectum-bladder fossae between rectum and bladder; in the female, with the posterior wall of the vagina, and the rectum-uterus fossa between rectum and uterus. The rectum is found on the pelvic diaphragm through by its fibrosheath, and fixed by the lateral ligament and anococcygeal ligament.

十四、肛门和直肠的生理功能
XIV. The Anorectal Physiology

肛门和直肠的主要生理功能是排便。直肠位于消化管的末段,没有消化作用,只能吸收少量水分、葡萄糖、氨基酸及经胰液处理过的牛奶等。另外,直肠能分泌黏液,使黏膜滑润,以利粪便排出。直肠内通常没有粪便存留。正常的直肠壁对压力刺激相当敏感,当粪便增加到一定容积时,即产生扩张性刺激,引起便意。但是,如对这种感觉经常给予制止,就会渐渐使直肠的容量增大,以致达到一定压力时仍不会引起便意。

Defecation is the main physical function of anus and rectum. The rectum is the distal portion of the alimentary canal, has no digestive function, but only absorbs a little water, glucose, amino acid, arranged milk by pancreatic juice, etc.

肛门和肛管位于直肠下段,主要作用是管理排便。当粪便移入直肠时,肛门括约肌(直肠环)就会收缩,使肛门紧闭;待粪便蓄积增多,直肠壁感受足够的刺激后会产生冲动,传入神经中枢。由于传导反射作用,又促使直肠收缩;肛门括约肌舒张,粪便才会排出。排便过程有随意运动和不随意运动之分。结肠和直肠蠕动,肛门内括约肌舒张,属于不随意运动。粪便排出时,肛门外括约肌随人的意识而收缩或舒张;肛提肌收缩,以及膈肌、腹肌收缩,以增加腹压协助排便等,均属于随意运动。当然,如此复杂的活动有赖于神经系统各级中枢的协调;而这种协调过程,又可以形成条件反射,即建立定时排便习惯。

Physiologically, the defecation is best explained on the basis of a modified somatic autonomic reflex, normally under cortical control, and in which the desire to defecate may be conveniently distinguished from the act of defecation. The initial sensory stimuli arise and produce the desire to defecate, are probably in the rectal musculature as well as in the anorectal line. The stimuli arises normally from the anorectal junctional area and are conveyed by the spinal sensory nerves to initiate the active phase of defecation. The distention of the rectal wall also gives rise to some extent, to the desire to defecate through the sympathetic afferent nerves. This results reflexively, in a relaxation of the anal sphincters, particularly the internal, and a contraction of the rectal musculature. The act may be inhibited by the will. On the other hand, voluntary relaxation of the anal sphincters with voluntary contraction of the colon and its complimentary muscles, with the expulsion of the rectal contents, is the actual act of defecation. In adult life, defecation is no longer a reflex, but normally becomes a voluntary act, once the summation of sensory stimuli is affected. It becomes a purely reflex act, in the autonomic innervated rectum, following destruction of its cerebral connections. The broad subject of constipation is directly related to the sensorimotor response of the entire gastrointestinal tract as well as those of the rectum. The sensory and motor dispersions, before, after, and during the act of defecation are complex and may be reflected throughout the entire nervous system, e. g. , fainting, abdominal cramping, orgasms, and neurocirculatory phenomena, are common clinical observations. Defecation may also be entirely a cortical response. Central stimulation of the vagus nerve produces the defecation reflex, a contraction of the rectum and a relaxation of the anal sphincters. In this regard, it may be observed that the segmental movements of the intestines are considered myogenic in origin. The autonomic system subserves a regulatory function. Diarrhea may be entirely an intrinsic myogenic basis.

第2章 肛肠科检查方法

Chapter 2 Proctological Examination

一、全身检查

I. Systemic Examinations

根据中医四诊和西医物理检查方法,初步整理出全身检查的方法。

A preliminary systemic examination should be made through the four methods of diagnosis by traditional Chinese medicine and physical ones by modern medicine.

1. 中医检查

1. TCM Examinations

(1)望诊:望诊的目的是观察病人的色、形、态、苔。①色是反映机体健康状况的表象。中医认为五脏气血外荣,健康者气血旺盛。②形,指身体形态,体质的强弱胖瘦。③态,指病人的动作、姿态。④苔,指舌苔,正常舌质色为淡红,润泽,不滑不燥。

(1) Observation: Play attention to expression, posture, color and tongue fur. ①Color, the color of skin is of great reference value to an overall analysis of the illness and the patient's condition. The health shows the luster of his eyes, speaking clearly and active reaction. ②Expression, the body's model is strong or weak, fat or thin. ③Posture, various posture in different diseases, worthy reference will be obtained with careful observation. ④Tongue fur, normal coating is tongue texture pink, lubricating, unsmooth and not dry.

(2)闻诊:即通过听觉和嗅觉辨认病情。

(2) Auscultation or olfaction: To differentiate diseases by senses of hearing and smell.

(3)问诊:即通过询问病人或家属等,了解病史,判断病情性质。

(3) Interrogation: To understand the patient's history and decide illness and the patient's condition through inquiring about illness from the patient and his family.

(4)切诊:即触摸脉搏,了解脉象,如血虚型会出现沉细或见芤的脉象。

(4) Pulse feeling: To feel pulses and understand pulse conditions, for example, the patients with blood asthenia are felt pulse sunken and thin, or hollow.

2. 体格检查 检查血压和心、肺,看是否正常,并检查腹部及肝、脾等。

2. **Physical Examinations**   To check blood pressure, heart, lungs, liver and spleen, etc.

二、局部检查
II. Local Examinations

1.检查姿式
1. Positions of Examination

(1)侧卧位:病人左或右侧卧,使肛门充分露出(图2-1)。

(1) Lateral recumbent posture:Be left or right lateral recumbent, anus is fully revealed (Fig. 2-1).

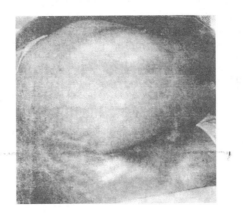

图2-1 侧卧位

Figure 2-1   Lateral recumbent position

(2)跪卧位(膝胸位):病人跪伏在床上(图2-2)。

(2)Kneeling posture (knee-chest position):Kneel on bed (Fig. 2-2).

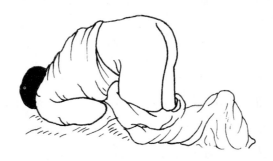

图2-2 跪位

Figure 2-2   Lateral kneeling position

(3)蹲位:病人蹲在地上(图2-3),查脱肛、息肉及内痔脱出。

（3）Kneeling-squatting posture：To squat on bed or on floor（Fig. 2 – 3）. To check up prolapse of the anus or internal hemorrhoids and polypus.

（4）截石位：病人仰卧，双膝屈起，两足上举（图 2 – 4）。

（4）Lithotomy position：To lay on back, curl up both knees with feet raised（Fig. 2 – 4）.

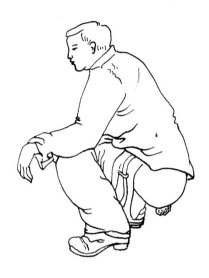

图 2 – 3　蹲位

Figure 2 – 3　Kneeling-squatting position

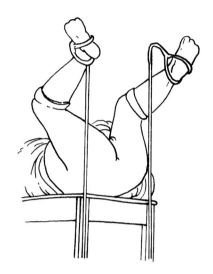

图 2 – 4　截石位

Figure 2 – 4　Lithotomy position

2. 检查方法

2. Methods of Examination

（1）视诊：查看有无红肿、瘢痕、外痔、湿疹、脱出的内痔和瘘管外口等病变，以及肛门外形。

（1）Observation：To look up whether or not red and swollen, engorged with blood, scar, external hemorrhoids, eczema, prolapse of internal hemorrhoids, external opening of fistula and external anal shape.

（2）指检：检查肛管直肠是否狭窄，有无硬结，肿瘤波及范围，或瘘管内口（触到有如豆大之较硬凹陷，即为瘘管内口）肛管直肠腔异物，肠套叠，肛门括约肌功能，鉴别男性前列腺或女性子宫颈疾病等。最后将手指抽出，观察指套上有无血迹或恶臭的黏液（指诊早期发现直肠癌或鉴别疾病的必查）。

（2）Digital examination：To examine whether or not narrow rectum, hard nodes, tumor and site, internal opening of fistulae（to feel hard pit like a bean）, foreign body in the lumen, rectal intussusception, anal sphincter pressures, prostate in male and cervices in female, etc.. To help finding the cause of symptoms such as rectal bleeding（blood in the stool）or mucus with stench

(many anorectal conditions may be successfully discovered by primary care). Growths such as hemorrhoids , polyps, tumors, or abscesses, may be found in the lower rectum.

(3)窥肛器检查:查直肠瓣状态,查看黏膜颜色,注意有无溃疡、息肉、肿瘤及异物;随后再将窥肛器慢慢退至齿线上方,检查有无内痔;在肛管上端查看有无肥大肛门乳头和发炎的肛窦、瘘管内口等。

(3)Anoscopic examination:To examine rectal valves, mucosal color, whether or not ulcer, polyp, tumor and foreign body are there; slowly draw back the anoscopy to look about whether internal hemorrhoids, hypertrophy of anal papilla, inflammation of crypts and internal opening of fistula, etc..

三、特殊检查
III. Special Examinations

1.光导纤维结肠镜检查　仅能观察肠腔内疾病。

1. **Fiberoptic Colonoscopy**　Limited to observe diseases in enteric cavity.

2.超声检查　直肠腔内超声检查,对肠管肿瘤定位准确,可早期发现黏膜下层癌。

2. **Ultrasound Examination**　The endoanorectal ultrasound can check accurate location of tumor in lumen for discovering early submucosal cancer.

3.CT检查　肛管、直肠CT检查不仅可见发现肠管腔内癌肿,而且可发现肠管壁内及邻近器官或组织病变。

3. **Computerized Tomography（CT）Examination**　This examination can discover not only cancer in intestinal lumen, but also lesions in intestinal wall and nearby organs or tissues.

4.磁共振成像检查　可发现肛肠肿瘤肠系膜疾病。多平面扫描可了解肿瘤的范围或是否转移,尤其是可以早期发现肿瘤。

4. **Magnetic Resonance Imaging Examination**　It can find out mesenteric pathologies of anorectal tumor and region of tumor and metastasis of cancer, especially early tumor.

5.放射性核素检查　主要是放射免疫分析,如测定肿瘤标志物。

5. **Radionuclide Tests**　They are mainly radioimmune analyses, such as the test of tumor markers.

6.肛瘘检查

6. **Anal Fistula Examination**

（1）探针检查：如探知瘘管方向、深度、长度，是否弯曲、有无分支，与肛管、直肠是否相通等。检查方法：以银制探针自瘘管外口徐徐插入，同时以另手示指带上指套（涂油），插入肛门内协助寻找内口。探针在肛门内顺利通过口，即为内口（图 2－5）。

（1）Probe examination：To explore the fistulous track，length，flexion and branch，communication with the cavity of the anal canal or rectum．In this way it may be possible to find out both openings of the fistula．The examination method：a silver probe may be slowly inserted into the sinus to look for internal outlet，the lubricant gloved finger（inunction）should be gently inserted into the rectum to help finding out the internal orifice of the sinus，the tip point of the probe can be felt waltz through the internal opening（Fig 2－5）．

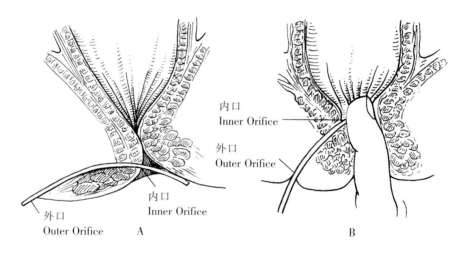

图 2－5　肛瘘探针检查
A. 探针伸入瘘管由肛门拉出；B. 探针检查瘘管内口（手指伸入肛门，探针伸入瘘管）
Figure 2－5　Anal fistula probe examination
A. The probe is injected into the fistulous tract and drawn from the internal opening；
B. Examine the internal opening with the probe（introduce the finger into the rectum，and the probe along the fistulous tract ）

（2）注射色素：为了证实瘘管有无内口，以保证顺利进行手术。其方法是：在肛门内放一块纱布（通过窥肛器放入），将 5% 亚甲蓝溶液由肛瘘外口注入，然后将纱布取出。如纱布染为蓝色，即证明为完全瘘（有内口）。但因瘘管弯曲及括约肌收缩，有时亚甲蓝溶液不能通过内口。因此，纱布没有染为蓝色，也不能武断地认为没有内口。遇到这种情况，还应做进一步检查。

（2）Injection of pigment：To find whether internal opening or not so as to perform the operation favorably．The method：to put a gauze into the anus（through anoscopy），the outer orifice of the sinus to inject with 5% methylene blue solution．If there is an internal opening the appearance of colored fluid within the bowel and the gauze will set the question at rest，making sure that the fistula is a complete one（there is an internal opening）．But sometimes the methylene blue cannot be passed through internal opening because of bended fistulous track and the sphincter contraction. The doctor must not arbitrarily make decision of there are not internal opening. If a doubt still exists as to the completeness of the track, the other methods may be introduced into the examinations as follows.

(3)X 线检查:对复杂的肛瘘,管道复杂,支管多,弯弯曲曲,不能确诊者,可用碘油造影检查。其方法是:注射碘油于瘘管内(或用次硝酸铋 1 份、丹士林 2 份,做成糊状,加温注入瘘管内),然后摄 X 线片,可以看到瘘管部位及分支情况。

(3)X-ray examination:For complex fistulae, complex tracks, many branches with winding. The diagnositic method of fistula has already been sufficiently detailed for complex fistulae, complex tracks and a few branches with winding. Through the outer orifice of the sinus a solution of Iodipin can be injected, if there be an internal opening the appearance of the colored fluid within the bowel, tracks and branches will be seen by X-ray.

(4)肛钩检查:检查瘘管内口位置,便于手术时正确找到内口。其方法是:常规消毒后,用鸭嘴窥肛器扩开肛门,然后用肛钩探钩肛窦。肛窦深度一般约为0.3cm,如超过这个深度,即可能是瘘管的内口。

(4)Anal hook examination:Look for the internal opening of fistula so as to find out the correct position in surgery. The method to sterilize as usual, then to dilate the anus with a duck-mouth anal dilator or anoscope, and then to probe and hook the anal crypts. The anal crypt's depth is about 0.3cm, if the depth is over, the internal opening of fistula may be there.

四、检查记录
IV. Records of Examinations

详见图 2 - 6。

To give a minute description in Fig. 2 - 6.

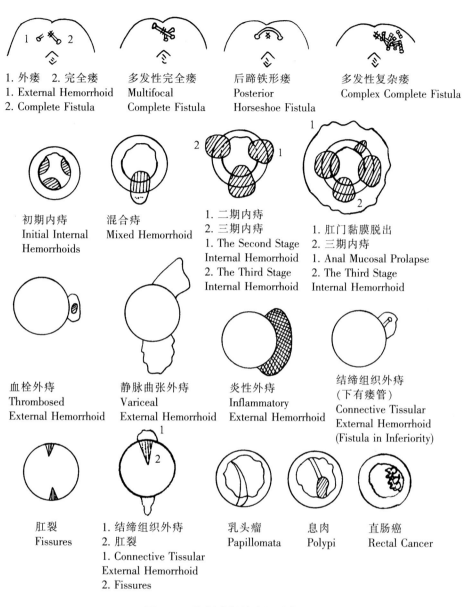

图 2－6　肛门直肠检查记录方法

Figure 2－6　Recordable method about anal rectal examination

第3章 肛肠疾病小针刀疗法概论

Chapter 3 An Introduction to Acupuncture Scalpel Therapy in Coloproctology

一、发展简史

I. Brief History on Development

1. 汉代 从公元1~2世纪起,文献记载的365种药物中,用来医治痔瘘的就有槐实等21种,其中有6种药都可治疗"五痔"。由此可见,在汉代不仅有了对痔的病证鉴别和治疗药物,也有了初步的分类。

1. Han Dynasty From the beginning of AD 1~2 Centuries the documents recorded that 21 kinds of Chinese herbs among 365 ones were used to treat hemorrhoid and fistula-in-ano, while 6 herbs from 21 ones could treat 5 types of hemorrhoids. So in Han dynasty the hemorrhoids could be not only diagnosed by differentiation of syndromes, but also treated by herbs with type classification initially.

2. 晋代 皇甫谧已开始用针刺方法治疗痔瘘,在《针灸甲乙经》里记载有"痔痛,攒竹主之;痔,会阴主之……。脱肛,下刺气街主之"。说明当时已将针刺疗法用于治疗痔瘘(图3-1)。

2. Jin Dynasty Huang Pumi had begun to treat hemorrhoids and fistulae with acupuncture through <ZhenJiu JiaYi Jing> (acupuncture meridian and channel)in which recorded：The pain of hemorrhoids is treated by acupuncturing Zanzhu point; while hemorrhoids, by acupuncturing HuiYin point…… The anal mucosal prolapse, by acupuncturing Qi Jie point. So that hemorrhoids and fistulae could have been treated by acupuncture therapy at that time(Fig. 3-1).

3. 隋代 巢元方在他所著《诸病源候论》里,总结了前人的经验,提出"五痔",并扼要地阐述了"五痔"的特征,包括了现代内痔、外痔、混合痔及肛瘘等概念。在治疗方面,当时创造了类似现代体育疗法的"导引法"(图3-2)。其方法是:一足踏地,一足屈膝,两手抱犊鼻下急挽向身极热,左右换易四七,去痔五劳,三里气不下(《诸病源候论》:诸痔疾)。"五痔"的特征如下。

3. Sui Dynasty As in the book <ZhuBing YuanHou Lun> (Etiology, Symptom and Sign)edited by Chao Yuanfang, he summed up predecessors' experience, and mentioned "the five types of hemorrhoids" and explained simply the different features, included internal hemorrhoids, external hemorrhoids, mixed hemorrhoids and fistulae, and etc.. In treatment he created "Dao Yin

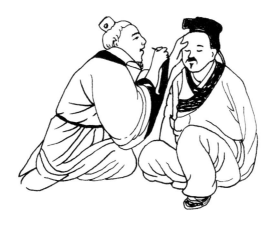

图 3 - 1　针刺法
Figure 3 - 1　Acupuncture Therapy

Fa（guiding method）" similar to modern physical exercise therapy（Fig. 3 - 2）. The method was that the patient stands on one foot, holds up the other foot, bends the knee and carries it in his arm, and rounds it to the chest. The patient should exercise again and again till sweating, then moves the other foot, the left and the right changed to act each other 4 ~ 7 times, so that the five signs of hemorrhoids could be treated（from ＜ ZhuBing YuanHou Lun ＞ : every kind of hemorrhoids）. The feature of the five signs of hemorrhoids is as follows :

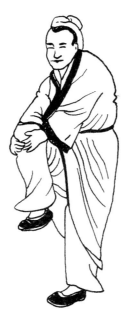

图 3 - 2　导引法
Figure 3 - 2　Guiding Method

（1）牡痔:肛边生鼠乳出在外者,时时有脓血者。

（1）MuZhi：In anal region there is an exit from which sanious pus outflows any time.

（2）牝痔：肛边肿生疮而出血者。

（2）PiZhi：In anal region there are swelling and sore with bleeding.

（3）肠痔：肛边肿核痛，发寒热而出血者。

（3）ChangZhi：In anal region there is a furuncle with bleeding accompanying with pain，shivers with cold and fever.

（4）脉痔：肛边生疮，痒而复痛出血者。

（4）MaiZhi：In anal region there is a sore with bleeding accompanying with itch and repeated pain.

（5）血痔：因便而清血随出者。

（5）XueZhi：Bright red blood covers the stool.

4. **唐代**　孙思邈《千金要方》中，在原有五痔的基础上，又增加了"燥湿痔"和"外痔"两种。在治疗上又有了应用蛇蜕、鳖甲、猬皮、猪蹄甲、蜂房五种药物，分别治疗气、牡、牝、肠、脉五痔的方法，并记载有以药物熏洗痔瘘的方法（图3－3）。王焘的《外台秘要》中，又提出了"酒痔"、"气痔"等分类，以及"灸痔"、"熨痔"等疗法（图3－4，图3－5）。

4. **Tang Dynasty**　Sun Simiao added"dry and damp hemorrhoid" and "external hemorrhoid" based on the five signs of hemorrhoids from his work ＜QianJin YaoFang＞（very important prescriptions）. In the treatment he added to 5 kinds of herbs, Snake slough, Turtle shell, Erinaceus europaeusl, Pig nail and Hive, to treat the five signs of hemorrhoids respectively, and recorded method of treating hemorrhoids and fistulae with fume and steep by herbs（Figure 3 － 3）. Wang Zhu, in ＜WaiTai MiYao＞（secret prescriptions）, classified signs of hemorrhoids again and put forward "Jiu Zhi（alcohol leading to hemorrhoids）and Qi Zhi", etc., meanwhile raised therapy, such as moxibustion and iron treating hemorrhoids（Figure 3 － 4, Figure 3 － 5）.

5. **南宋**　魏岘的《魏氏字藏方》记载"枯痔疗法"。

5. **South Song Dynasty**　＜WeiShi ZiCangFang＞（collected prescriptions）worked by Wei Xian, recorded "drying up hemorrhoid therapy".

6. **明代**　徐春甫著的《古今医统》介绍了"挂线疗法"。在内治法方面遵照李东垣的湿、热、风、燥四治法，以及朱丹溪的补阴凉血为主的疗法。

6. **Ming Dynasty**　＜GuJin YiTong＞（ancient and modern medicine）worked by Xu Chunpu introduced "ligation method". The therapy of oral herbs, should be conformed to both Li Dongyan and Zhu Danxi. Li had four kinds of therapy：wet, hot, winded, and dry, and Zhu was to invigorate Yin and cool blood mainly.

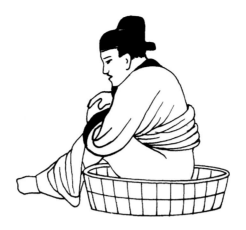

图 3 - 3　熏洗法

Figure 3 - 3　Fuming and washing

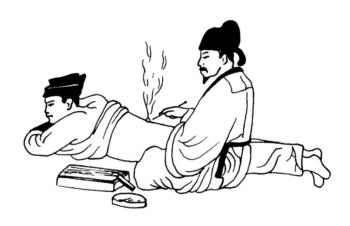

图 3 - 4　灸痔法

Figure 3 - 4　Moxibustion

7.**清代**　《医宗金鉴》记载："此证系肛门生疮,有生于肛门者,有生于门外者。初起成垒不破者为痔,易治;破溃而出脓血,黄水侵淫,淋漓久不止者为漏难愈。"并发明了探肛筒、过肛针、弯刀等器械,用来治疗痔、瘘。

7. **Qing Dynasty**　< YiZong Jinjian > (appreciation of medicine) recorded: "The symptoms show that there are sores on the inside of anus or the outside. They are called piles when they form hard nodes, however they are called anal fistulae when they can be broken easily by treatment, then they are festering, bleeding, dripping, and then the wound heals slowly and difficultly." The appliances to treat piles and fistulae were invited such as a tube for probing the inside of anus, a needle for going into anus, and a crooked knife for surgery, etc.

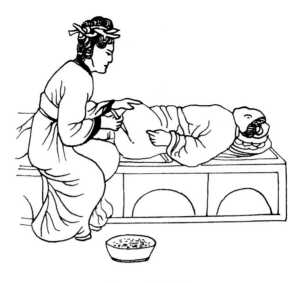

图 3 - 5　熨痔法

Figure 3 - 5　Method of iron treating hemorrhoids

二、中医对肛肠生理病理的认识

Ⅱ. The Cognition of Traditional Chinese Medicine

1.《内经素问》

1. < NeiJin SuWen >

(1)《金匮真言论》:"胆、胃、大肠、小肠、膀胱、六腑皆为阳。"

(1) < JinGui ZhenYan Lun >:"The six hollow organs such as the stomach, large intestine, small intestine and bladder, etc. are all Yang."

(2)《阴阳应象大记》:"故清阳出上窍,浊阴出下窍。"

(2) < YinYang YingXiang DaJi >:"The cleaning is superior, the fouling is inferior."

(3)《良兰秘典记》:"大肠者结道之宝,变化出焉。"

(3) < LiangLan MiDian Ji >:"The large intestine is the passway, and the matter after being assimilated is excreted from here."

(4)《六节脉象记》:"脾胃大肠小肠三者膀胱者,仓廪之本,营之居也,名曰器。能化糟粕,转味而入出奇也。"

(4) < LiuJie MaiXiang Ji >:"The spleen, stomach, large intestine and small intestine are like warehouses and can digest and absorb and metabolize."

(5)《王腑制记》:"胃大肠小肠三膀胱此五者,天气之所生也,其气象天,故泻而不藏,此受五脏浊气,名曰结化之府,此不能久泻,输泻者也,魄门变为五脏,使水谷不得久存……六腑者,结化物而不藏,故实而不能满也,所以然者水谷入口,则胃实而肠虚。食下则肠实而胃虚。故曰实而不满,满而不实也。"

（5）＜WangFu ZhiJi＞:The stomach, large intestine, small intestine, and bladder have drainable function.

2.《灵枢》

2. ＜Ling Shu＞

（1）《胀记》:"大肠胀者,肠鸣而痛(强者)的,冬日重形于寒,则餐泄不化。"

（1）＜ZhangJi＞ :"The abdominal distension and pain may result from catching cold, and the patient feels the body heaviness, excreting indigestible food. "

（2）《本藏记》皇帝曰:"愿闻六腑之应。"岐伯曰:"肺合大肠,大肠者,皮其应。"皇帝曰:"应之奈何。"岐伯曰:"肺应皮,皮厚者大肠厚,皮薄者,大肠薄。皮缓肤是大者,大肠大而长。皮急者大肠急而短。皮滑者,大肠直,皮内不相离者大肠结。"

（2）＜BenZang Ji＞ An emperor said:I want to listen to the correspondence relationship about viscerae. Qi Bo said:"The large intestines interrelate the lungs each other over inside and outside, and the skin corresponds with them. " The emperor said again:"How about correspondence?" QiBo said:"The person whose skin is thick has thick large intestine, and it's the same the other way round. The skin is soft while the large intestine is large and long; the skin is tight, the large intestine is short, smooth, straight, inseparable and obstructive. "

（3）《难经》四十四难:"七冲门何在。然唇为正门。齿为户门。会状为吸门。胃为贲门。大仓下口为出口。故曰七冲门也。""丁曰……大肠小肠会出阀门,会者合也,大肠小肠合会之处分阑水谷,精血各有所归,故曰阑门也。下极为魄门,大肠者肺之腑也,藏其魄,大肠下名肛门,又曰魄门者。杨曰,人有七窍是五腑之门户,皆出于面,今七冲门者亦是脏腑之所出,而内外廉有征焉……。大肠小肠会为阑门。阑门者遗火之义也,言大小二肠皆输泻广畅,即受传而出之。是遗失之义也。故曰阑门。下极为魄门,魄门者下极肛门也。肺气上通喉咙,下通于肛门,是肺气之所出也。肺藏魄,故曰:魄门焉,仲者通也,出也,言脏腑之气通出之所也(难经集注)。"

（3）＜NanJing＞ the 44th Nan:Where are 7 Chong doors? Here the lips are front gates; the teeth are house door; the epiglottis is entrance of respiratory tract; the stomach's inlet is cardia; inferior opening of the large intestine is outlet… " Ding said:"…there is a valve in the communicating part of large intestine and small intestine. It's ileocecal valve, and the appendix is here. The terminal potion of the large intestine is soul gate. The large intestine is a hollow organ, and its interactive solid organ is lungs. They are in relationship of exterior and interior, and the large intestine saves the lungs' soul. The inferior end of large intestine is anus with another name as soul gate. Yang said:there are 7 apertures in the human body which are the doors of viscerae while 7 Chong doors are the outlets of viscerae, so that the 7 apertures and 7 Chong are also in relationship of exterior and interior ······. The appendix of the communicating part of large intestine and small intestine is a lost and forgetful organ, that's so called appendix. The lungs' outlet is upward throat, downward is anus(<Annotation of NanJing >). "

(4)《医学入门》:"痔非外邪,乃脏腑注热风燥,因时相合而成。"

(4) < Elementary Medicine > :" To form hemorrhoids have something to do with that wind and dryness affecting the body, then they transform heat in viscera. So the formation of hemorrhoids is totally with actual situation of climate change, except that the body is invaded directly by pathogeny from exterior.

(5)《丹溪心法》:"痔者皆因脏腑本虚、外防风邪内靠温毒⋯⋯致气血下坠于肛门,宿滞不散而为痔。"

(5) < Study of DanXi > :"The hemorrhoids have something to do with visceral inherent weakness, and the body is affected and invaded by external wind evil and internal warm toxin⋯⋯ leading to the anal tenesmus with gas and blood detained. So unhealthiness influences from internal and external environment cause the disease.

(6)痔术后脱落出血,补中益气汤。

(6)The postoperative bleeding:May be treated by BuZhongYiQi decoction (tonify blood and Qi).

三、中医五脏与大肠功能的关系

Ⅲ. The Relationship between 5 Viscerae and Large Intestinal Function in Traditional Chinese Medicine

《素问·五脏别论》有"魄门亦为五脏,使水谷不得久藏"之说。说明人体脏腑之间功能上相互联系又相互制约,才能保持体内外环境的统一。它们与大肠功能的关系如下:

< SuWen · 5Viscerae >:"The soul gate also belongs to 5 viscerae, in which the contents from transformed water and gain can't be stored for long time. The book explained that the human body keep the relation and condition each other among visceral function so as to integrate between internal environment with external one. The fullness follows:

1. 肺主气、主宣、发肃降 肺与大肠,即表与里、脏与腑相结合。肺气肃降,则大肠传导顺利,肺气虚则便秘,肺热下血,大肠可致脱肛;反之,大肠传导失司,则肺气不通。魄门不能排泻浊气,则影响肺气肃降,产生咳喘,故在泻白承气,温治肺热

喘咳。

1. **The Lungs Govern Gas（Qi）, Diffusion and Depuration**　The relation of lungs and large intestine is like connection of interior and exterior. Depurative downbearing of the lung gas will make conveyance of large intestine without a hitch; vacuity of lung gas will lead to constipation, precipitation of blood of lung; heat will cause anal desertion; conversely, large intestine can't convey, and the lung gas flow stops. It influences depurative downbearing of the lung gas and produce cough and panting that the soul gate can't excrete turbid gas, so that the prescription of XieBaiChengQi can treat the diseases from lung heat.

2. **脾主运化,主升清**　脾关连大肠的传导,脾气有升清固脱作用,故脾虚产生腹泻,脱肛。脾虚则大肠传导无力而产生气虚便秘,脾统血如统摄失常,则可出现便血,例如沈月南在《金匮要略注》中说"五脏六腑之血,全赖脾气统摄"。若脾的统摄失调,则可造成便血。

2. **The Spleen Governs Transformation and Upbearing the clear**　The spleen has something to do with conveyance of large intestine and acts on upbearing the clear and steming desertion so that the spleen vacuity causes either diarrhea and anal desertion or constipation of deficiency. Another action the spleen is to command blood. If it doesn't work, bleeding may be occurring in patient's stool. It's just like "All blood coming from viscerae is controlled by the spleen." From ＜Annotation of JinGui YaoLue＞ worked by ShenYuenan.

3. **肾开窍于二阴,主魄门与小便开与闭**　若肾阳虚损不能温煦下元可致五更泻。魄门不利,则引起便秘,肾的封藏失调、关门不利,则引起久泻滑脱。

3. **The Kidneys Govern Urine and Soul Gate**　If the kidneys Yang is weak they can't warm downwards, so that the diarrhea will occur in the early morning. The soul gate doesn't work well then constipation will take place; the function of kidney's preservation is maladjustment, and the downward desertion and diarrhea for a long time will come.

4. **肝主疏泄,调气机**　人体气机升降,出入疏通畅达,其魄门才可运行正常。肝气不和,其魄门开闭不利,则腹满胀气、大便涩燥。

4. **The Liver Governs Dredge and Adjustment**　The soul gate acting relies on liver dredging. The liver Qi doesn't cooperate in work, then abdominal distension and the constipation will occur.

5. **心藏神,主魄门的开闭**　心神正常,则魄门开闭有序。心神不宁,则魄门开闭无序,引起大便失禁。

5. **The Heart Stores Soul and Spirit, and Governs the Opening and Closing of the Soul Gate**　The spirit is normal while the soul gate opens and closes regularly; conversely, disorderly. The heart doesn't work well while incontinence of defecation will occur.

四、小针刀治疗肛肠疾病的应用
Ⅳ. Application of Acupuncture Scalpel to Coloproctology

小针刀治疗肛肠病是"针眼外科"范畴。它通过试验,寻找出病变关键部位,以微创外科为基础,以微小的灵巧器械选择性地改变组织结构,以最小的创伤达到最佳的治疗效果。它可以保持局部结构基本完整,不伤及正常组织,不留瘢痕。

Applying acupuncture scalpel to treat coloproctology belongs to "needlepoint surgery", based on finding out critical part of pathology by experiment. The therapy uses small ingenious surgical appliances to change selectively the structure of tissues so as to arrive at best effect going through with minimal trauma, and keeps local structure intact, neither injuring normal tissues, nor leaving scar.

自配合小针刀疗法以来,不但将许多复杂的肛肠开放性手术变为简单、闭合性手术,而且疗效好,是中西医结合的结晶。小针刀治疗肛肠病,是以西医解剖学和诊断学知识为基础,对病变定性、定位,再运用中医小针刀的刺、切、钩、割和挑拨手法解除病痛的方法。因而手术创面小,不损伤正常肛肠组织,不会导致肛门失禁。它将针刺疗法的针和手术疗法的刀融为一体,即中医针灸疗法与西医手术疗法结合,因而既是传统医学发展的新成果,也是中国的特色疗法。该疗法的许多创新之处,不仅获得多项专利,也获得不少国内外大奖,好评如潮。

The therapy of acupuncture scalpel surgery is a crystallization of integrated TCM and WM that the therapy not only changes many complex open surgeries to be simple close one for treating ano-rectal diseases, but also gets good effect. The therapy relies on the knowledge from WM anatomy and diagnostics to decide position and quality of the lesion, and then makes use of TCM puncturing, slicing, hooking, cutting and pricking to remove the disease. So with the method the wound of surgery is small and light, and normal tissue is not injured, and the incontinence of feces will not be a question. It's the fusion of needle from acupuncture and knife from surgery that's the integrated therapy of both TCM and WM. So it's a new achievement, of being either modern or traditional. This therapy brings forth new ideas, and wins many patents and prizes at home and abroad, and is well accepted by the doctors and patients.

小针刀疗法闭合性手术,有其独特的理论基础,操作简单,技法灵巧,可做到无切口,不出血,且局部麻醉安全可靠,无后遗症,无并发症和无不良反应。患者治疗前与后,均可以照常饮食、排大便和活动。

The therapy of acupuncture scalpel is a simple operation, with clever skill, least trauma, least bleeding, and local anesthesia, safe, no complications, no side effects and no sequelae. The patients can have meal, defecate stool and take action as usual in the peri-operative period.

　　可以说,小针刀治疗肛肠疾病的诊断基础是西医,而治疗基础是中医,两者结合的优点是:①西医先确定诊断,中医再进行辨证,缩小中医辨证范围,便于摸清中医辨证规律,从中医辨证的角度掌握病变的实质;②中西医结合诊断,弥补了彼此的不足,创造了新的有利条件,丰富了现代诊断方法,提高了治疗效果;③推动了中西医结合治疗的发展,进而产生了新疗法和新理论。

　　The basis of diagnosis comes from WM while that of treatment from TCM in arranging anorectum with acupuncture scalpel. The advantages of integrated WM and TCM are:①To diagnose first with WM, then to take differentiation of syndromes by TCM, reduce the scope of differentiation by TCM, and to master the crux of disease from angles of differentiation by TCM. ②The diagnosis of WM and TCM have counteracted their own weaknesses each other, created new good conditions,enriched modern diagnosis and improved the treating effects. ③The therapy improves the development of treatment with integrated WM and TCM so as to produce new therapy and theory.

第4章　肛肠疾病中医非手术疗法

Chapter 4　Nonoperative Therapies by Traditional Chinese Medicine for Coloproctology

肛肠疾病中医非手术疗法,本不属本书介绍范围,但是由于这些疗法对于小针刀治疗肛肠疾病的围手术期准备和处理非常重要而有效,因而特别介绍如下。

The nonoperative therapies by traditional Chinese medicine for coloproctology is very important and effective for preparation and arrangement around surgery to treat diseases of the anus and rectum with acupuncture scalpel.

第一节　气病及其治疗

§ 1　Qi Disease and Treatment

理气开郁疗法是肛肠病常用八法之一,有着广泛应用范围。

Regulating Qi and dispelling stasis is one of the eight common therapies on proctology, with a broad application scope, should be used extensively.

【基本概念】

[Fundamental Conception]

气的名称散见于中医的各种著作和历代医案之中。例如,张景岳说:"生化之道以气为本,天地万物莫不有之……四时万物得以生长收藏,何非气之所为,人之有生全赖此气。"又如《杂病广要》中说:"阴阳虽大,未离乎气,故通天下一气耳,一吐纳,一动静,何所逃哉,与气通而已。故气平则宁,气不平则病。"说明"气"在维持正常生理活动中有着重要意义。

Qi shows cases of TCM in every medical work in every dynasty. For example, Zhang Jingyue said: "Qi is a foundation of physiology. There is nothing on the earth without Qi…… All living matter can grow and reap all the year round, why not for Qi to do? The reason why the human being can live and act here is to rely on the Qi." In ＜ZaBing GuangYao＞ "Yin and Yang should never for a moment deviate from Qi although they are very important, so that Qi links up all over the world. Only by keeping Qi going can all living things metabolize. So Qi goes free, the person is healthy, conversely, Qi doesn't work well, the disease falls down." So Qi is very important to keep normal physiological activities.

总的来说,中医对气的认识包含着两方面内容:①指物质而言,如大气、营气;

②指功能而言,如心平、肝气。像《灵枢·邪容篇》说:"营气者,泌其津液,注之于脉,化以为血,以荣四末,内注五脏六腑。"说明营气是血液中的营养物质。该篇又说:"宗气积于胸中,出于喉咙,以贯心脉,而行呼吸。"说明宗气有主司呼吸,又有促进血液循环的功能。总之,中医学对气的认识,不论是指功能的或物质的,均说明机体之所以能够维持正常的生命活动,保持各器官的生理平衡,是由于气的正常流通生化的结果。因此,人体气的生化有着重要的意义。

In general there are two contents of Qi from TCM:①material Qi such as gas and air;②functional Qi such as liver Qi. In <LingShu·XieRong Pian>:"Ying Qi can secrete body fluid, then pour into vessels, and then transform into blood, in order to supply outwards the four limbs, and irrigate inwards viscerae. So it explains, that Ying Qi is a nutrition in the blood." In this book there is another record:Zong Qi stores in the chest, and goes out of throat, and runs through the heart and vessels, and performs or practices respiration. It explains that Zong Qi either governs respiration, or facilitates blood circulation. In a word, whether functional Qi or material Qi, the recognition about Qi from TCM is a significance on maintaining normal physiological action and balance.

【病因病理】

[Etiology and Pathology]

中医认为,不论七情内伤,外感六淫,或房事劳倦,均可伤气而致病。凡气的盛衰、急缓和乱结等都可以发生不同的病变。张景岳说:"气之在人,和则为正气,不和则为邪气。"如在内伤七情的病变中,有怒则气上,喜则气缓,悲则气消,恐则气下,惊则气乱,劳则气耗,思则气结等。在外感六淫的病变中,有风伤气为疼痛,寒伤气为战栗,暑伤气为热闷,湿伤气为肿满,燥伤气为闭结等。

TCM holds emotional disturbances, external invasive causes and sexual intercourse which all injure Qi and cause diseases. For Qi, prosperity and decline, acuteness and slowness, irregularity and obstruction, etc. all cause diseases. Zhang Jingyue said:The person with even-tempered and good-mood will accompany with healthy trends and normal metabolism, conversely, bad mood will lead to unhealthy trends. In the syndrome, differentiation of etiology from external courses, cold Qi (air) brings about pain and tremble; summer Qi, hotness; damp Qi, edema and fullness; dry Qi, constipation; etc.

总之,由于病因的不同,出现不同的病理变化和证候,其性质可有虚、实、寒、热的差异,变化多端。但其根本原因,皆为气不通调所致。

Different causes lead to different pathologic changes and syndrome. Although there are variations such as virtual, real, cold and hot, the basic cause is that Qi isn't freely moving.

【临床表现】

[Clinical Manifestations]

由于气机失调所在部位的不同与症状的差异，常将气病分为气滞、气郁、气逆和气陷四大类。

Because the different portion of Qi imbalance and the different symptoms, Qi diseases can be divided into 4 categories.

1. 气滞　病在经络，症状多表现为疼痛阵发，时发时止，得热即缓。气聚则痛而见形，气散则平而无迹，痛无定所，往来走窜。脉弦，涩或紧。

1. **Qi Stagnation**　The disease is in superficial layer of the body, and the symptoms are intermittent pain mainly, sometimes occurring, sometimes stopping. Hardly do meet heat with alleviated pain. The pain is at undefined position. Pulses string are hesitant or tense.

2. 气郁　病在脏腑，症状多为胁肋疼痛，痞塞胀闷，饮食不化，神志忧郁。脉弦细。

2. **Qi Stasis**　The disease in viscera often shows chest pain and hypochondriac pain, abdominal distention and fullness, dyspepsia and melancholy. Pulses string are thin.

3. 气逆　病在上，多为呕吐、喘满、气晕、头痛、耳鸣、面红。如肺气上逆可致咳喘，胃气上逆可致呃逆、呕吐等。脉弦紧有力。

3. **Qi Adversity**　The disease in superior part of the body often shows vomiting, heavy breath or asthma, dizzy, headache, tinnitus, being red in the face. For example, the lung Qi is adversity that can cause the pulmonary diseases, such as cough or heavy breath; the stomach Qi is adversity that can cause gastric diseases, such as nausea, vomiting, etc. Pulses string are tense and excess.

4. 气陷　病在下，常表现为少气懒言、面黄白、自汗、腹泻、脱肛、崩漏、子宫下垂、尿频、四肢无力。脉沉细无力。

4. **Qi Depression**　The disease in inferior part of body often shows laziness to speak, yellow and white face, night sweat, prolapse of anus, uterine bleeding, prolapse of uterus, frequent micturition and fatigued limbs. Pulses are sunken, thin and feeble.

气病脉象以沉弦为多见。古人云："手下脉沉便知是气，大凡气病轻者，肺脉独沉，重者六脉俱沉。"又气病轻者，肝脉独弦，重者脾脉亦弦。

The pulse in Qi disease is often sunken. The ancient doctor said: "the hand feels pulse sunken, that's Qi disease. Being a mild disease, lung pulse is felt sunken only; in severe ones all the pulses are sunken." Another doctor said: "in the mild case, the liver pulse is strict only, and in severe case, the spleen pulse is strict too.

【治疗】

[Treatment]

如前所述,气机失调可导致各种疾病,常采用行气、开郁、降气、补气等治法。前三者适用于气病之实证,如气滞、气郁、气逆;后者适用于气虚、气陷等虚证。

Qi imbalance can cause various diseases. The common treating method consists of moving Qi, dispelling stasis, reducing and depressing Qi, invigorating Qi, etc. The first three methods are managed in excess syndrome of Qi disease, such as Qi stagnation, Qi stasis, Qi adversity; the latter is managed in deficiency syndrome, such as Qi deficiency and Qi depression, etc.

1.**气滞治法**　宜行宜破,多用辛香行气止痛之品,如香附、苏叶、木香、川楝子、延胡索、乳香、没药、枳壳、厚朴等。代表方剂有木香顺气丸、金铃子散。

1. **Method for Treating Qi Stagnation**　To let Qi going and break up stagnation, frequently to use aromatic and analgesia, such as Rhizoma Cyperi, Perillae, Folium, Fructus Meliae Toosendan, Chinaberry Fruit, Rhizoma Corydalis, Mastic, Myrrha, Fructus Aurantii and Mangnolia Officinalis, etc. The representative prescriptions are MuXiangShunQi Pill and JinLingZi Powder.

(1)木香顺气丸

(1)MuXiangShunQi Pill (qi-regulating pill of aucklandia)

①组成:木香、厚朴、青陈皮、苍术、半夏、茯苓、泽泻、益智仁、草蔻仁、吴茱萸、干姜、柴胡、升麻、当归。

①Components:Folium, Mangnolia officinalis, Dried tangerine, Rhizoma atractylodis, Tuckahoe, Rhizoma alismatis, Semen amomi amari, Semen alpinae katsumadai, Evodia rutaecarpa, Rhizoma zingiberis, Radix bupleuri, Rhizoma cimicifugae.

②功用:调中顺气,益脾消胀。

②Function:Regulating middle energizer to harmonize vitality(Qi), invigorating spleen to relieve flatulence.

③适应证:胸膈痞闷,胁肤胀满,气不宣通。

③Indication:Thoracic fullness and rib-side distention.

(2)金铃子散

(2)JinLingZi (Fructus Toosendan) Powder

①组成:川楝子、延胡索。

①Components:Fructus Meliae Toosendan, Chinaberry fruit.

②功用:疏肝行气止痛。

②Function：Dispersing stagnated hepato-Qi, analgesia.

③适应证：心肤胁肋诸痛,时发时止。脉数、舌红、苔黄。

③Indication：Heart and rib-side pain, sometimes occurring, sometimes stopping. Pulse is rapid; tongue is red texture, yellowish fur.

2. 气郁的治法　宜疏宜散,多用行气解郁止痛健胃的药物,如香附、郁金、柴胡、蔻仁、砂仁等。常用代表方有柴胡疏肝丸。

2. Method for Treating Qi Stasis　To evacuate stasis, frequently to take herbs of dispersing Qi stasis, analgesia and invigorating stomach, such as Rhizoma Cyperi, Radix Curcumae, Radix Bupleuri, Fructus Amomi Rotundus and Fructus Amomi, etc.

（1）组成：柴胡、枳实、杭芍、川芎、枳壳、香附、生甘草。

（1）Components：Radix Bupleuri, Fructus Aurantii Immaturus, Radix Paeoniae Alba from Hangzhou, Ligusticum Wallichii, Fructus Aurantii, Rhizoma Cyperi and Liquorice. The common representative prescription is ChaiHu ShuGan（dredge stasis）Pill.

（2）功用：调和肝脾。

（2）Function：Reconciling liver and spleen.

（3）适应证：胁肋疼痛,寒热往来。

（3）Indication：Rib-side pain, sometimes cold and sometimes hot.

3. 气逆治法　宜降宜缓,采用降逆重镇之品,如苏子、旋覆花、半夏、代赭石、沉香、炒莱菔子等。用于气机上逆,见有恶心、呃逆、喘咳等症者。其代表方如旋覆代赭汤。胃虚而气逆者,可配人参、甘草,以益胃气;痰湿内郁者可配半夏、厚朴以化痰湿;有热者可用清降之品,如竹茹、桑皮等;有寒者可用温降之品,如丁香、柿蒂等。

3. Method for Treating Qi Adversity　To reduce adversity, take the herbs of moving downward, such as Perilliaseed, Inula flower, Pinellia Ternate, Ruddle, Linalool and Stir-baked semen Raphani, etc. To treat symptom of adversity, such as nausea, hiccup, cough and heavy breath, the representative prescription is Inulae and Ochrae Decoction. For stomach asthenia with Qi adversity, to add Ginseng and Liquorice to nourish stomach Qi; for sputum, to add Pinellia ternate and Mangnolia officinalis to reduce sputum; for heat, add reducing heat herbs by cooling nature such as Bambusae caulis im taeniam and Cortex mori, etc. ; for coldness, add reducing coldness herbs by warm nature such as Clove and kaki calyx, etc.

（1）组成：旋覆花、人参、生姜、代赭石、甘草、半夏、大枣。

（1）Components：Inula flower, Ginseng, Ginger, Ruddle, Liquorice, Pincllia ternate, Fructus ziziphi jujubae.

（2）功用：扶正益气，降逆化痰。

（2）Function：Nourishing Qi and reducing sputum.

（3）适应证：胃气虚弱痰浊内阻，心下痞硬，时嗳气，大便秘，苔浊腻，脉弦虚者。

（3）Indication：Stomach Qi asthenia, sputum, eructation, constipation, damp greasy fur, pulse is spring and asthenia.

4.**气陷治法**　常用补气益气之法，故宜升宜补。如用升麻、柴胡、党参、黄芪、白术、桂枝等。其代表方为补中益气汤。

4. **Method for Treating Qi Depression**　To promote and nourish Qi commonly, such as Rhizoma cimicifugae, Radix bupleuri, Codonopsis pilosula, Astragalus mongholicus, White atractylodes, Rhizoma and Cassia twig, etc. The representative prescription is BuZhongYiQi(nourishing)Decoction.

（1）组成：黄芪、人参、甘草、白术、当归、陈皮、升麻、柴胡、大枣。

（1）Components：Astragalus mongholicus, Ginseng, Liquorice, White atractylodes Rhizoma Angelica, Dried Tangerine, Rhizoma cimicifugae, Radix bupleuri, Jujubae.

（2）功用：升阳益气，调补脾胃。

（2）Function：Promoting and nourishing Qi, nourishing spleen and stomach.

（3）适应证：劳倦伤脾、清阳下陷、中气不足、自汗、泄泻、子宫下垂、脱肛等。

（3）Indication：Overworked, spontaneous perspiration, diarrhea, hysteroptosis, prolapse of rectum, and proctoptosis.

以上是对于气机失调而常采用的治疗方法（表4-1）。在治疗气病使用理气药时，要注意以下几点：①理气药多为辛温香燥之品，用之不可过量或连续使用时间太长，否则会有耗气伤阴之流弊；②气郁而见津伤者，忌用理气药；③虚人和孕妇对破气、降气药须慎用。

All the above methods treating Qi imbalance are shown in Table 4-1. In making use of regular herbs to treat Qi diseases, some points for attention should be noticed：①The nature of many regulating Qi herbs is pungent warm, aroma and dry. Whatever happens, never take an overdose or overtime of these herbs, or there will be depleting Qi and damaging Yin；②The patient with body fluid losing must abstain from these herbs；③Patients with deficiency or pregnancy should take care in using these herbs of breaking up and reducing Qi.

表4-1 气病的分类与治法

Table 4-1 Categories and therapy about Qi diseases

分类 Categories	病位 Location	症状 Symptoms	治法 Therapy	方剂 Prescription	药物 Components
气滞 Qi stagnation	病在经络 Disease in surfacelayer of body	疼痛阵发、时发、时止、得热可缓、气聚则痛而见形、气散则平而无迹、痛无定所往来走窜。脉弦紧涩 Intermittent pain; sometimes occur and stop; meet heat, pain alleviate; pain of undefined position. Pulses: string, hesitant, tense	宜行宜破 Qi go, stagnationbreak up	木香顺气丸 Regular Qi Pill of Costusroot	川楝子、延胡索、乳香、没药、木香、枳壳、厚朴、乌药 Toosendan, ambigua, mastic, myrrh, costusroot, fructus aurantii, magnolia officinalis, linderae
气郁 Qi stasis	病在脏腑 Disease in viscera	胁肋疼痛、痞满胀闷、食不化、神情忧郁。脉弦细 Chest, hypochondriac pain; distensible & full abdomen;dyspepsia & melancholy. Pulses are string and thin	宜疏宜散 Evacuate stasis	柴胡疏肝丸 Dredge liver Qi Pill of Bupleuri	香附、郁金、柴胡、砂仁、豆蔻 Curcumae, bupleuri, fructus amomi rotundus, etc.
气逆 Qi adversity	病在上 Disease in super part of body	为呕为吐、喘满头晕、头痛、耳鸣、面红。脉弦紧有力 Vomiting, heavy breath, asthma, dizzy, headache, tinnitus, red in the face. Pulses:string, tense, excess	宜降宜缓 Reduce adversity	旋覆赭石汤苏子降气丸 Inula Decoction Perilla seed Pill	半夏、代赭石、杭芍、旋覆花、竹茹、苏子、炒莱菔子、沉香 Pinellia, rubble, paeony, inula, caulis bamboo, perillaseed, stirraphani, agalloch
气陷 Qi depression	病在下 Disease in down part of body	少气懒言、面黄白、自汗、腹泻、脱肛、崩漏、子宫下垂、尿频、四肢无力。脉沉细无力 Lazy speech, yellow-white face, night sweat, prolapse of anus, uterine bleeding,prolapse of uterus, frequent micturition fatigued limbs. Pulses: sunken, thin, feeble	宜升宜补 Nourishtion& promotion for Qi	补中益气丸 BuZhong Yi Qi Pill (nourish and promote)	升麻、柴胡、党参、黄芪、白术、桂枝 Cimicifuga, bupleuri, codonopsis pilosula, astragalus, atractylodesrhizome and cassia twig

5. 理气开郁疗法

5. The Therapy of LiQi KaiYu (Regulating Qi and Dispelling Stasis)

(1)急性肛瘘:中医认为,其病因病理是肝、胆失疏泄,湿热滞结,热壅阳亢。根据临床症状、舌苔、脉象,分为气滞型、湿热型与实火型。方剂组成:柴胡、黄芩、半夏、枳壳、香附、郁金、延胡索各9g,木香9g,杭芍15g,生军15g(后下),川楝子9g。

(1)Acute anal fistulas:In traditional Chinese Medicine etiology and pathology are that Qi can't disperse stagnated liver and gall so as to form damp heat and pyretic promotion. According to clinical manifestations the disease is divided into 3 categories: stagnation, damp heat and sthenia heat. The components of prescription: Bupleuri, Scutellaria Baicalensis, Pinellia Ternate, Fructus Aurantii, Cyperi, Curcuma Aromatica, Corydalis, each 9g, Saussureae 9g, Paeoniae from Hangshao 15g, Radix Rhizoma Rhei 15g (decocted later), Toosendan fruit 9g.

（2）急性肛门脓肿：根据肛门脓肿的病理发展过程，参照临床症状、脉象、舌苔，将它分为三个阶段，即气滞血瘀期、蕴热期与毒热期。对气滞血瘀期用行气活血的方法进行治疗。方剂组成：木香 10g，川楝子 10g，延胡索 6g，桃仁 10g，牡丹皮 10g，金银花 30g，大黄 20g（后下），红藤 20g。

（2）Acute anal abscess: According to pathologic changing courses and clinical manifestations the disease is divided into 3 stages: Qi stagnation and blood stasis, fever and toxic fever, Moving Qi and activating blood. The components of prescription: Saussureae 10g, Toosendan 10g, Corydalis 6g, Peach seed 10g, Peony bark 10g, Honeysuckle 30g, Radix et Rhizoma Rhei 20g (decocted later), Sargent Gloryvine 20g.

（3）急性肠阻塞：肠阻塞的发生是气机失调，主要是恢复气机的正常运行，以行气、攻下为主。不论哪一类方剂，行气的药物都不可缺。方剂组成：川朴 9g，木香 9g，乌药 9g，炒莱菔子 9g，桃仁 9g，赤芍 9g，芒硝 6g（冲），番泻叶 9g。

（3）Acute intestinal obstruction: The pathologic changing course is that Qi can't be regulated so that the treating method is to recover Qi function, that's mainly activating Qi and purgation. Whatever prescription is, the herbs of moving Qi is absolutely necessary. The components of prescription: Officinalis 9g, Saussureae 9g, The root of three-nerved spicebush 9g, stir-baked Semen Raphant 9g, Peach seed 9g, Peony 9g, Mirabilite 6g (take after mixing it with water), Folium Sennae 9g.

对气胀较重的肠阻塞可用复方大承气汤。方剂组成：川朴 9g，炒莱菔子 9g，枳壳 9g，桃仁 9g，赤芍 9g，川军 30g（后下），芒硝 6g（冲），木香 9g。

For the disease with severe Qi distension, Compound DaChengQi decoction can be used. The components of prescription: Cortex Magnoliae Officinalis 9g, stir-baked Semen Raphant 9g, Fructus Aurantii 9g, Peach seed 9g, Rhizoma Peoniae 15g (decocted later), Mirabilite 6g (take after mixing it with water), Saussureae 10g.

从上述应用情况可以看出，中医学的理气开郁疗法在中西医结合治疗肛肠病中有着广泛的应用适应证，并占有重要的地位。如何用现代科学的方法，加以整理研究，进一步指导临床治疗，是摆在我们当前的一项重要任务。

The therapy of LiQi KaiYu (regulating Qi and dispelling stasis) from traditional Chinese medicine has extensive indications and significant position in coloproctological treatment by integrated traditional Chinese medicine and Western medicine.

第二节 瘀血及其治疗

§ 2　Blood Stasis and Management

气血学说是中医学病理生理的重要学说之一。过去对气血的关系,以及瘀血的认识是不够的。王肯堂指出:"夫人饮食起居,一失其宜,皆能使血瘀滞不行,故百病由污血者多,而医书分门类证,有上气而无蓄血,予故增著之此说为是,然古人间有为蓄血立类者但不多见耳。"在肛肠病非手术治疗中也广泛应用逐瘀疗法,收到了较满意效果。

Qi and blood theory is one of the important theories of pathophysiology from traditional Chinese medicine. Wang Kentang pointed out:"If the life of human being is disorder and imbalance, it will cause blood stasis, then lead to various diseases. " The method of dispelling stasis is extensively carried on nonoperative therapies for coloproctology, and get to comfortable curative effect.

【基本概念】

[Fundamental Conception]

1. 气　是机体一切功能活动的动力,因作用及分布部位不同而有不同名称。

1. **Qi**　Qi is the dynamic about all functional activities in the human being.

(1)大气:亦称阳气或正气,是由元气、心阳气与谷气在气海中经气化而成。

(1)Atmosphere:It's also called Yang Qi, vital energy, health atmosphere, to encourage health treads.

(2)谷气:亦称胃气,是水谷在胃中经腐熟而产生。

(2)Essence:It's also called Stomach Qi, derives from the transformed vital energy after food is digested and absorbed in the alimentary canal.

(3)元气:是先天元阳之气,在后天是由右肾相火与左肾水精相合而成。

(3)Archaeus:It's congenital.

(4)心阳气:是心阳热吸收天阳气而成。

(4)Heart-yang.

(5)天阳气:是天地间大气,由天阳热和地之水气交蒸而成。

(5)TianYang Qi.

(6)经气:行于十二经中的大气。

(6)Meridian-Qi:It's also called the function of meridian.

（7）精气：藏于脏腑之大气也叫脏气，计有肺气、肝气、心气、肾气、脾气等。

（7）Energy：It's spirit, stored in the viscerae, including Lung-Qi, Liver-Qi, Heart-Qi, Kidney-Qi, and Spleen-Qi, etc.

2. 血　是水谷精微中的浊液，经十二经最后受心阳热锻炼而成。在《灵枢·决气篇》说："中焦受气，取汁变化而赤，是谓血。"血属阴，行于脉中，周流不息，营养全身，外注四肢百骸，内灌五脏六腑。"是故血和则经脉流行，营复阴阳，筋骨劲强，关节清和矣"。"肝受血而能视，足受血而能步，掌受血而能握，能受血而能摄"。总之，血是最重要的生命物质之一。

2. Blood　Oxygen from air and nutrition from food such as amine, protein, iron, etc. mix and then form blood. In < LingShu · JueQi Pian > it is said："Marrow and spleen can produce blood, and the main component in blood is hemoglobin containing iron, and so the blood is red." Blood belongs to Yin, to move in the vessels, to provide nutrition to all over the body, to flow to four limbs and hundred bones, to irrigate inside vital organs, never to stop circulation. "Only by blood normal flow in the vessels can the body get nutrition, physique be strong, joints act free". "When blood is full and sufficient, the person has vigorous strides and good eyesight(liver corresponds to apertures in the human face are eyes). In general, the blood is one of the most important life materials.

3. 气血关系　气与血，一阴一阳，气可生血，血可化气。气为血帅，气行则血行，血为气守，血宁则气平。气血同源而并行，互相资生、相互促进。故唐容川说："人身气为阳，血为阴，阳无阴不符，气无血不留。"

3. The Relationship of Qi and Blood　Qi and blood, one is Yang and the other is Yin. Qi can transform blood, and it is the same the other way round. Qi is a commander of blood. Qi goes while blood follows; blood is a guarder of Qi; blood flow is normal and so do Qi. Qi and blood have the same resource, and they promote and help each other forward. So Tang Rongchuan said："In the human being Qi is believed as Yang, while blood is Yin."

【病理变化】

[Pathology]

1. 气病对血的影响

1. Qi Disease Influences Blood.

（1）气虚而血虚：心、肝、脾气虚可引起血虚，治疗这类血虚宜用益气的方法，如用当归补血汤。

（1）Qi asthenia leads to blood asthenia：Heart, liver, or spleen Qi asthenia can lead to blood asthenia. To treat these blood asthenia can use the method of invigorating Qi, such as Angelica Invigorating Blood Decoction.

(2)气虚不能统血:在大气下陷或脾气虚损时,可发生崩漏、便血等症,宜用提升方法补气健脾,如用补中益气汤。

(2)Qi asthenia can't control blood:Spleen Qi asthenia can cause uterine bleeding, bleeding with defecation, etc.. To treat these conditions can use raising method of invigorating Qi and spleen, such as Center-supplementing Qi-boosting Decoction.

(3)气滞而血瘀:气为血帅,气滞不行可造成瘀血,宜行气以活血。

(3)Qi stagnation, then blood stasis:Qi is a commander of blood. Qi stops moving, causing blood stops; we can treat blood asthenia by moving Qi to activate blood.

(4)气逆或气盛:可迫血妄行而出血,引起吐血、呕吐、咯血等症,宜用降气顺气方药。

(4)Qi adversity or blood plenty:To make the blood go disorderly and informally which leads to vomiting with blood, cough with blood, etc.; to treat these diseases can use the prescription of reducing adversity and going in order.

2. 血病对气的影响
2. Blood Influences Qi

(1)血脱气散:大出血后造成"营血暴竭,卫气无依",出现气散虚脱。治疗上有"有形之血不能速生,无形之气法当急固"之说,宜用独参汤、升脉散等。

(1)Blood losing leads to Qi dispersing:After a lot of bleeding the body shows collapse. "The tangible blood can't retain to normal quickly, invisible Qi should be filled at once. " So Decoction of only Ginseng or Powder for restoring pulse should be used.

(2)血瘀而气滞:血瘀在经阻遏气机而导致气机不利。治疗此类气滞当以活血为主。

(2)Blood stasis leads to Qi not free going, so to treat this condition the method of activating blood mainly should be taken.

【病因】
[Etiology]

六淫、七情、饮食不节、暴急奔走,打扑损伤、产后败血不尽均可造成瘀血。经书常谓"气血者喜温而恶寒,寒则泣不能流"。其实六淫除寒以外,风湿成痹,湿热成痈,无一不造成气血郁滞。气病是瘀血的重要原因之一,尤其是肝郁气滞更为常见,肝气不疏血行不畅而胁痛。肝气犯胃,脾胃气血郁滞而胃脘痛。外伤也是造成瘀血的一个原因,《订补明医指掌》一书中谓"跌仆损伤或被人打踢,或物相撞,可取闪肭,或奔走努力,或受困屈,或发恼怒,一时不觉,过至半日,或一二三日而发者有之,十数日或半月一月而发者有之。一般寒热交作,其心胸肋下小腹满痛,按之手不可近者,此有瘀血也"。因此,瘀血的病因相当广泛。

Six kinds of bad external causes, seven kinds of internal feeling, eating and drinking without temperance, overtired, injury, losing blood of postpartum, all lead to blood stasis. The classical medical book recorded that "The patient with Qi-blood diseases likes warm and detests cold, and cold can lead to stasis". Wind and damp cause rheumatism; wet and heat cause carbuncle and abscess; most external factors can cause Qi and blood stasis. Qi disease is one of the important causes of blood stasis. Especially, liver stasis with Qi stagnation is more often seen. Liver Qi doesn't go and blood doesn't go, either, leading to pain at the side of chest. Liver Qi influencing stomach leads to Qi-blood stasis of spleen and stomach, with stomach pain. Injury is also another cause of blood stasis. From falling or broken injury one may feel chest or abdominal fullness or pain, lasting for a few days or even one month, together with tenderness, chilly and fever. That's blood stasis.

【临床表现】

[Clinical Manifestations]

1. **疼痛**　后世医家李念莪曾说:"通则不痛,痛则不通。"概括了疼痛是因气血不通所致。究竟以气滞为主还是以血瘀为主,需要从疼痛性质上加以鉴别。

1. **Pain**　Doctor Li Nianer ever said:"There will be painless when the tunnel is smoothly running, and there will be pain whenever the tunnel stops running."So that the pain is caused by that Qi-blood can't move normally. What exactly may be Qi stagnation or blood stasis, it needs to be differentiated by the character of pain.

(1)气痛:时痛时止,痛无常处,气聚则痛而见形,气散则平而无迹,如肠痉挛。

(1)Qi pain:Sometimes pain, and sometimes painless, and the pain hasn't fix position. Qi goes together while pain has a shape, and Qi disperse which shows quite mild, such as spasm of intestine.

(2)血痛:痛无休止,痛有定所,血积则成肿块,如血栓外痔。

(2)Blood pain:Sustained pain has a fixed position, and blood gets together and forms a mass, such as external hemorrhoids.

(3)痛有虚实寒热之分,亦可详辨(表4-2)。

(3)Pain may be asthenia and sthenia, cold and heat (Table 4-2).

表4-2 实热病与虚寒病的鉴别

Table 4-2 Differentiation of sthenia hot diseases and asthenia cold diseases

鉴别要点 Differentiation	实热痛 Sthenia hot pain	虚寒痛 Asthenia cold pain
是否胀痛 Distension and pain, or not	痛而胀 Pain and distension	痛而不胀 Pain and no distension
是否喜按压 Like being pressed, or not	痛而拒按 Pain, refuse being pressed	痛而喜按 Pain, like being pressed
是否喜温热 Like warm and heat, or not	痛而喜冷 Pain, like cold	痛而喜热 Pain, like heat
是否与饥饿有关 Reaction of hungry and full	饱而痛甚 Full with pain even more	饥而痛甚 Hungry with pain even more
是否腹泻 Diarrhea, or not	痛而闭 Pain and constipation	痛而泻 Pain and diarrhea

可分以下几种情况：①梗阻或痉挛引起的疼痛,特点是阵发性绞痛,多以气为主,如肛门内括肌病。②炎症或肿胀引起的疼痛,特点是持续性跳痛或胀痛,多以血为主,如肛门脓肿。③腹膜受刺激引起的疼痛,特点是持续性,起始重,逐渐减缓,化学性刺激所致刀割样者多以气为主。内出血所致针刺样痛者,多以血为主,如肠穿孔。④缺血所引起的腹痛,呈持续性,活动后加重,多表现为气血相兼,如嵌顿痔。

The pain can be divided into some states as follows: ①Pain from obstruction or spasm, and its feature is intermittent colic pain to take Qi as the dominant factor, such as diseases of anal internal sphincter. ②Pain from inflammation or swelling, and its feature is continued throbbing or distended pain to take blood as the dominant factor, such as anal abscess. ③Abdominal pain like cutting and sting from peritoneum being directly irritated by chemical and internal hemorrhagic effusion, and its feature is sustain and continued pain to take Qi or blood as the dominant factor, such as perforation of alimentary canal. ④Abdominal pain from ischemia, the feature is sustain pain and worsen action later to take both Qi and blood as the dominant factors, such as incarcerated hemorrhoids.

2. 肿块　中医学关于肿块的论述很多,最早见于《内经·灵枢五变篇》,其后又有癥瘕疣癖等说。在认识上总离不开气血(表4-3)。

2. Mass　There are many theories about mass in traditional Chinese medicine which were recorded first in the initial work <Neijing Lingshu WuBian Pian> (Table 4-3).

表 4 - 3　肿块的鉴别

Table 4 - 3 Differentiation of masses

鉴别要点 Differentiation	积(癥)有形可证 Real mass and his shape	聚(瘕)假物成形 Spurious mass and his shape
气血 Qi blood	属血 Belong to blood	属气 Belong to Qi
脏腑 Viscera	属脏 Belong to organ	属腑 Belong to hollow viscera
阴阳 Yin Yang	阴 Belong to Yin	阳 Belong to Yang
主要特点 Main feature	有形可循,固定不移,痛有定处 Pain has fix shape and position	聚散无常,往来浮动,疼痛走窜 Gather and disperse irregularly,undefinite pain
病情 Diseases' degree	较重,如肠肿瘤 Severe, such as intestinal tumor	较轻,如肠痉挛 Mild, such as intestinal spasm

3. **发热**　《金匮》:"病者如热状,口干燥而渴,其脉反无热,此为阴伏是瘀血也。"《医林改错》中曾说:"心里热名曰灯笼病,身外凉心里热,为内有瘀血。"另外,疳痨类疾病,午后发热至晚尤甚。还有人认为,时发寒热而无外感者为内瘀血。

3. **Fever**　In ＜ Jin Gui ＞:"It's blood stasis that the patient who has a fever and dry mouth and thirsty but with no bouncing and range pulse." The ＜ Correct Mistakes in Medicine ＞ ever recorded:"Inner body being hot and outer body being cold, it's lantern disease that blood stasis is inside of the body." The diseases of malnutrition and consumption (including tuberculosis) showed fever in afternoon especially at night. Other doctors thought that the patients who had sometimes cold and hot would not catch cold, but they were inner blood stasis.

4. **热血**　吐血、鼻出血、便血、漏血诸症均有瘀血,有因瘀血而出血者,亦有因出血而瘀血者。一般认为,大便黑亮如漆似胶有异臭者为内瘀血;皮下有青紫斑为外瘀血;经前腹痛,月经有血块为内瘀血。

4. **Heat Bleeding**　Vomiting with blood, nosebleed, having blood in stool and uterine bleeding, all have blood stasis. There is bleeding because of blood stasis while blood stasis because of bleeding. Generally speaking, the patient with black bright stool sticking to each other like glue or lacquer and offensive smell is internal blood stasis; the patient with purplish red spot or strain in subcutaneous tissue is external blood stasis; the patient with abdominal pain before menstruation and mass in menstruation is internal blood stasis.

5. **精神神经症状**　《医林改错》中说:"瞀闷"为瘀血。

5. **Psychiatry**　＜ Correct Mistakes in Medicine ＞ recorded:Terrible upset is blood stasis.

6. 舌与脉 舌色发紫或舌质有紫斑为瘀血。脉以弦紧涩为主,但也有沉细者。"弦而紧,胁痛脏伤,有瘀血"。"挟血者脉来乍涩乍数,闪烁明灭"。

6. Tongue and Pulse The patient with purplish red tongue or ecchymosed texture is blood stasis. Pulses are mainly string, tense and unsmooth, sometimes sunken thin. "The patient with string and tense pulses are blood stasis", or "hesitant and rapid pulses".

7. 其他 面色黧黑,尤以眼眶口唇暗黑者为瘀血。皮肤有蛛纹丝缕如蟹足者为瘀血。

7. Other Signs Dark black face, especially at eye socket and lips is blood stasis. The patient with skin grain like the thread of spider web and like crab feet is blood stasis.

【治疗】

[Treatment]

1. 治疗原则 无论何种原因所引起的瘀血,治宜祛瘀为先,轻者用消散之法,重者用逐破攻坚之法。但欲使其气血循经恢复正常,一定还要掌握气血兼顾,因为气为血帅,气行则血行。

1. Principles of Treatment No matter what causes induce blood stasis, the disease should first be treated by the method of relieving stasis, mild by dispersing, severe by breaking up gradually, and consideration must be given to both Qi and blood at the same time, because Qi is a commander of blood, and Qi goes while blood follows.

(1)磨平饮:治死血成块。方用:红花、桃仁、山楂、苏木、三棱、莪术、枳壳、香附、乌药。

(1)MoPing Decoction:To treat fixed blood mass. The components of prescription:Safflower, Peach seed, Whitethorn, Sapanwood, Rhizoma Sparganii, Curcuma Zedoary, Fructus Aurantii, Rhizoma Cyperi, Root of three-nerved Spicebush.

(2)大黄散:治瘕结两胁胀痛。方用:川大黄、京三棱、鳖甲、槟榔、木香、赤芍、桃仁、生姜。

(2) Powder of Rhubarb:To treat pain. The components of prescription:Rhubarb Rhei Sichuan, Rhizoma Sparganii from Beijing, Turtle shell, Areca, Radices Saussureae, Radix Paeoniae Rubrathe, Peach seed, Ginger.

治疗早期肛门脓肿以行血为主,辅以行气药,组成化瘀汤。反之,欲行其滞气也需理血佐之,如肠梗阻治疗应用桃仁、红花、牛膝等。

Moving blood is the main method to treat initial anal abscess, and moving Qi is adjuvant method. The prescription is Decoction Hua Yu (dispelling stasis). Conversely, for Qi stagnation moving Qi is the main method, and moving blood is the adjuvant method, for example, to treat intestinal obstruction with Peach seed, Safflower and Hyssop, etc.

2. 辨证施治　瘀血本为实邪,血实宜决之。另外,还应注意人体正气的盛衰,以及引起瘀血的原因和因瘀血产生的后果。因此,在治疗上必须辨明虚实证。实证指邪气,虚证指正气,做到祛邪不伤正,扶正以祛邪。

2. Differential Treatment　Blood stasis is sthenia disease, and blood sthenia should be solved at once. Otherwise pay attention to prosperity and decline about Qi, and to cause and result from blood stasis. One must differentiate asthenia and sthenia. Eliminate diseases while the body can't be injured, and nourish the body while the disease can be treated.

(1)病急,正盛,邪实:可用速战,专事攻消,邪祛再调正。

(1)Acute disease, the body is strong and the disease is sthenia:Treat the disease quickly, then regulate the body.

(2)病急,正虚,邪实:可用攻补兼施的办法治疗。

(2)Acute disease, the body is deficiency and the disease is sthenia:Treat the disease and at the same time nourish the body.

(3)病缓,正虚,邪实:可用扶正以祛邪,补中有行的办法。

(3)Chronic disease, the body is deficiency and the disease is sthenia:Nourish the body while gradually treat the disease.

(4)病缓,正未伤,邪实:可用祛邪与扶正交替的办法,病已久不可图速功,宜消磨之。

(4)Chronic disease, the body isn't deficiency and the disease is sthenia:Treat the disease and nourish body alternatively, and the treatment should be done gradually, and not quickly as the disease last long.

(5)除以上虚实辨证外,还需根据瘀血原因和结果,分别运用止血祛瘀、清热祛瘀、散寒祛瘀、通里祛瘀及渗湿祛瘀诸法。

(5)Besides the above differentiation of sthenia and asthenia, the treatment according to the cause and result of blood stasis should be arranged separately by use of the method of hemostasis and eliminating stasis, relieving fever and eliminating stasis, dispelling cold and eliminating stasis, purgation and eliminating stasis, infiltrating and eliminating stasis.

3. 代表方剂　(录自《医林改错》)。

3. Representative Prescriptions　(From < Correct Mistakes of Medicine >)

(1)血府逐瘀汤:治上焦瘀血诸症。

(1)XueFu ZhuYu Decoction:Treating chest diseases and diseases above the chest with blood stasis.

①处方:当归、生地黄、桃仁、红花、枳壳、赤芍、桔梗、川芎、牛膝各 9g,柴胡 6g,甘草 3g。

①Prescription:Angelica, Dried Rhamnnia root, Peach seed, Safflower, Fructus Aurantii, Radix Paeoniae Rubrathe, Platycodon Grandifiorum, Ligusticum Wallichii, Hyssop, each 9g, Radix bupleuri 6g, Liquorice 3g.

②主治:a. 头痛:患头痛,无表证,无里证,无气虚痰饮等症,忽犯忽好。b. 胸痛:胸痛在前木金散可愈,后通背亦痛用瓜蒌薤白白酒汤可愈。有忽然胸痛,前方皆不应用此方。c. 呃逆:俗名打咯忒,无论伤寒、瘟疫,杂症一见呃逆速用此方。d. 饮水即呛。e. 不眠:夜不能睡用安神养血药治之不效者。

②Indication: a. Headache:Paroxysmal pain. b. Chest pain:Anterior chest pain, the prescription is MuJin Powder; posterior chest pain, the prescription is distilled spirit Decoction of Trichosanthes Kirilowii Maxim and Allii Macrostemi Bulbus. c. Hiccup. d. Choke over water. e. Insomnia:The patient who has a sleepless night and needs to take medicine, but it is of no effect that he takes herbs of invigorating blood.

(2)膈下逐瘀汤:治中焦瘀血诸症。

(2)GeXia ZhuYu Decoction:Treat various abdominal blood stasis diseases.

①处方:五灵脂、当归、川芎、桃仁、赤芍、乌药、延胡索、香附、红花、枳壳各 9g,牡丹皮 6g,甘草 3g。

①Prescription:Excrementum Pteropi, Angelica, Ligusticum Wallichii, Peach seed, Radix Paeoniae Rubrathe, Root of three-nerved spicebush, Rhizoma Corydalis, Rhizoma Cyperi, Safflower, Fructus Aurantii, each 9g, Bark of tree peony root 6g, Liquorice 3g.

②主治:a. 积块、小儿痞块(肚大青筋)、痛不移处。b. 卧则腹坠:病人夜卧,腹中似有物,左卧向左边坠,右卧向右边坠,为内有血瘀。c. 五更泻:二神、四神无效者。d. 久泻:泻肚日久,百方不效者。

②Indication:a. Mass, also seen on children's abdomen, the pain with fixed position. b. Abdominal distension and falling. There is blood stasis in cavity. c. Loose stool in early morning. d. Diarrhea long time, even treated with many prescriptions but of no effect.

(3)少腹逐瘀汤:治下焦瘀血诸症。

(3)ShaoFu ZhuYu Decoction:To treat pelvic cavity blood stasis diseases.

①处方:小茴香七粒炒,干姜 3 片,延胡索、没药、当归、川芎、赤芍、蒲黄、五灵脂各 9g,官桂 3g。

①Prescription:Roasted 7 seeds with Cumin, Rhizoma Corydalis, Myrrha, Angelica, Ligusticum Wallichii, Radix Paeoniae Rubrathe, Cattail Pollen, Faeces Tragopterori, each 9g, Cortex cinnamomi 3g.

②主治：a. 小腹积块疼痛或不疼痛或疼痛而无积块，或少腹胀满；b. 经血见时先腰酸少腹胀。

②Indication：a. A mass in pelvic cavity with pain, or without pain, or pain without mass, or lower abdominal distension. b. Feel soreness of waist and distension of lower abdomen before having menstruation.

第三节　热病及其治疗
§3　Heat Diseases and Treatment

《素问·至真要大论》说："治热以寒"、"温者清之"是清解热邪的一种治疗方法。由于热在表里，与虚实不同，在此大法之下设有清热解表、清解里热、里热成实当以攻里下热。此外，还有甘寒养阴的清解阴虚内热之剂等。

The ＜SuWen·ZhiZhenYaoDaLun＞ recorded：It's a method of clearing heat and detoxication that "to treat high hot diseases relying on cold herbs", "low hot relying on cool herbs". According to the method, on the base of heat in inner or outer, there are clearing and relieving superficial heat, clearing and relieving interior heat, purgating heat downwards, in addition to clearing Yin deficiency and interior heat.

【基本概念】

［Fundamental Conception］

中医学认为，人体热证有四种来源。

In traditional Chinese medicine it is believed that there are four kinds of sources about hot syndrome in the human being：

1. **天阳气有余**　人身的阳气，在正常情况下，本身有养神柔筋、温照脏腑经络的生理作用，称之为"少火"。但如果阳气过元，必致伤阳耗精，失去生理功用而成病理状态，被称为"壮火"。所以《素问·阴阳应象大论》说："壮火散气，少火生气"是指此而言。

1. **The Rest of Human Energy**　The vitality in human, in normal condition, can keep repost, relax the muscles and joints, maintain visceral physical actions; but if even more, it may reduce the energy and make physical function changing into pathologic station.

2. **外感六淫，内伤积滞郁结**　外感风、寒、燥、湿之邪，均能郁而化热。如寒湿均为阴邪，寒邪外来，阳气不得宣泄，郁而发热。湿邪阻滞阳气，郁久化热。燥火均为阳邪。侵袭人体，骤然病热。再者内伤食积，虫积等皆郁而化热。

2. Six External Causes Leading to Internal Stagnation and Stasis The external factors such as wind, cold, dry, damp, all can lead to stasis, then turn to fever. For example, cold and damp can press down Yang Qi, and they make Qi won't break out and do stasis so as to be stasis forming heat, further the long time stasis can produce heat. Dry heat strikes person, and the person may catch the disease suddenly. Other reasons: eating more food, bacterial or viral infection, etc., also can cause heat from stasis.

3. **情志拂郁，郁热化火** 称五志之火，如《素问·生气通天论》说："大怒则形气绝、而血菀于上"此为怒伤肝，郁而化热、化火，阳气不下，使气血并病之例。

3. **Emotion Causing Stasis and Stasis Causing Heat** The heat is called the fire of five emotion. < SuWen · ShengQi TongTian Lun > recorded: The human's figure and quality will be exhausted as being very angry, and it's called angry injuring liver, and makes liver Qi stasis, then the stasis transforms heat, so as to cause diseases of both Qi and blood.

4. **精亡血少，阴虚阳亢而生内热** 谓之虚热、虚火，如《素问·生气通天论》说："阳气者烦劳则张，精绝，辟积于夏，使人煎厥。"就是由于劳伤过度，精血亏耗，阳气被扰，虚火上炎的见证。

4. **Yin weak and Yang exciting causing internal heat** It's called weak heat, for example: in < Su Wen · ShengQi TongTian Lun > : The person being overtired and exhausted easily fall on the ground in a faint, especially in summer.

【病理变化】

[Pathology]

上述由六淫、七情、内伤等所发生的热，在人体的病理变化，中医学有如下认识：

Heat from the six external causes, seven emotion and internal causes, etc., is recognized by traditional Chinese medicine in human body's pathological changes as follows:

1. **热主开泄** 如热在皮肤，则腠理开，汗大泄，阳气得泄，热也随之消减。若阳气不得泄越，内热便由此产生。热在不同脏腑发展，产生不同病理变化。

1. **Heat Reacting in the Center of Regulating Temperature** The center of regulating temperature governs nerves and hormones, and through them the center can regulate skin sweat gland secretion. The skin even breaks out a lot of sweat so as to reduce fever and the body temperature, or internal heat grows up and the temperature continues to cause different pathological changes in normal functional viscera.

2. **热在血脉** 则脉流薄疾，甚至追血妄行。

2. **Heat in Circulation** The pulses are floatable and rapid, even in severe cases causing

hemorrhage.

3. 热在筋肉　则泄纵不收,热郁腠理肌肤,则为痤痱。

3. Heat in Muscles and Joints　Easily cause acne and prickly heat.

4. 热盛　则血聚肉腐,发为痈肿。

4. Heat Being Very High　Having a high fever shows in the severe infectious diseases, blood and muscles decompose, causing carbuncle and abscess.

5. 热郁脘腹肠胃之间　则使传化功能失常。所谓"诸胀腹大,皆属于热"、"诸病有声,敲之如鼓,皆属于热"均指此而言。

5. Heat in Stomach, Intestine and Abdominal Cavity　Abdominal visceral malfunction lead to abnormal digestion and absorption. That's called "abdominal distension which belongs to hot diseases", "beating swollen abdomen like beating a drum belonging to heat diseases".

6. 大热不上,热盛化火,火盛神动　则出现神昏谵语,烦躁不宁,挛急抽搐,胡言乱语,行动超越正常,即所谓"诸症冒瘈皆属于火"、"诸躁狂越皆属于火"。

6. High Heat Influencing Neuropsychiatric System　Coma and delirium, dysphoria, spasm, twitched, rave, abnormal acting, which is so-called that "every spasm syndrome belongs to heat", "every mania syndrome belongs to fire".

总之,"阳胜则为热"或为"气实者热也"。就是说热的基本病理是"阳盛"或"气实"。"阳盛"就是"气实"。中医讲阴阳,是一种朴素的唯物主义思想。实指阴,代表精、血、津、液等有形之体,是物质基础。阳代表气,如元气、营气、卫气、宗气等无形之用,是发挥功能的基础。所以阴阳、气血,是指质与功能,体与用的关系。如"阴平阳秘"的阴阳平衡协调,处于正常生理状态,则达到"精神乃治"的健康状况。如"阳盛"或"气实"则功能作用过盛而出现病理状态。因此,可以说热是人体功能病理性亢奋的现象(表4-4)。

In general, Yang is strong and healthy, but this is only exterior phenomenon. In fact Yang from traditional Chinese medicine participate in every part in the human being, and hyper-diseases are commonly seen in the clinic. For those patients to be treated nonoperatively by integrated medicine, differentiation of syndrome, typing and staging should be made based on references from Yin and Yang. Yin Yang coming from traditional Chinese medicine is a frugal materialism thought. Yin is the base of material that stands for things corporeal such as blood, fluid, juice, semen, etc. Qi is the base of function that stands for intangibles such as archaeus, so that Yin and Yang, Qi and blood are the relationship between Yin and Yang. Yin and Yang in equilibrium can keep normal physical station, leading to normal healthy condition with good spirit. While 'High Yang' or 'Full Qi' means over function or the appearance of pathologic conditions. High or low Yin or Yang will cause pathological changes. Therefore, heat can be said to be a pathologic phenomenon of extremely excited human function (Table 4 – 4).

表 4 – 4　热证特点及亢奋表现
Table 4 – 4　Heat syndrome features and hyperfunctional phenomena

热证特点 Feature	亢奋表现 Violable organ and system
烦而多言 Dysphoria, spasm, twitched, rave	热扰神明,致使多动多语功能亢奋 Heat violate neuropsychiatry:over speaking and moving
脉浮洪急数 Pulses:floating, bouncing, tense, rapid	为营气功能亢奋致脉流诸疾 Heat violate circulation system:pulses being rapid
大便秘结 Dry feces or constipation	大肠燥化功能亢奋 Translating malfunction of large intestine:dry feces
小便赤短 Oliguria and red color	小肠化火过亢,泌别清浊失司 Malfunction:intestinal organ and urine secreting system
消谷善饥 Often eating more and feeling hungry	胃腐熟水谷亢奋 Often eating more and feeling hungry

　　凡属人体功能病理性亢奋的表现均属热证。其范围较西医广,包括体温升高的热病,也指体温不升高的热病。如《灵枢·师传篇》说:"胃中热,则消谷,令人悬心善饥",也许是指一部分糖尿病病人,或甲状腺功能亢进症病人。

　　All pathological hyperfunction of human being belongs to hot syndrome. This hot syndrome is not only having a fever, but also it includes metabolism problem and heat disease with low body temperature. For example < LingShu·ShiChuanPian > recorded:The patients like to eat a lot, as heat being in stomach, may be the part of diabetes or hyperthyroidism.

【临床表现】

[Clinical Manifestations]

　　1. 基本证型表现　热是八纲中的一纲,因此用八纲辨证是最基本的辨证方法。临床上凡是出现口渴饮凉、潮热、烦躁、面红目赤、小便短赤、大便闭结、舌苔黄燥、脉速等,便可以认为是热证。联系表里、虚实四纲可分为表热、里热、虚热、实热,进而又分表热虚、表热实、里热虚、果热实,表里俱熟……。

　　1. Basic Syndrome Manifestations　In traditional Chinese medicine the syndrome differentiation by eight principles is the most basic and the first step. With the eight concepts of Yin and Yang, interior and exterior, cold and heat, asthenia and sthenia (deficiency and excess), the nature, position, bodily resistance and severity of the disease can be summarized for laying a foundation of further syndrome differentiation. Heat is one kind of the eight concepts. In clinic it's the hot syndrome:thirsty and drinking cold things, tiding heat, dysphoria, being red in the face, oliguria and red color, constipation, yellow and dry fur of tongue, rapid pulses, etc. According to interior and exterior, asthenia and sthenia, the hot syndrome is divided into exterior heat, interior heat, asthenia heat and sthenia heat, further divided into exterior asthenia heat, exterior sthenia heat, interior asthenia heat, interior sthenia heat, exterior and interior heat, etc.

（1）表热：发热、恶风、有汗或无汗、头痛、口渴，舌尖红苔薄白不润，脉浮数。

（1）External heat：Having a fever, being disgusted with wind, sweat or no sweat, headache, thirsty, red tongue tip, tongue fur being white thin, not moist, pulses floating and rapid.

（2）里热：壮热、口渴、目赤唇红、小便短赤。舌质赤红苔黄脉沉数。

（2）Internal heat：Pyretic syndrome, thirsty, being red in the face including eyes and lips, oliguria and red color, bright red tongue with yellow fur, rapid sunken pulses.

（3）虚热：午后发热或热无定时，心烦、盗汗、咽喉干痛，舌红降无苔，脉细数无力。

（3）Asthenia heat：Tiding heat in the afternoon and pain of undefinite position, feeling vexed, sweat in the night, swelling and dry pain in pharynx and larynx, bright red tongue without fur, thin rapid and weak pulses.

（4）实热：在表与表热证相同；在里高热、烦渴、声粗、腹满、便秘，舌苔黄燥，脉实数。

（4）Sthenia Heat：heat in the surface and the same as exterior syndrome; heat inside with a pyretic, thirsty, a deep gruff voice, abdominal distension, constipation, dry yellow tongue fur, rapid sthenia pulses.

（5）里热虚：多由肝肾阴虚引起，掌心热、头晕、口渴、心烦不眠。

（5）Internal asthenia heat：Mainly caused by Yin asthenia of liver and kidneys, heat in the centre of palm, dizzy, thirsty, feeling vexed, insomnia.

（6）里热实：外邪化热传里，壮热、口渴烦躁、腹满便秘、腹痛拒按，甚者神昏谵语。

（6）Internal sthenia heat：External disease transmits to interior, pyretic, thirsty and dysphoria, abdominal distension, constipation, abdominal pain with tenderness, even coma and delirium speech.

（7）表热虚：即阴虚潮热一类，午后肌热、掌心热、自汗出。

（7）External asthenia heat：Belong to Yin asthenia tiding heat, having a fever in the afternoon, the heat in the center of the palm, free breaking out sweat.

（8）表热实：外感温痛初起，同表热证。

（8）External sthenia heat: External diseases leading to low fever and pain, which belong to initial disease, the same as external hot syndrome.

（9）表里俱实：表邪化热传里，发热不退，反而增剧，类似里热实证。

（9）External and internal sthenia：External disease transmits to internal fever. The temperature is not decreasing, but rapid, increasing, like internal sthenia heat.

2. 真热与假热表现 热是一种症状的归纳方法，不能单凭某一个证候就做出热的判断，而必须结合证候，如舌苔、脉象等全面分析，才能做出判断。然而，证候浮于表面现象，有时难免给人以假象，造成辨证错误，这就要求我们必须善于分辨真热与假热。

2. Appearances of Real Heat and False Heat The heat syndrome can't be diagnosed only by one simple symptom, and the doctor must diagnose the disease relying on comprehensive analysis. The local pathologic changes and general reaction status should be recognized. A proper qualitative and quantitative diagnosis of definite localization should be made through utilization of diagnostic techniques.

（1）真热：应当脉数有力，滑大而实，症见烦躁、喘粗、胸闷腹胀，口渴饮凉，大便闭结小便短赤，发热不欲盖被。

（1）Real heat：Pulses being powerful and smooth and excess; the symptoms showing agitated, boredom, rapid breath, abdominal distension, thirsty and drinking cool liquid, constipation, oliguria and red color and having a fever without liking quilt.

（2）假热：则外虽热内却寒，脉微细或虚数浮大无根，身上发热而神态安静，言语谵妄而声音低微，或似狂妄但禁之即止或皮肤有假斑而浅红细碎、或喜凉饮而所用不多或少溲多利，大便不闭结。这种热象并非真热而是假热实属寒证，即所谓寒极反兼热化，又叫阴盛格阳。

（2）False heat：Although surface of body feels heat, while feels cold inside of the body, very thin rapid float pulses without having root, having a fever and being perfectly calm, skin having false light red spots, drinking cool liquid but drinking not much, having no constipation. These symptoms are not real heat diseases, but false heat which belongs to cold syndrome.

（3）肛肠病急性期，绝大多数病人表现为里热证或里实热证。

（3）Acute anal rectal diseases mostly show internal hot syndrome or internal sthenia hot syndrome.

3. 其他辨证方法下的热证表现 应用八纲辨别热证只能解决一个总纲领或大方向问题，要解决一个完善的证还应与六经、卫气营血（包括三焦）、脏腑、病因辨证结合起来，六经、卫气营血辨证是辨证热病的传统主要方法。

3. Manifestations of Hot Syndrome in Other Differential Methods The hot syndrome being carried on eight concepts can only solve the question of general principles and direction so that the differentiation must combine with other differentiations including six Jing, Qi, blood, viscerae and causes, etc. , in order to solve total syndrome. One can have an overall recognization only by combining organically total differentiations. Six Jing differentiation and WeiQiYingXue differentiation are traditional main methods of differentiating hot diseases.

(1)六经辨证:六经指太阳、阳明,少阳、太阴、少阴,厥阴。三阳经证均表现功能亢奋现象,即热证。肛肠病常见表有阳明证和少阳证。阳明脉证指外邪在太阳经未解,向里发展,此时无形热邪弥漫胃肠,但肠内糟粕尚未结成燥屎,热而未实,热盛。症见大热、大渴、大汗、脉大,称阳明经证。若肠内燥粪成形,更见便闭结,腹满,腹痛拒按,烦躁谵语,甚至神志不清,热而兼实,邪已化火,具有一派热象,称为阳明腑证。肛门脓肿或肠梗阻常表现为阳明经证和阳明腑证。少阳证指病邪传至半表半里,出现寒热往来,口苦咽干,目眩心烦,呕不欲食,脉弦数有典型少阳证,另外少阳与阳明合疾也最为多见,如肛门脓肿、门静脉炎、肝脓肿。

(1)Syndrome differentiation of Six Jing (six main and collateral channels, regarded as a network of passages through which vital energy circulates along which the acupuncture points are distributed. Three Yang Jing syndrome shows hyperfunctional phenomena of hot syndrome, such as constipation, abdominal distension and pain and tenderness, agitated acting, even losing consciousness; also showing bitter taste in the mouth and dry throat, rexation, vomiting, etc.

(2)卫气营血、三焦辨证:是六经辨证的发展,可以辨出发病部位和热病的轻重浅深。在肛肠病某些发展阶段也具备这一辨证的特点。常见有气分热和血分热。气分热,症见壮热、口渴、舌苔黄、脉滑数,基本同中焦阳明经证如肛肠病感染。血分热指热邪入血,症见狂妄,神昏谵语痉抽,外有斑疹,内有吐、鼻出血、便血舌质深降少液,脉细数或弦数,如严重的感染性门静脉炎败血症、内痔硬化注射后感染等。

(2)Syndrome differentiation of WeiQiYingXue: The syndrome shows a high fever, thirsty, yellow tongue fur, rapid smooth pulses, even spasm, spots, endohemorrhage, nosebleed, stool with blood, deep bright red tongue, rapid thin and rapid string pulses.

(3)把三焦与六经辨证做一对比,不难看出三焦自上而下,是一个纵的关系,六经从表走里,是一个横的关系,纵横之交点,在三焦为中焦,在六经为阳明太阴原是一处。因此三焦、六经辨证在热证辨证中经常结合应用。

(3)Syndrome differentiation of the combination of WeiQiYingXue and Six Jing. Although these conditions belong to the same kind in WM diagnosis, because of the different local pathologic changes and different physical reactions, they may belong to different kinds in TCM syndromes so that they should be treated by different methods. That's so called "The same disease is treated by different methods. "

(4)脏腑、病因辨证:亦应明确热在脾应还是在肝胆,热由何种病因引起或与何种病因合而致病。如脾胃实热主要表现为脘腹胀满、腹痛拒按,大便闭结,脉滑大;肝胆实热主要表现为胸脘烦闷、肋痛、口苦、易怒、脉弦数。两者均为实热,不分脏腑,可以知病在脾胃或肝胆。又如热从湿邪所化,或与湿邪合而为病,则临床除热象外,必有湿象,如口淡无味胸脘痞闷、腹胀、食少、苔黄腻或黄厚腻、脉滑数。湿与热合,成为湿热证,治法不离清化湿热。由此不难理解分析脏腑、病因的实用价值。

(4) Syndrome differentiation of viscera and etiology: Visceral syndrome differentiation is actually a determination of the diseased position. It is mostly common that the liver, spleen, stomach, large and small intestine are affected and commonly more than two viscerae. During the development of the disease, the translocation of the diseased organ is in a regular order. In the theory of traditional Chinese medicine the functions of the six hollow organs are mainly passage ways of material, also called transformation, but they are not storing houses. The six hollow organs prefer moving and expelling to stagnating and persisting. Moving downward, excretion, and purgation indicate their normal function, while moving upwards or stagnating means impaired function of them. Whatever etiology causes excretive difficulty, six hollow organs will mainly suffer from dysfunction such as pain (abdominal pain), vomiting (nausea and vomiting), distension (abdominal distension), constipation (dry feces) and fever (running a temperature). In short, there will be abdominal pain whenever one hollow organ running. After distinguishing etiology and identifying the main diseased position, the treatment of purgation adaptable to etiology and pathogeneses through alleviating the obstruction, eliminating the accumulating mass, should be given with expelling cold with heat herbs or expelling heat with cold herbs. To know where the heat is spleen or liver and gall, what reason the heat occurs, for example, sthenia heat in spleen and stomach shows abdominal distension, pain and tenderness, constipation, smooth pulses; sthenia heat in liver and gall show vexation and oppression, bitter in the mouth, irascibility, string pulse. Spleen-stomach and liver-gall are all sthenia heat showing all above symptoms. Another example, heat coming from damp showing bland taste in the mouth, chest and abdominal distension, less intake, thick yellow tongue coating and slippery rapid pulse. So the therapy should be clearing away damp-heat.

总之,热证的辨证应当以八纲为总纲,结合六经、卫气营血、三焦、脏腑、病因辨证,才能全面获得较正确的辨证结论。

In general, the hot syndrome differentiation should make eight concepts and general principles combining with other differentiation so as to get correct answer and result.

【治疗】

[Treatment]

热证治法主要是清热,即《内经》所说"热者寒之",亦称清解法,属于"正"的范围。清热法最适用邪在表已得汗热不退,或里热已炽而尚未结实之证。热有表里、虚实、气分、血分之分,脏腑偏盛之殊,因此,清热法亦分数种。

The treating method of hot syndrome is mainly clearing heat, so that ＜ NeiJing ＞ recorded "Heat diseases should be treated by cold-natured herbs". This therapy is also called clearing heat and detoxication, in the field of "Positive or Correct Therapies". There are several kinds of clearing heat methods.

1. 清热解表 用于清表(卫)分热,如银翘散、桑菊饮之类。

1. Clearing Heat and Resolving the Exterior For treating exterior heat, to take Powder of Lonicera and Forsythia, and Decoction of Mori and Chrysanthemi.

2. 清热泻火 用于清里热、实热,热在气分的用白虎汤。例如,阳明腑实者用大承气汤,治骨盆直肠间隔脓肿。

2. Clearing Heat and Interior-Fire For treating internal heat, sthenia heat, and heat in Qi, to take BaiHu Decoction, DaChengQi Decoction, etc. , to treat thc pelvirectal space abscess.

3. 清热解毒 用于毒热炽盛病症,如高热、头面咽喉肿痛,用普济消毒饮;如胃肠积热,疮疡肿毒,高热狂躁,则用三黄解毒汤、清解汤。

3. Clearing Heat and Detoxication For treating pyretic syndrome, such as having a high fever, sore swollen throat, to take General Antiphlogistic Decoction; for treating heat in stomach and intestines, swelling and ulcer on the body surface, having a high fever and mania, to take Decoction of SanHuang detoxication, QingJie Decoction.

4. 清热生津 用于气分热盛,津液伤耗,余热未清之证,用竹叶石膏汤(竹叶、生石膏、半夏、人参、麦冬、甘草、梗米)。

4. Clearing Heat and Producing Liquid For treating pyretic and depleted liquid, and what the rest of fever have not yet been cleared completely, to take Lophatherum and Gypsum Decoction (Lophatherum, Gypsum, Pinellia ternate, Ginseng, Ophiopogon root, Liquorice, Rice).

5. 清热凉血 用于清里热、清营血分热。营分热用清营汤(犀角、生地黄、玄参、竹叶心、金银花、连翘、黄连、丹参、麦冬),血分热用犀角地黄汤(犀角、生地黄、芍药、牡丹皮)。治肛门感染、败血症。

5. Clearing Heat and Cooling Blood For treating internal heat syndrome, anal region infection and septicemia to take QingYing Decoction (Rhinoceros horn, Unprocessed Rehmannia root, Radix Scrophulariae, Lophatherum, Honeysuckle, Fructus Forsythiae, Coptis, Red-rooted Salvia, Ophiopogon root); heat in blood, to take Comus Rhinoceri and Rehmanniae Decoction (Rhinoceros horn, Unprocessed Rehmannia root, Herbaceous Peony, Bark of tree Peony root).

6. 气血两清 用于热邪侵入气分与血分,所谓"血气两燔",用清瘟败毒饮(生石膏、犀角、川连、栀子、桔梗、黄苓、知母、赤芍、玄参、连翘、甘草、牡丹皮、竹叶)。

6. **Vigorous Heat at Qi-Blood Phase** For treating heat in Qi-blood phase, to take QiWen-BaiTu Decoction (Gypsum, Rhinoceros horn, Coptis from Sichuan, Gardenia, Platycodon Grandifiorum, Scutellaria Baicalensis, Rhizoma Anemarrhenae, Radix Paeoniae Rubrathe, Radix Scrophulariae, Fructus Forsythiae, Liquorice, Bark of tree Peony root, Lophatherum).

7. **清热腑热** 用于热邪偏盛于某一脏腑。清肝胆经热用龙胆泻肝汤(龙胆草、黄芩、栀子、泽泻、木通、车前子、当归、柴胡、甘草、生地黄),清胃肠热用清胃散(黄连、生地黄、牡丹皮、当归、升麻)。

7. **Clearing Visceral Heat** For treating pyretic in some viscerae, clearing liver and gall heat to take Decoction of Gentian to purge the liver (Radix Gentianae, Scutellaria Baicalensis, Gardenia, Rhizoma Alismatis, Akebia Quinata Decne, Plantago seed, Angelica, Radix Bupleuri, Liquorice, Unprocessed Rehmannia root); clearing stomach and intestine heat to take Powder of clearing stomach (Rhizoma Coptidis, take processed Radix Rehmanniae, Bark of tree Peony root, Angelica, Rhizoma Cimicifugae).

8. **滋阴清热** 用于虚热证,久热伤阴者。如热病后期余热未清,阴液已伤,用青蒿鳖甲汤养阴透热(青蒿、鳖甲、生地黄、知母、牡丹皮)。阴虚火旺,骨蒸潮热,盗汗用秦艽鳖甲汤滋阴养血,清热除蒸(地骨皮、柴胡、秦艽、知母、当归、鳖甲)。

8. **Clearing Heat and Enrich Yin** For treating asthenia syndrome, and injured Yin from long time heat, for example, the rest of fever have not yet been cleared completely in the later stage of hot disease, but Yin liquid had been depleted, to take Decoction of Southernwood and Turtle shell; for treating Yin asthenia with heat, tiding heat, and sweat in the night, to take Decoction, enrich Yin and invigorating blood; and another Decoction of clearing heat.

【注意事项】

[Note]

(1)清热法应用范围广泛,应当辨证选用;清脏腑热要按脏腑虚实辨证施治,才恰当。

(1)Clearing heat method have extensive arrangement, so treatment should be done after differentiation of syndrome; clearing visceral heat must accord with visceral asthenia and sthenia.

(2)热证兼表证当解表以清热;半表半里则和解以清热;热解腑实者通里以清热;毒热炽盛者则清热凉血或清热降火并用,热与湿合当清化湿热。

(2)Hot syndrome with exterior syndrome, should clear heat and resolve exterior; half of exterior and interior syndrome, allaying fever by regulation; visceral sthenia and heat, clear heat and purge downwards; pyretic syndrome, very pyretic syndrome, clear fever and cool blood.

(3)使用清热法,必须辨明热证真假,勿为假象所迷惑。

（3）To distinguish real heat and false heat, don't be misled by false appearances.

（4）清热药应当根据热势轻重、体质强弱,投以适当药量,若用量太过和使用过久则可损害脾胃,影响消化。

（4）Take care of heat diseases being light or severe, and human body strong or weak, so we should take care if doses are over and long time being taken, that injures spleen and stomach thus influences digestion.

（5）屡用清热泻火法热仍不退,如王太仆所说:"寒之不寒,是无水也"之证,应改用滋阴壮水之法,阴多则其热自退。配合输液纠正水电解质平衡。

（5）If the heat has not retired, as Wang Taipu said:"If the cold natured herbs can't reduce the body temperature, that's short of liquid". So the doctor should change over to enriching Yin and increasing fluid with venous infusion to correct water and electrolyte balance.

（6）于毒热炽盛阶段,服清热药入口即吐者,可于清热剂中少佐辛温之药剂或凉药热服,此即《素问·五常政大论》所谓"热因热用"之法。

（6）In pyretic if the patient vomits the herbs, the doctor should take warm natured herbs, it's that hot syndrome can be treated by hot natural herbs.

（7）清热之法对体质虚弱而有里寒者禁用,妇女产后慎用。

（7）The method of clearing heat is forbidden. for old, weak persons, is taken care of using in postpartum.

第5章　肛门直肠常用麻醉

Chapter 5　The Common Anorectal Anesthesia

一、肛门外麻醉

Ⅰ. External Anal Anesthesia

【适应证】

[Indication]

单纯肛门病,直肠深部手术效果欠佳,肛门括约肌松弛不理想。

The surgery is performed only for anal region diseases, but the operational effect for the deep part of rectum is not good because the anal sphincters can't be relaxed very well.

【常用药物】

[Common Drugs]

(1)1% 利多卡因 20~25ml。

(1)1% Lidocaine 20~25ml.

(2)1:1000 肾上腺素 2~3 滴(高血压心脏病不用)。

(2)1:1000 Epinephrine 2~3drops (except in patients with high blood pressure and heart diseases).

【麻醉方法】

[Anesthetic Method]

(1)取截石位,安尔碘消毒,2 点、6 层注射法;于 3 点和 9 点分别先皮丘注射,起点进针。

(1)Taking lithotomy posture, with Iodide skin sterilization and injection at 2 o'clock point, to use 6 layers injection method; the first injection to form skin hillock in 3 o'clock and 9 o'clock points separately, then go into continually from the points.

(2)朝肛管方向皮下及深层各注射 4ml 局麻药(勿刺入肛管腔)。

(2)Towards anal canal take subcutaneous layer and deep tissue injection 4ml of local anesthetic separately (don't go into anal canal cavity).

（3）朝尾骨方向皮下及深层各注射 4ml 局麻药。

（3）Towards coccyx take subcutaneous layer and deep tissue injection 4ml of local anesthetic separately.

（4）朝会阴方向皮下及深部各注射 4ml 局麻药,勿刺入尿道(图 5 – 1 ~ 图 5 – 3)。

（4）Towards perineum take subcutaneous layer and deep tissue injection 4ml of local anesthetic separately（don't go into urethra）(Fig. 5 – 1 ~ Fig. 5 – 3).

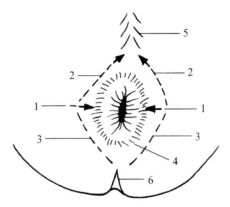

图 5 – 1　肛门区麻醉给药方向
1 – 肛门方向;2 – 会阴方向;3 – 尾骨方向;4 – 肛门区;5 – 会阴区;6 – 尾骨
Figure 5 – 1　Anesthetic injection directions of anal region
1. To anus; 2. To perineum; 3. To coccyx region; 4. To anal region; 5. To perineum region; 6. To coccyx

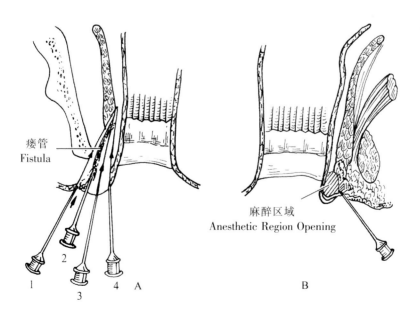

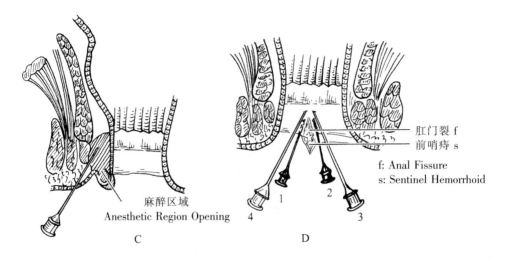

肛门裂 f
前哨痔 s

f: Anal Fissure
s: Sentinel Hemorrhoid

麻醉区域
Anesthetic Region Opening

C   D

图 5 - 2　肛管外麻醉

A. 肛瘘手术时局部麻醉；B. 外痔麻醉部位；C. 内痔脱出麻醉部位；D. 肛裂手术时局部麻醉

Figure 5 - 2　External anal canal anesthesia

A. Local anesthesia for fistulae；B. Local anesthesia for external hemorrhoid；

C. Local anesthesia for protruding internal hemorrhoid；D. Local anesthesia for anal fissure

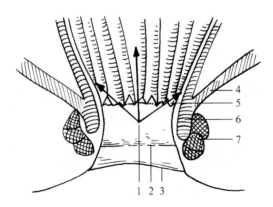

图 5 - 3　肛管内麻醉注药方向

1 - 肛管内局麻针眼；2 - 白线；3 - 肛门；4 - 提肛肌；5 - 齿线；6 - 内括约肌；7 - 外括约肌

Figure 5 - 3　Anesthetic injection directions of internal anal canal

1. Anesthetic puncturing points；2. White line；3. Anus；4. The levator ani muscle；

5. Dental；6. Internal sphincter；7. External sphincter

二、肛管内麻醉

Ⅱ. Internal Anal Canal Anesthesia

【适应证】

[Indication]

肛管直肠深部手术和肛门括约肌痉挛者。

Deep anal canal and rectum, and spasm of anal sphincter.

【常用药物】

[Common Drugs]

同"肛门外麻醉"。

The same as external Anal Anesthesia.

【麻醉方法】

[Anesthetic Method]

取截石位(安尔碘消毒)1点,6层用细长针头;注射法。采用圆头缺口电池灯肛门镜,看到直肠内腔,于齿线下1cm(第1步)先于6点处,进针,继往前上,黏膜下层及深层肌肉有肌性感,各注射麻药3ml,第2步朝3点方向黏膜下层及浅层肌肉层各注射麻药3ml。第3步朝9点方向黏膜下层及浅层肌肉层各注射麻药3ml(图5-3)。

Taking lithotomy posture (with Iodide skin sterilization) and injection at 1 o'clock point, to use 6 layers injection method with long and thin syringe needle. By using optical anoscopy to observe the rectal cavity, the first step is to inject under dental line at the 6 o'clock point, then go towards anterosuperiorly to inject into submucosa and deep muscularis 3ml anesthetic separately; the second step is towards 3 o'clock point into submucosa and shallow muscularis 3 ml anesthetic separately; the third step is towards 9 o'clock point to inject the same layers and dosages(Fig. 5-3).

肛管内麻醉优于肛门外麻醉,因为肛管肌肉松弛,无牵拉和坠胀感注意预防感染。

Internal anal canal anesthesia is performed easier than external anal anesthesia, because there are relaxed muscles in anal canal, and there are no senses of sinking and distending. The doctor should pay attention to guard against infection.

三、骶裂孔阻滞麻醉

Ⅲ. Sacral Hiatus Block Anesthesia

【适应证】

[Indication]

适用于各种肛门直肠手术。

Every surgery of analrectum.

【常用药物】

[Common Drugs]

2%普鲁卡因20ml,加1∶1000肾上腺素2滴或1%利多卡因20ml,加1∶1000肾上腺素2滴。高血压、心脏病病人不用肾上腺素。

To 2% 20ml Parocaine add 1∶1000 Epinephirine 2 drops or 1% Lidocaine 20ml with 1∶1000 Epinephirine 2 drops. Don't use Epinephrine in patients with high blood pressure and heart diseases.

【麻醉方法】

[Method of Giving Anesthesia]

(1)侧卧位(患侧)屈膝。

(1)Patient in lateral recumbent position.

(2)左手拇指由骶骨棘突正中线往下,摸到两个结节(骶骨侧角)与骶骨顶角呈等腰三角形凹陷,即是骶裂孔。

(2)The doctor places his left thumb at the sacral spine and move downwards. He touches two tubercles (lateral corners of the coccyx and sacral tip). These three points form a triangle in which is the sacral fissure foramen.

(3)右手持针管垂直刺入,通过骶尾韧带即有刺空感,到骶管腔。如再深刺遇到发硬的骶骨,要稍后退,回抽没回血,即可缓缓(约15分钟)推入麻药。部位准确时有刺空感,推药无阻力(图5-4,图5-5)。

(3)His right hand takes a syringe with needle, and inserts the needle vertically till a feeling of cavity, which is the sacral canal cavity. He retracts the syringe a little, if no blood is seen, then the anesthetic can be injected very gently in (in 15 minutes) (Fig 5-4, Fig 5-5).

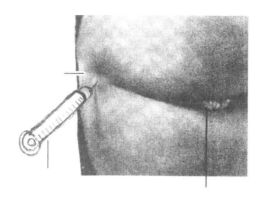

图 5 - 4　骶裂孔阻滞麻醉

Figure 5 - 4　Sacral fissure block anesthesia

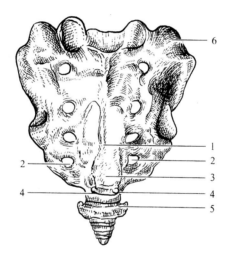

图 5 - 5　骶骨背面

1 - 顶角;2 - 骶孔;3 - 骶裂孔;4 - 侧角;5 - 尾骨;6 - 骶骨

Figure 5 - 5　Backside of Sacrum

1. Spine tip;2. Sacral foramen;3. Sacral fissure foramen;

4. Lateral corner;5. Coccyx;6. Sacrum

【不良反应】

[Adverse Reactions]

仅少数病人发生,多因推入麻药过多、过快,或将血管刺破,使麻药迅速吸收造成。主要表现为普鲁卡因中毒或脑压增高反应,如头晕、气短、心悸、乱语、烦躁、血压升高或下降,心率、脉搏加快。紧急处理包括:停止推药;给予苯妥英钠 0.2g,或氯丙嗪加异丙嗪各 25mg(肌内注射),或地西泮,输液,吸氧;一旦发生窒息,用注射器针,气管穿刺给氧或使用呼吸机。

Few adverse reactions occur, mostly due to too much anesthetic or too fast injection, or breaking blood vessels leading to rapid absorption of anesthetic. The main manifestations of intoxication of procaine or increased intracranial pressure, includes high blood pressure or decreased blood pressure, fainting, short breath, palpitation, jargon, dusphonia, increased heart rates and pulse rates. Urgent treatment includes stopping pushing in anesthetics, giving Bentoina 0. 2 g i. m. or Choractil 25 mg + Isomethazine 25 mg i. m. , or Demoxepam i. v. infusion, and giving oxygen inhalation. Once asphyxia happens, intratracheal oxygenation should be given or respiration machine be used.

第6章 肛门直肠常见疾病

Chapter 6 Common Diseases of Anorectum

第一节 痔

§ 1 Hemorrhoids

痔是一种最常见的肛门病,是由于种种原因而使直肠下部、肛管或肛门边缘的静脉曲张扩大而形成柔软的静脉团块,肛垫病理性肥大下移。

The hemorrhoids are the most common anal disease. The term hemorrhoids refers to a condition in which the veins around the anus or lower rectum are swollen and inflamed, and the anal cushions of pathological hypertrophy are stretched with the tendency to prolapse outside the anal canal.

【病因病机】

[Etiology and Pathology]

痔是由于机体内部调节功能失常(阴阳失调、抗病能力减低)和解剖生理缺陷,以及各种各样的外在诱因而引起的一系列病变。其中,机体内在因素是其发生、发展的决定性因素。

Hemorrhoids may result from the body's regulating malfunction (Yin and Yang imbalance, diseases resistance reduced), anatomic and physiological defect and various external inducer, while the internal problems are decisive factors that hemorrhoids take place and develop.

1. **大便干燥或便秘** 因为粪块的直接压迫和刺激痔静脉丛,因而血流发生障碍,引起痔静脉充血扩张;或因大便时用力过甚,使静脉破裂而出血瘀滞在皮下,则形成血栓性外痔。

1. **Constipation** Large or small volume stools press and strain directly the venous plexus so that the blood flow is obstructed, to make veins swollen, straining during defecation and the passage of hard stool results in breaking of veins to form blood stasis and clot in subcutaneous tissue. This condition is known as a thrombosed external hemorrhoid.

2. **饮食不节** 饮酒过量,经常吃辛辣刺激性食物,使盆腔脏器充血,影响静脉回流,同时刺激性食物往往可以引起便秘。

2. **Dietary Irregularities** To drink excessive consumption of alcohol, and to often eat pungent and irritant food, make pelvic organ become engorged with blood so as to form obstruction of venous return, meanwhile the food may usually lead to constipation, so hemorrhoids may result

from straining to move stool.

3. **久坐久站**　由于重力影响,盆腔静脉的回流迟滞,肠的蠕动减少,粪便下行缓慢,压迫静脉,造成血液回流困难。

3. **Sitting or Standing Long Time**　Especially the erect position of the human being, gravity affects pelvic venous return flow.

4. **妊娠与分娩**　妇女怀孕后期,子宫膨大,压迫盆腔静脉,使腹压过度增加,这些都可以影响痔静脉的血液回流。

4. **Pregnancy and Childbirth**　Hemorrhoids are also common among pregnant women. The pressure of the fetus on abdomen, as well as hormonal changes, causes the hemorrhoidal vessels to enlarge. These vessels are also placed under severe pressure during childbirth. The pelvic venous return flow is influenced.

5. **局部刺激**　肛门受湿受热,慢性直肠炎,久泻久痢,都可以使痔静脉丛血管壁弹性减弱;经常刺激局部使其感染发炎。以上诱因都可使局部血液回流受阻,循环不畅,血管内压增高,静脉壁变薄,弹力减弱,静脉瘀血,肛垫的黏膜下肌纤维组织断裂使下移衬垫组织脱垂形成痔疮,是肛垫的病理性肥大。肛外静脉纡曲扩张容易发生炎性外痔。

5. **Other anal Diseases**　Many factors have been implicated in the causation of hemorrhoids, including the erect position of the human being, the absence of venous valves, obstruction of venous return, and hereditary weakness of the vessels. These factors are all present in the normal physiologic status of the vascular arrangement of the anal canal, and they bear no direct relationship to the disease state, straining during defecation and the passage of hard, small-volume stools, however, results in tense engorgement of the anal cushions. This may cause injury to the mucous membrane, resulting in bright red bleeding from the capillaries of the lamina propria. With repeated straining, the anal cushions are damaged so that the normal supports are stretched and the tendency is to prolapse outside and the anal canal develops.

【临床表现】

[Clinical Manifestations]

1. **全身症状**

1. **Systemic Symptoms**

(1)血滞型:由于痔核初起,偶有便血。

(1)Blood stasis type:The occurrence of blood stool in initial hemorrhoids.

(2)湿热型:表现口苦、胃部痞满、大便干燥或秘结、小便色黄。

(2)Damp heat type:Bitter taste, stomach full, dry defecation or constipation.

（3）热毒型：有恶寒发热、口干咽燥、食欲缺乏、尿短赤；局部多有剧痛。

（3）Heat toxin type：Chill and fever, bitter taste and dry pharynx, poor appetite, dark reddish brown urine；very pain in location.

（4）血虚型：表现头晕、目眩、心悸、耳鸣、盗汗、四肢无力等症状。

（4）Blood deficiency type：Dizziness, palpitation, tinnitus, night sweat, weak, etc.

（5）气虚型：多表现有心跳、气短、自汗、精神疲倦、肛门部有下坠感等症状。

（5）Qi deficiency type：Palpitation, pant, spontaneous perspiration, weariness, tenesmus, etc.

2. 局部症状

2. Local Symptoms

（1）外痔：发炎肿胀，而有剧烈疼痛。①血栓性外痔的症状是病人感觉灼热、疼痛，肿物表面呈青紫色，触之感到疼痛；②静脉曲张性外痔的症状是有时刺痒作痛；③炎性外痔的症状是肛门红肿，疼痛剧烈；④结缔组织性外痔的症状是局部胀痛而发痒。

（1）External hemorrhoids：To be inflamed, swelling and twinge. ①The symptoms of thrombus external hemorrhoids are violaceous color mass going with flaming pain and serious tenderness. ②The symptoms of varicose external hemorrhoids are itching pain sometimes. ③The symptoms of inflamed external hemorrhoids may include painful swelling and red and swollen signs around the anus. ④The symptoms of connective tissue external hemorrhoids are painful swelling with itching.

（2）内痔：内痔生于肛门内部，齿线之上。①流血：在大便时或大便后有血流出。②内痔脱出：大便时向下推动，而脱出肛门之外。有时内痔脱出，发生嵌顿，称为绞窄性内痔。③黏液流出：因为直肠黏膜受到痔块刺激，分泌物增多。④疼痛：痔块内有血栓形成时，特别是内痔嵌顿于肛外。

（2）Internal hemorrhoids：Above dental line, inside of anus. ①Bleeding：bleeding as purging stool or post-stool. ②Internal hemorrhoids coming off or projecting：to strain and push downwards till projecting out from anus. Sometimes incarcerated, it's called strangulated internal hemorrhoid. ③Mucus flowing from anus：the mucosa of rectum is influenced by hemorrhoids to cause increasing secretion. ④Pain：internal hemorrhoids may have the pain which accompanies thrombosis, especially being incarcerated internal hemorrhoids projecting from anus.

（3）混合痔：兼内痔与外痔的表现。

（3）Mixed hemorrhoids：Having symptoms either in internal hemorrhoids or external hemorrhoids.

【诊断】

[Diagnosis]

根据中医学的望、闻、问、切四诊和局部检查确定。

The diagnosis relies on the four methods by traditional Chinese medicine:observation, auscultation or olfaction, interrogation, pulse feeling or palpation, and local examination.

1.定型
1. Types

(1)血滞型:脉象多为平脉或弦脉;舌苔薄白或少苔;局部病变多属于静脉曲张性或结缔组织性外痔。初期内痔。

(1)Blood stasis:Pulses are mild or string; tongue fur white thin or a little fur; local lesion being external hemorrhoids with varicosity or connective tissue. These are initial hemorrhoids.

(2)湿热型:脉象多见弦数;舌苔黄腻而厚,舌尖多带红色;局部病变多为静脉曲张性外痔初起,血栓性外痔,或初期、中期内痔较重者。

(2)Damp heat:Pulses are often rapid string; tongue fur is yellow with greasy and thick, the tip of tongue is usually red; local forms are initial variceal external hemorrhoids, thrombosed external hemorrhoids, or initial and mild internal hemorrhoids.

(3)热毒型:脉象多见弦数或洪数或弦紧;舌苔黄燥,舌质红赤;局部病变为大型血栓性外痔,嵌顿性内痔。

(3)Heat toxin:Pulses are often rapid string, rapid bouncing, string tense; bright red tongue with yellow-dry fur; local forms are big thrombosed external hemorrhoids and incarcerated internal hemorrhoids.

(4)血虚型:脉象细而无力或见芤象;舌苔薄白,舌质淡;局部病变多为初、中期内痔。

(4)Blood deficiency:Pulses are feeble and thin, or hollow; pale tongue with white thin fur; local forms are often initial and mild internal hemorrhoids.

(5)气虚型:脉象沉细无力或微脉;舌苔薄白或无苔;局部病变为中期内痔较久或中期内痔并有痔核脱出。

(5)Qi deficiency:Pulses are sunken, feeble and thin; tongue fur, white thin or without fur; local forms are mild stage internal hemorrhoids with long time, or mild stage internal hemorrhoids with prolapse of hemorrhoids.

2.分类
2. Classification

（1）外痔

（1）External hemorrhoids

①血栓性外痔：在肛门皮肤上有椭圆形青紫色肿物（图 6 – 1）。

①Thrombosed external hemorrhoid：Elliptical violaceous color，swelling lump under the skin around the anus（Fig. 6 – 1）.

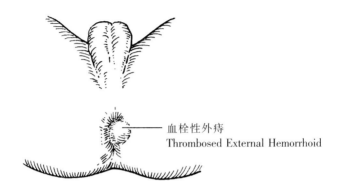

图 6 – 1 血栓性外痔

Figure 6 – 1 Thrombosed external hemorrhoid

②静脉曲张性外痔：在肛门皮肤皱襞处，有囊状肿物（图 6 – 2）。

②Varicose external hemorrhoid：sacciform swelling lump in skin fold around the anus（Figure.6 – 2）.

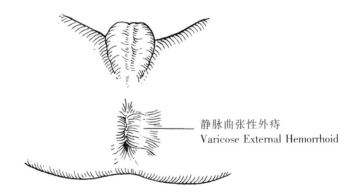

图 6 – 2 静脉曲张性外痔

Figure 6 – 2 Varicose external hemorrhoid

③炎性外痔：在肛门皱襞表面有炎症肿物（图 6 – 3）。

③Inflamed external hemorrhoids：Inflammatory swelling lump in surface skin fold around the anus（Fig.6 – 3）.

④结缔组织性外痔（也称前哨痔）：在肛门前、后两部分，生有大小不同而较硬的肿物（图 6 – 4）。

④Connective tissue external hemorrhoids: Commonly seen in front or behind anus, and they are masses around the anus, sometimes big, sometimes small(Fig. 6 - 4).

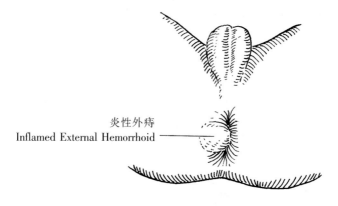

炎性外痔
Inflamed External Hemorrhoid ——————

图 6 - 3　炎性外痔

Figure 6 - 3　Inflamed external hemorrhoid

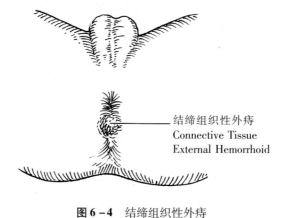

—————— 结缔组织性外痔
Connective Tissue
External Hemorrhoid

图 6 - 4　结缔组织性外痔

Figure 6 - 4　Connective tissue external hemorrhoid

(2)内痔

(2)Internal hemorrhoids

①初期内痔:有时便血,通过窥肛器检查才能发现。这种痔是在齿线以上(图6 - 5)。

①Initial internal hemorrhoids: Bleeding associated with defecation, above the dental line, can only be discovered by proctoscopy (Fig. 6 - 5).

②中期内痔:在大便用力时会脱出在肛门的边缘,其颜色红紫,黏膜表面常有出血点(图6 - 6)。

②Mild internal hemorrhoids: The lump prolapse fringe of anus, and may result from straining to move stool. There are bleeding points in the mucosal surface (Fig. 6 - 6).

③嵌顿性内痔:痔核脱出肛外不能送其中央,为嵌顿痔核(图6-7)。

③Incarcerated internal hemorrhoids:The internal hemorrhoids come off anus and can't be carried out (Fig. 6-7).

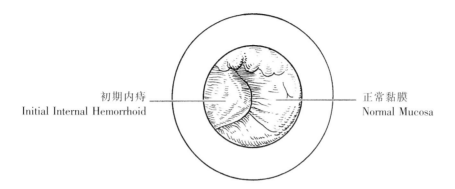

初期内痔　　　　　　　　　　　正常黏膜
Initial Internal Hemorrhoid　　　Normal Mucosa

图6-5 初期内痔

Figure 6-5 Initial internal hemorrhoid

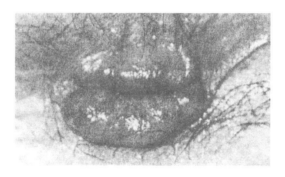

图6-6 中期内痔(脱出肛外)

Figure 6-6 Mild internal hemorrhoids

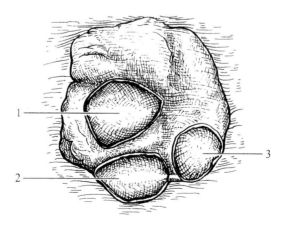

图6-7 3个嵌顿性内痔

Figure 6-7 Three incarcerated internal hemorrhoid

(3)混合痔:内痔外痔连在一起的叫混合痔,也叫中间痔(图 6 - 8)。

(3)Mixed hemorrhoid:It is a combination of an external and internal hemorrhoid(Fig. 6 - 8).

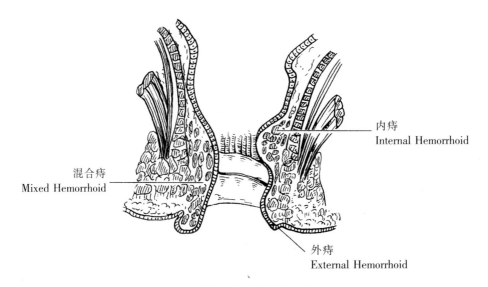

图 6 - 8　混合痔

Figure 6 - 8　Mixed hemorrhoid

【鉴别诊断】

[Differential Diagnosis]

1. **直肠脱垂**　黏膜脱出肛外,其下垂之黏膜呈均匀鲜红色,旋形而有层次。

1. **Prolapse of Rectum**　The mucosa come off anus, and there are spiral layers with bright red mucosa.

2. **脱肛**　是在肛门边缘有一圈堤样突起,而外痔为个体散在之肿物。

2. **Rectocele**　There is a round of dyke style protuberance hanging over the anus, however, the external hemorrhoids are sporadic projecting.

3. **直肠息肉**　有一乳头状的圆形小瘤,带有长蒂,呈朱红色。

3. **Rectal Polypus**　There is a round tumor of papillae shape, red color with thin and long root-shape base.

4. **直肠癌**　可触到大小不同硬性肿物,边界不整,表面凹凸不平,后期者直肠肛门直肠狭窄。

4. **Rectal Cancer**　Feeling hard tumor, it's of different shapes, disorder edge, uneven surface, and it can cause rectal stenosis in the later stage.

5. **肠内出血**　血色较深(黑紫色),而且与粪便混合;内痔出血,则为鲜红色,且常于大便之前流出。

5. **Bleeding in the Intestinal Cavity**　The color of bleeding is from black red to bright red gradually accompanying with the part of bleeding downwards.

6. 肛裂　肛裂流血不多,但十分疼痛。

6. **Anal Fissure**　The hemorrhage is of a little quantity or adhere to only at surface of excrement, accompanying with the knife cutting pain.

【治疗】

[Treatment]

根据辨证施治的原则,采用标本兼治、局部治疗与全身治疗相结合的医疗方案。

According to the principle of treatment relying on syndrome differentiation, combined local and systemic treatments can be carried out.

1. 全身治疗

1. **Systemic Treatment**

(1)血滞型:一般不做全身治疗。

(1)Blood stagnation:Not indicated in this treatment.

(2)湿热型:以清热通便为主。常用槐角丸、麻仁滋脾丸,以及双醋酚汀等药物。

(2)Damp heat:Mainly to clear heat and purge stool, the common using Pill from the pod of Chinese scholartree, Pill of MaRen ZiPi Isophen, etc.

(3)热毒型:以清热解毒,消肿止痛为主。常用消肿止痛汤或其他抗生素等药物。

(3)Heat toxin:Mainly to clear heat and detoxication, commonly using Decoction of subsidence of swelling and reducing pain or antibiotics.

(4)血虚型:以补血、止血、和血为主。常用四物汤。

(4)Blood deficiency:Mainly to invigorate blood, hemostasis and to activate blood, commonly using Decoction of Four Kinds of Herbs.

(5)气虚型:以健脾补气为主。常用补中益气汤。

(5)Qi deficiency:Mainly to invigorate Qi and spleen, commonly using Decoction of BuZhongYiQi.

2. 外痔局部治疗

2. **Local Treatment**

(1)简易疗法:适用于不宜手术的痔疮患者。可内服消肿止痛汤,外用祛毒汤熏洗,洗后敷入九华膏外痔贴中药膏,但不能根除。

(1) Simple therapy: Indicated in those surgery not being performed, taking Decoction of subsidence of swelling and reducing pain, tub baths with decoction, application of a hemorrhoidal cream suppository to the affected area, such as Cream of JiuHua. This therapy can't effect a radical cure.

(2)小针刀切开法

(2) Incision of applying acupuncture scalpel

①适应证:静脉曲张性外痔、血栓性外痔、结缔组织性外痔,以及混合痔的外痔。

①Indication: The varicose, thrombosed, connective tissue and mixed external hemorrhoids.

②操作方法:嘱患者侧卧,剃净肛门周围的阴毛,然后常规消毒皮肤,并在痔核周围应用1%利多卡因10ml,亚甲蓝注射液2ml。进行长效浸润麻醉。距肛门缘0.5~1cm,再用小针刀自外痔基底部,纵行切开部分外痔的前层皮肤。用小针刀钩,将外痔内的静脉曲张、血栓块或结缔组织钩出部分。其切口,用痔瘘粉棉球,创可贴压迫(图6-9)。

②Arrangement: Lateroflexion position, with a clean pubes-cut, sterilize the skin, 1% Lidocain 10ml local anesthesia around hemorrhoids and Methylene blue 2ml, taking a long effect infiltrative anesthesia. From 0.5 ~ 1 cm to anal edge, to take acupuncture scalpel vertical incision on the anterior layer of external hemorrhoids, then to take the hook of acupuncture scalpel hooking out the pan of varicose veins, thrombosed masses and connective tissue, then to press the incision using cotton ball with Powder treating hemorrhoids and fistula from herbs, then using adhesive plaster. (Fig. 6-9).

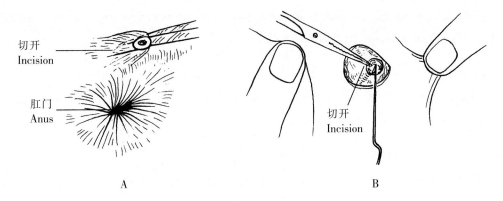

图6-9 外痔小针刀治疗

A.切口;B.切开痔核

Figure 6-9 Acupuncture scalpel treating external hemorrhoids

A. Incision; B. Cutting the hemorrhoid

（3）小针刀针孔法

（3）Needle point hole method

①适应证：血栓、静脉曲张外痔。

①Indication：The varicose and thrombosed external hemorrhoids.

②治疗方法：取侧卧位，局麻下以血栓外痔的外侧边缘基底部为进口处。右手持钩状小针刀顺血栓外痔相平行方向，从点状局麻针眼进口处刺入。然后潜行性插割直达血栓块的上缘，不要刺破外痔（皮肤）其他处皮肤，并以"血栓块"为中旋转钩状小针刀 1 圈，将其血栓块与外痔的周围粘连组织切割开，再从原进口处将血栓块钩出来，给予塔形纱布加压包扎（图 6 - 10）。

②Arrangement：Lateroflexion positure, local anesthesia, to go in from lateral basic edge of thrombosed external hemorrhoids, and this is the inlet. The right hand handles the hook style acupuncture scalpel in the direction of paralleling thrombosed external hemorrhoids, to puncture from needle point hole of local anesthesia, then to insert and cut till above edge of the thrombosed external hemorrhoid in moving under skin. Don't injure the skin of external hemorrhoids, then to spin the hook style acupuncture scalpel one round in taking "the thrombosed mass" as the center, to cut off adhesive tissues around thrombosed mass, then hook out the thrombosed mass, to press tower-shape gauze and pack up（Fig. 6 - 10）.

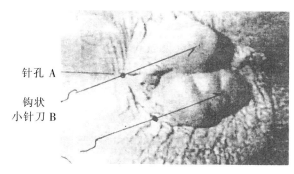
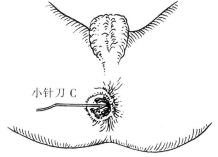

针孔 A

钩状
小针刀 B

小针刀 C

A: Puncture Hole of Acupuncture Scalpel
B: Hook Style Acupuncture Scalpel

C: Acupuncture Scalpel

图 6 - 10　血栓外痔

Figure 6 - 10　Thrombosed external hemorrhoids

③体会：钩状小针刀治疗是刺破血栓外痔钩出血栓块，并无切口。若血栓块与外痔皮肤粘连或钩状小针刀一旦刺破外痔或其他外部皮肤，也可顺其形状，而钩割成小洞式切口，然后顺之钩出血栓块后；如血栓块过大，也可钩切碎块，再从针眼钩出外痔的血栓块，用同法加压包扎，一般不用换药。

③Realization：The method of hook style acupuncture scalpel is to puncture the thrombosed external hemorrhoids and to hook out thrombosed masses, without skin incision. If the thrombosed masses adhere to skin of external hemorrhoids, leading to the scalpel puncture the external hemorrhoids broken of the skin, continue to cut and hook forming a small hole conveniently, then hook out thrombosed masses. If the thrombosed masses are too big, the doctor can also hook and cut, and make them broken, then hook out the thrombosed masses of external hemorrhoids from needle hole, and then press gauze and pack up with the same method.

(4)钩状小针刀法
(4)The method of the hook style acupuncture scalpel

①适应证:治疗静脉曲张性外痔。

①Indication:The varicose external hemorrhoids.

②治疗方法:取侧卧位,局麻下以静脉曲张性外痔的外下侧边缘为进口处。右手持钩状小针,钩刀与其曲张性外痔相平行方向,从点状局麻针眼进口处刺入。然后潜行性皮下切剥静脉曲张团的前侧粘连,直达曲张外痔的上缘,再旋切至对侧面,即切一圈。随即边退钩状小针刀,边钩出已离断的静脉曲张团于痔外。给予塔形纱布加压包扎。

②Arrangement:Lateroflexion position, local anesthesia, to go into from edge of lateral inferior varicose external hemorrhoid, and this is the inlet. The right hand handles the hook style acupuncture scalpel in the direction of paralleling varicose external hemorrhoids, to puncture from needle point hole of local anesthesia, then to insert and cut till above anterior of varicose external in moving under skin, to cut off adhesive tissues and turn round to the opposite, that's cutting one round, then to pull back the hook style acupuncture scalpel at the same time hook out the varicose masses, to press with tower-shape gauze and pack up(Fig 6 – 11).

③体会:钩状小针刀治疗只是刺破静脉曲张性外痔的皮肤,将其内静脉曲张团钩出来,并无切口。治疗中一旦钩切破静脉曲张团,也无碍,仍将其残碎的静脉尽量钩出来。若切破外痔的皮肤则顺其钩割成小洞口,作为引流,用同法加压包扎,一般用外痔贴换药(图6 – 11)。经临床证实,该疗法可以代替手术,并且简单易行,疗效可靠。

③Realization:The method is to puncture the hemorrhoids and hook out varicose masses. If the varicose masses adhere to the skin, easily puncture the hemorrhoids or the outside of skins broken, then continue to cut and hook forming a small hole conveniently, then hook out varicose masses from the hole, it can also be a draining hole, to press with gauze(Fig. 6 – 11). The clinical experiences prove that the method can replace surgery and it's easy to do and curative effect is reliable.

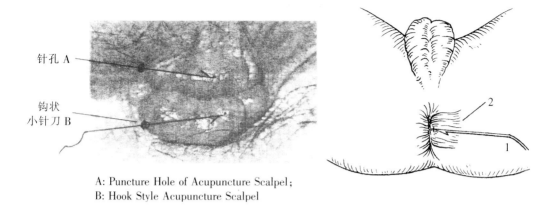

针孔 A

钩状
小针刀 B

A: Puncture Hole of Acupuncture Scalpel；
B: Hook Style Acupuncture Scalpel

图 6 - 11　静脉曲张外痔

1 - 钩状小针刀；2 - 静脉曲张外痔

Figure 6 - 11　Varicose external hemorrhoid

1. Hook Style Acupuncture Scalpel；2. Varicose External Hemorrhoid

3. 内痔局部治疗

3. Local Treatment for Internal Hemorrhoids

（1）简易疗法

（1）Simple and easy therapy

①适应证：不宜手术的内痔患者。可以防止内痔脱出肛外，并能减少流血，但不能达到根治目的。凡无明显症状之初期内痔，或因某种原因不能手术，均可采用此法。

①Indication：The patients of internal hemorrhoids who are not suitable for surgery，without obvious clinical symptoms. This method can reduce bleeding，but doesn't effect a radical cure of hemorrhoids.

②调理大便：要使大便通畅，减少对痔核的刺激。如大便干时可内服槐角丸、脏连丸、五仁润肠丸、液状石蜡等。如果痔核已有脱出，应及时送回肛内，以免发炎或嵌顿。还纳时应先挤压较小的痔核，使痔内血液回流而缩小，逐渐全部缩入肛内。若内痔发炎红肿胀大，嵌顿于肛外，疼痛剧烈时，应内服消肿止痛汤，以及用中药外痔贴，熏洗坐浴，每日 2～3 次，然后在肛内注入九华膏。

②Regulation of defecation：The patients can keep free movement of the bowels so as to reduce the stimulation for nucleus of the hemorrhoid. If the patient has dry stool，he should take Pill of the pod of Chinese scholartree，ZangLian，Five seeds smoothening intestinal cavity and Paraffin，etc.. If the hemorrhoids are protruding，they should be pushed back inside the anus lest infection or getting stuck. As returning，to press the hemorrhoids to squeeze blood back，the hemorrhoids reduce the scope, and so gradually return to inside of anus. If the internal hemorrhoids are inflamed and red swollen, protruding outside of anus, very pain, the patients should take decoction of reducing inflammation and pain, plaster of herbs, baths with warm water or herbs soup, 2 ~ 3 times every-day, then squeeze JiuHua cream into the anus.

(2)小针刀挑痔法

(2)Method of pricking hemorrhoids with acupuncture scalpel

①寻找穴位:在第 3 腰椎至第 2 骶椎之间,从上至下纵行,在其椎体外缘,再离开 1.5 ~ 3cm 寻找痔点穴位。

①Looking for points:To look for hemorrhoidal acupuncture points between the third lumbar vertebra and the second sacral vertebra downwards, the distance from the external later fringe of vertebral body being 1.5 ~ 3cm.

②寻找皮肤痔点:在前述穴位周围皮肤范围内寻找其皮肤肛门"内痔点"的内投影。其特点是形似丘疹,稍隆起皮肤表面;或针头或小米粒、圆形,略带光泽,颜色有的呈灰白色、棕褐色或淡红色。

②Looking for skin hemorrhoidal acupuncture points:Looking for inner skin projection of internal hemorrhoidal acupuncture points, and the feature is similar to papula, a little projecting on skin, the size of needle point or millet, round shape with a little luster, and the color is pale, brown drab or light red.

③区分开是痔点与色斑或痦子。痔点手指压迫不褪色,而色斑或痦子手指压迫则是褪色或变淡。

③Differentiation of hemorrhoidal acupuncture points from spot or mole:Being pressed by finger the points of hemorrhoidal acupuncture don't fade, while spots fade or change light.

④小针刀手法:患者平躺卧位,背朝上,将其痔点的皮肤消毒,用 1% 丁卡因涂抹在皮肤表面止痛。先用挑穴小针刀,如同针灸一样垂直由上自下刺入皮肤深处 0.2 ~ 0.3cm,深达皮下为止,勿刺入脂肪层。然后用挑穴小针刀的刀尖挑出白色纤维物 5 ~ 6 条,继用小针刀的前端刀刃切断。该穴位内的每条被挑到的纤维条索均要挑割断开,或钩断。挑割同时上下提插,如同针灸发挥针灸"得气"与小针刀"切断纤条"的作用。然后依次类推,照前法从第 3 腰椎至第 2 骶椎;从腰或骶椎的外缘起至腰大肌缘止,凡在此范围内的"痔点"均一一挑割切断。有少许渗血或出血点稍用干棉球压迫即可(图 6 - 12)。

④Method of acupuncture scalpel:The patient lies on the back with the prone position. The doctor sterilizes the skin of hemorrhoidal acupuncture points, and scribbles 1% Amethocaine on the skin for stopping pain. Firstly, the doctor takes pricking point scalpel like acupuncture to puncture vertically 0.2 ~ 0.3cm, not to put into fat layer; then takes the scalpel point to prick out white fibers 5 ~ 6 strips, then cut off them by the anterior edge of scalpel; in the point every fiber must be cut off; at the same time takes scalpel up and down just like using the acupuncture to treat diseases. According to the method, he pricks hemorrhoidal acupuncture points from the third lumbar vertebra to the second sacral vertebra, from outer fringe of lumbar vertebra and the second sacral vertebra to psoas major muscle, and in the area all hemorrhoidal acupuncture points need to be cut off. To take a dry cotton ball and to press the points in case of a little oozing blood or bleeding(Fig 6 – 12).

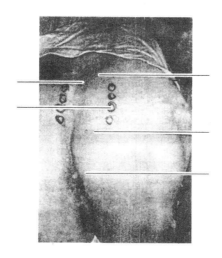

图 6 – 12　小针刀挑痔法(跪位)

1 – 脊柱;2 – 痔点;3 – 第 3 腰椎;4 – 第 2 骶椎;5 – 肛门

Figure 6 – 12　Method of pricking hemorrhoids with acupuncture scalpel(kneeling chest position)

1. Vertebra;2. Hemorrhoidal acupuncture points;

3. The third lumbar vertebra;4. The second sacral vertebra;5. Anus

⑤疗效评估:挑治后 1 周内内痔出血、肛门疼痛消失,内痔变小变软,为临床治愈。

⑤Effect:The bleeding and pain will disappear in one week, and internal hemorrhoids change into small and soft, and that's all clinic cure.

用小针刀对内痔体表投影点的挑割法,只是临床治愈,并未根治,只是改善临床症状,为今后进一步治疗做好准备,或为年老体弱难以接受手术者的对症疗法。

The method of cutting skinny projection of internal hemorrhoidal acupuncture points is only clinic cure of reducing symptom, not radical cure, but makes a preparation for further treatment, and it's a symptomatic treatment for old persons and weakness who can hardly be surgically treated.

（3）内痔普通注射疗法

（3）Injection therapy

内痔注射是将药物注入痔块的黏膜下组织内,使淋巴凝固,引起轻度无菌性炎性反应;进一步有结缔组织增生,阻塞曲张的静脉,使血管硬化,减少出血机会,并可使痔核缩小或消失而治愈。

To inject the medicine into the submucosal tissue above hemorrhoid to sclerose lymphatic tissue and induce to no-bacillus inflamed reaction; and further to cause proliferation of connective tissue , to obstruct veins and make the vessels sclerosed, reduce bleeding chance, decrease hemorrhoid nuclear even disappear, to arrive at the aim of cure.

①常用药物:a. 石炭酸甘油,由石炭酸与甘油混合而成,通常用5% ~10% 。因该药为油剂,注入较困难。b. 鱼肝油酸钠,为血管硬化剂,注入比较容易,且比石炭酸甘油效果更好。c. 消痔灵:为硬化粘连剂。

①Common drugs:a. Phenol in glycerine, the mixed drug from phenol and glycerine, common dose of 5% ~10%. Since the drug is oil shape, injection is difficult. b. Sodium morrhuate, vessel sclerosant, injection is easier, and with better result than phenol in glycerine. c. XiaoZhiLing(eliminate hemorrhoids), is an adherent sclerosants.

②器械:1ml 注射器、12 号针头、圆筒窦肛器、长镊子等。

②Appliance:1 ml syringe, 12# syringe needle, cylinder anal endoscopy, a long forceps.

③适应证:适用于初期内痔,可达到临床治愈效果。对有结核病、心脏病或年老体弱,或因某种原因不宜做手术或枯痔法的内痔病人都可采用。注射以后,症状可以减轻,如流血停止,痔块缩小,不再脱出肛外,有治愈的可能;或只能减轻症状,不易根除。但内痔如配合整体治疗也可以达到基本临床治愈目的。

③Indication:Initial internal hemorrhoids, to arrive at clinical cure, effect for patients who suffer from tuberculosis, heart disease, old and weak patients, and can't be performed surgery for some reasons. Effect:the symptom relieves, the swelling mass reduces, no prolapse from anus, may be cured but not easy to be radically cured. If the patient coordinates integral treatment, the internal hemorrhoids can arrive at the aim of clinical cure.

④禁忌证:有显著纤维增生者,或有并发症,如发炎、溃烂、血栓和有肛裂、肛窦炎直肠炎,或其他感染者。

④Contraindication:Patients who have obvious fiber tissue hyperplasia, or complication such as inflammation, fester, thrombus, anal fissure, anal sinusitis, rectitis, and other infections.

⑤操作方法:注射前嘱病人先排便。注射时采用侧卧位或跪位均可。将肛门局部清洁消毒,以窥肛器涂滑润剂插入肛门,选择较大的痔核,涂安尔碘液,随后将针由痔核的顶部刺入于黏膜下层(图6－13,图6－14),再次刺入痔核体内,不要将药液注射到血管内。一般只注入 0.3 ~ 1.0ml, 至痔核黏膜胀大变白为止(图6－15)。再将窥肛器退出一些,抽出空针头。用安尔碘棉球堵在针孔,当窥肛器退出时,括约肌收缩,这样可避免由针孔内出血。注射时病人并不感到疼痛,疼痛多因注射部位太低(侵及齿线以下),如针头刺入时感觉疼痛,可以将针抽出,再

向较高位置刺入，即可免去疼痛。如果痔核脱出肛外，应先推回，然后注射。每次最好注射一个较大的痔核，如痔核均较小，可注射两个。每周可交替注射，每个痔核平均注射 2～4 次即可使其缩小、硬化或消失。

⑤Method of arrangement：The doctor orders the patient defecate before injection. In injection the patient lays on side or kneeling chest position，and the doctor sterilizes patient's anal area，analscopy with lubricant is put into anus，look for bigger hemorrhoidal nucleus. Inject an iodide needle puncture into submucosa from hemorrhoidal top（Fig. 6 – 13，Fig. 6 – 14），then into hemorrhoidal centre，don't inject into the vessels. To inject only 0.3～1.0 ml，the hemorrhoidal mucosa turn white（Fig. 6 – 15）. To pull back the anoscope a little，taking the needle head off，stopping up the point of needle with an iodide cotton ball，then to retire the anoscopy completely，so that the sphincter can constrict gradually and press the point with least bleeding from the point. The patient won't feel pain，the pain due to too low injective position（ inferior dental line）. If the patient feels pain，the doctor should insert the needle，choose higher parts to puncture so that the pain disappears. When the hemorrhoid prolapses from the anus，injection should be done after the hemorrhoid being put back inside the anus，to inject one bigger hemorrhoid or two smaller hemorrhoids every time once a week. The hemorrhoids are sclerosed，gradually reduced to be disappearing after injecting two to four times for every hemorrhoid.

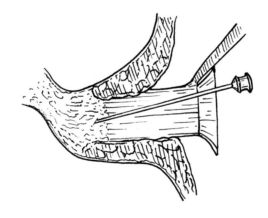

图 6 – 13　内痔注射法

Figure 6 – 13　Injection therapy for internal hemorrhoids

⑥注意事项：a. 必须注入痔核的黏膜下层，如注射过浅则痔核表面发生坏死；注射过深达到肌层，会引起化学性炎症狭窄，会使痔核因肿胀而脱出肛外，发生剧烈疼痛，甚至引起局部坏死；注入痔核静脉内，则可引起全身反应（如头晕恶心）或不良后果。b. 同一个痔核，应间隔 10 天以上再进行第 2 次注射，每次注射 1～2 个，交替注射。每次注射后，要详细记录，最好用图表记录痔核部位（图 6 – 16）。当痔核已纤维化时，可停止注射。

⑥Note：a. Injection must reach into submucosa of hemorrhoids，if it is injected superficial to

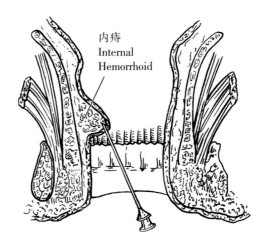

图 6 - 14 内痔注射法

Figure 6 - 14 Injection therapy for internal hemorrhoids

the hemorrhoid, then necrosis will be formed on the surface of the hemorrhoid; if it is deep in the muscle layer, the chemically inflamed narrow tissue will occur, and hemorrhoid will be swollen and prolapsing out of the anus, which is very painful even causing local necrosis; if be injected into hemorrhoidal veins, then systemic reactions will take place (such as dizzy, nausea)or bad consequences.

b. For the same hemorrhoid the second injection should be taken after over 10 days, 1 ~ 2 hemorrhoids every time. To take detailed record by the position of hemorrhoid nuclear using tables and figures (Fig. 6 - 16). When the hemorrhoids have been fibrosed, injection method can be discontinued.

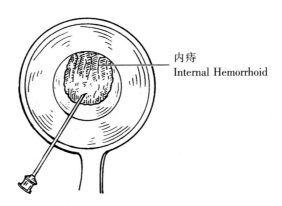

图 6 - 15 内痔注射法

Figure 6 - 15 Injection therapy for internal hemorrhoids

（4）网式注射和阻碍痔血供法,配合小针刀,治疗内痔和并发脱垂病。

（4）Method of injection of net style and obstruction of hemorrhoidal blood supply cooperate acupuncture scalpel to treat internal hemorrhoids and prolapse.

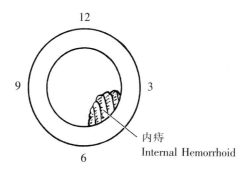

图 6 – 16 内痔注射记录

Figure 6 – 16 Recorder of injection therapy for internal hemorrhoids

目前,在内痔治疗中,尤其是环形痔治疗后复发率较高,其原因是只治疗内痔,对肛垫及伴有的直肠黏膜松弛没有治疗。采用网式注射疗法可解除肛门下坠及便意不净感,且可有效预防内痔复发,使松弛的直肠黏膜和肛垫,与直肠壁层和肌肉层产生粘连固定。实践证明,防止直肠黏膜和肛垫松弛,是治愈和防止内痔复发的关键。

Recently there is a high relapse rate in treating internal hemorrhoids, especially for annular hemorrhoids, the result from only treating internal hemorrhoids but not anal cushions and accompanying rectal mucosal relaxation; taking net style injection can relieve the feeling of falling anus and defecating, preventing the recurrence of internal hemorrhoids, making the relaxed rectal mucosa and anal cushions to adhere rectal muscle layer. The experiment proves that preventing rectal mucosa and anal cushions from relaxing is crucial to curing internal hemorrhoids, and to avoiding relapse.

①阻碍内痔血液供给:在母痔核上方,触及搏动痔上动脉及其下方及周围,给予 0.25% 利多卡因加入消痔灵液(1:1)1ml 封闭(注射前回吸没回血即可以注射),可以达到阻碍内痔血供的效果。如果采用手术结扎痔法,可用细丝线于痔上动脉贯穿缝合 1 针,同样可达到阻断内痔血流供给的效果(图 6 – 17)。

①Blocking the blood supply of internal hemorrhoids:Above the hemorrhoids, the doctor can touch pulsation of the superior artery , then in the inferior of the artery and around it, give Lidocaine and XiaoZhiLing(1:1)local anesthesia(Note:Injection as drawing back no blood). The arrangement can block the blood supply of internal hemorrhoids. Taking surgical ligation method is an effective procedure of blocking the blood supply of internal hemorrhoids. It's same that thin silk suture sew up through superior hemorrhoidal artery once(Fig. 6 – 17).

②网式注射:在圆头缺口电池灯肛门镜下,选择距齿线上分别在约 3 点钟、9 点钟、11 点钟位置,分别在直肠黏膜下层纵行向上部进针 4~6cm。回抽没回血即纵行由上往下,边退针(左右倾斜)边注入药液,形成网柱状,使药液弥散开,致使黏膜下层,包括肛垫产生无菌性纤维粘连,恢复原位肛门衬垫,即可起间接悬吊作用。再行消痔灵三层注射法(图 6 – 18)。

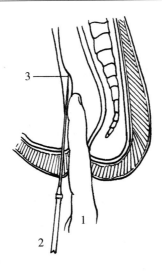

图 6 - 17 阻碍内痔血供给

1 - 手指;2 - 消痔灵皮试针管;3 - 痔上动脉区

Figure 6 - 17 Blocking the blood supply of internal hemorrhoids

1. Finger;2. Spyring;3. The area of superior hemorrhoidal artery

②Net style injection:Taking injection vertically upwards above the dental line 3,9,11 o'clock position separately in rectal submucosa by anoscopy, first inject and drawing back with no blood, then inject gradually as drawing back the syringe(tilted toward left and right), to forn net column style and to make drugs spreading over the submucosa. The method is forming fiber adhesion so as to return to anal cushion of original position to take part in indirect hanging. Then take the method of three layer injection by XiaoZhiLing(Fig. 6 - 18).

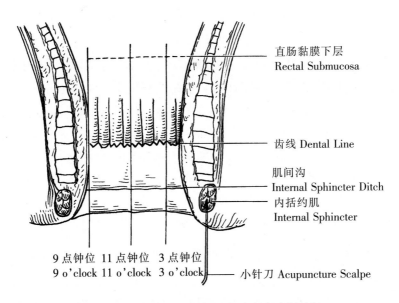

直肠黏膜下层
Rectal Submucosa

齿线 Dental Line

肌间沟
Internal Sphincter Ditch

内括约肌
Internal Sphincter

9点钟位 11点钟位 3点钟位
9 o'clock 11 o'clock 3 o'clock

小针刀 Acupuncture Scalpe

图 6 - 18 网式注射和小针刀闭合切断内括约肌

Figure 6 - 18 Net style injection and acupuncture scalpel cutting off internal sphincter

③三层注射法

③Three layer injection

第 1 层注射法：针头斜向痔基底部穿刺，总刺入深度 1～2cm，待有直肠肌性抵抗感后，稍退针约 0.1cm，以松解针头与组织的紧密接触，回抽无血后注药 1～2ml。

The first layer injection：To puncture obliquely towards the base of hemorrhoid to the depth of 1～2cm, meet the feeling of muscle resistance, then pull backward 0.1cm and aspirate no blood to be sure that syringe needle did not pierce into a blood vessel, then inject the drug 1～2ml.

第 2 层注射法：在第 1 层注射后针头退至黏膜下层，不取出针头，于黏膜下层刺入，可注药 1～2ml，使痔核胀大。

The second layer injection：After the first layer injection, to pull back the syringe needle to submucosa, continue puncturing from this layer, inject drug 1～2ml so as to enlarge the hemorrhoids.

第 3 层注射法，调整肛镜，使齿线上区的洞状血管区痔体暴露可以再调整针头，经近乎 85°斜角，再进针 0.5cm。注药 1ml，使痔核充盈（图 6－19）。

The third layer injection：To regulate the anoscope so as to expose hemorrhoids of hole style area of vessels above dental line, then regulate syringe to about 85° oblique angle correctly, then go into 0.5cm again, inject 1ml drug to enlarge the hemorrhoid (Fig. 6－19).

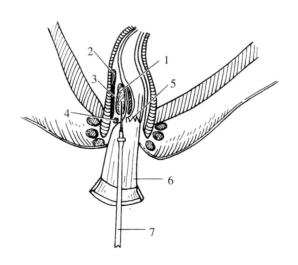

图 6－19　三层注射法

1－痔基底层；2－痔区黏膜层；3－痔区黏膜下层；4－洞状静脉区层；

5－齿线；6－圆头缺口肛门镜；7－消痔灵皮试针管

Figure 6－19　Three layer injection

1. Hemorrhoidal basic layer；2. Hemorrhoidal mucosal layer；3. Hemorrhoidal submucosal layer；

4. Veous area layer；5. Dental line；6. AnalscopX；7. Springe

注意正确选择早期内痔。对较大脱出的内痔,要辅助像皮圈套扎法,对伴有肛门瘘、肛门梳结者,不适单纯注射法。注药量及其部位的深浅要掌握好,黏膜固有层注药过多可引起坏死病灶,黏膜下层注药过多可致痔核早期坏死脱药;如注药量不足,可致痔核萎缩不愈合,注药量过于集中局部可形成硬结症;不慎将药注入尿道,可引起血尿、前列腺炎;不慎将药注入直肠壁范围过大,则可造成直肠狭窄。注意局部无菌消毒及术后给予甲硝唑和消炎药,否则易发生痔核病灶感染,甚至门静脉炎。

Pay attention to correctly choosing initial internal hemorrhoids. When meeting big protruding internal hemorrhoids, take the method of rubber band ligation as adjuvant therapy for the patient who take accompany with anal fistula and don't suit for injection. The doctor should control the dose and depth of the drug, and over dosages in mucosa can cause mucosal necrosis. If the drug is injected carelessly into the urinary tract, that may cause bloody urine or prostatitis; if the region of injected drug is too large, it can cause rectal stricture. Attention should be made to carrying on bacteria-free technology and taking metronidazole and antibiotics in postoperative period, or the infection will occur, even more portal phlebitis.

④小针刀配合治疗:在尾骨尖与肛门缘的中间,点状局麻,在左手食指伸入肛管导引,于右手持钩状小针刀自针眼插入将外括约肌皮下部分割断开。然后,拔出钩状小针刀,换斜面小针刀仍在左手食指导引下将内括约肌闭合性纵切1cm,以松解内括约肌层及外括约肌皮下,解除内括约肌痉挛,缓解直肠颈高压,使内痔的静脉血和淋巴液回流通畅(图6-18)。

④Acupuncture scalpel cooperated with treatment:In the middle between the tip of coccyx and the fringe of anus, the doctor takes local anesthesia. His left index finger enters the anal canal for introduction, and the right hand handles the hook style acupuncture scalpel to insert and cut subcutaneous muscle of external sphincter closely. Then the doctor takes the scalpel out, using incline scalpel instead, the same as inducing of left index finger going into the anal canal for introduction, cuts internal sphincter 1cm vertically and closely so as to relax the muscle of internal sphincter and subcutaneous muscle of external sphincter, to resolve the spasm of internal sphincter, to relieve the high pressure of rectal neck, to make the hemorrhoidal vein and lymph drainage free(Fig. 6 – 18).

(5)小针刀配合单纯结扎治疗内痔:适应证为内痔合并黏膜脱垂者。采用局麻或腰俞麻醉,取截石位,常规消毒。左手食指伸入肛内,摸清肌间沟,右手持小针刀选择距肛门左缘0.5cm处进针,深达外括约肌皮下部予以切断。在左手示指引导下,于肛管直肠左壁外继续潜行性插入小针刀,纵行切割部分内括约肌,以肛内左手示指有松解感为适度(图6-20)。将两叶肛门直肠镜插入肛管直肠腔,直视下在齿线上将内痔连同脱垂黏膜一同用弯角血管钳于基底部钳夹,用10-0粗丝线给予单纯结扎,再用7-0丝线重复结扎。同法依次结扎其余内痔及连同脱垂的黏膜。每个结扎点之间要留有 0.2 ~ 0.3cm 的黏膜桥,使结扎点不在同一水平,以防肛门狭窄(图 6 - 21)。

（5）Acupuncture scalpel cooperated with simple ligation treating internal hemorrhoids: The indication is that internal hemorrhoids take accompany with mucosal prolapse. With local anesthesia or lumbar anesthesia, lithotomy posture, sterilizing the skin as usual, the left index finger goes into the anus, touches clearly the ditch of internal sphincter, the right hand handles the acupuncture scalpel to insert from left anal fringe 0.5 cm till subcutaneous muscle of external sphincter and cuts it. The same as inducing of left index finger going into the anal canal, in the left side wall of anal canal, the right hand handles the acupuncture scalpel to insert and to cut vertically the part of internal sphincter until left index finger of staying inside anus feels relaxation (Fig. 6 - 20). The doctor inserts bifoliate anal speculum into anal canal and rectal cavity, and under direct vision, takes curved hemostatic forceps to hold the bases of internal hemorrhoid and falling mucosa above dental line, then ligates with 10 - 0 thick silk thread, 7 - 0 thread ligatures again. According to the same method to ligate the other base of internal hemorrhoid and falling mucosa. To reserve mucosa 0.2 ~ 0.3 cm between ligaturing points, and avoid the ligaturing points being on a horizontal plane so as to prevent stricture of the anus(Fig. 6 - 21).

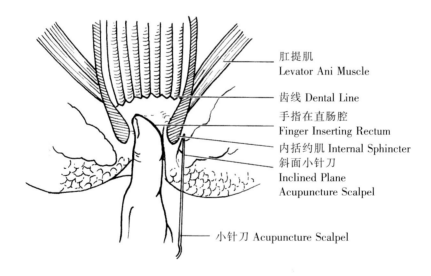

肛提肌
Levator Ani Muscle

齿线 Dental Line
手指在直肠腔
Finger Inserting Rectum
内括约肌 Internal Sphincter
斜面小针刀
Inclined Plane
Acupuncture Scalpel

小针刀 Acupuncture Scalpel

图 6 - 20　小针刀切断内括约肌

Figure 6 - 20　Acupuncture scalpel cutting internal sphincter

（6）负压吸力式弯头套扎枪治疗内痔

（6）Angle head loop ligaturing gun with vacuum suction treating internal hemorrhoids

①适应证:早期内痔、后期内痔或伴直肠黏膜内脱垂者。

①Indication: Initial, later internal hemorrhoids and rectal mucosal prolapses.

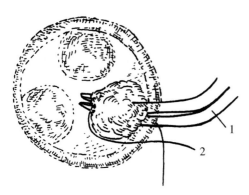
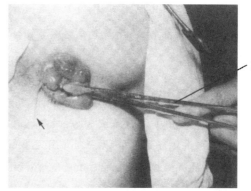

图 6 – 21　内痔单纯结扎

1 – 弯血管钳夹;2 – 丝线结扎

Figure 6 – 21　Simple ligation treating internal hemorrhoids

1. Curved hemostatic forceps hold the base;2. Silk thread ligatures below the forceps

②指肛检查:首先了解肛管腔内情况,尤其排除直肠癌。

②Digital rectal examination:First to understand the inside of the anal canal and how to exclude rectal cancer.

③将圆筒斜面缺口,带光源的肛门镜徐徐插入肛管中,不用麻醉其斜面口缺口,对准要套扎的内痔部位。例如跪位 3 点内痔,则斜口镜对其右侧肛管。拔出肛门镜芯(栓),在其内灯光照射下,观察确定是内痔,然后再用弯枪头口完全扣入其内痔基底部,即直肠黏膜基底层。勿只扣入一半,不完全扣入,易引起术后出血或复发。然后将弯枪的枪尾用 50ml 注射器,给予负压外吸,将内痔吸入弯枪口腔内,这时扣动扳机,通过其杠杆,将弯枪口外缘凹上预制的气门芯胶圈套入内痔基底部。在其被套扎后,其胶圈上的内痔,再注入 1ml 消痔灵致使痔核胀大。此后,产生套扎痔核枯死,5 ~ 7 天,枯死痔核组织自行随粪便脱掉。如不理想,一周后可以再重复套扎一次,此后再用上法分别套扎 9 点钟位,6 点钟位和 12 点钟位内痔。但套扎部位要超过齿线,以防术后疼痛。每次套扎 1 ~ 4 个为宜。最后肛门内挤入九华膏一类的药物,套扎后,次日再排大便,其饮食活动照常。

③The doctor inserts slowly the inclined opening optic anoscope into the anal canal, this technique does not require anesthesia, the inclined opening is aimed to define the internal hemorrhoid need to be ligated. For example, treating the internal hemorrhoid at 3 o'clock of knee-chest position, the doctor takes the inclined opening aimed to the right of anal canal, extracts the plug of the anoscope, in its light shining to observe to decide internal hemorrhoid or not, then takes the muzzle of the gun to loop completely the base of internal hemorrhoid:the base of rectal mucosa. Don't loop the half of hemorrhoid, if loop incompletely, it induces bleeding and relapse after having done this technique. The doctor takes the end of gun to connect 50 ml injector, the injector is taken negative pressure to breathe internal hemorrhoid into the bore of the gun, at the time touches trigger. According to lever principle, takes a little rubbcr circle which have been prepared on sunken outside of edge of muzzle loop the base of internal hemorrhoid (the little rubber circle is of minor diameter about 1~2mm that it's similar to a rubber valve inside of bicycle tyre), the rubber circle possesses high resilience and constriction. After the internal hemorrhoid is ligated, the doctor injects 1 ml XiaoZhi Ling (drug for treating hemorrhoids) to enlarge the hemorrhoid, then later the hemorrhoid necroses. Necrotic tissue sloughs following defecation in approximately 5~7 days. This technique should be done again in case it doesn't achieve the desired results in one week. According to the technique the internal hemorrhoids of 9, 6, 12 o'clock positions are separately ligated. The position of loop ligation is above dental line so as to be painless post-technique. The loop ligates 1~4 internal hemorrhoids each time, to squeeze a drug, such as JiuHuaGao(cream for treating hemorrhoids), etc., into the anus at the end of the technique.

④在圆头缺口电池灯带光源的肛门镜下,用弯头套扎枪,套扎早期内痔(图 6-22)。

④Angle head loop ligating gun with vacuum suction treating initial internal hemorrhoids by the inclined opening optic anoscope (Fig. 6-22).

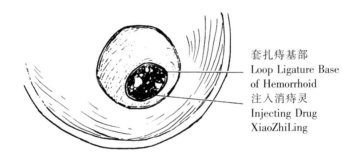

套扎痔基部
Loop Ligature Base
of Hemorrhoid
注入消痔灵
Injecting Drug
XiaoZhiLing

图 6-22　内痔套扎注入消痔灵

Figure 6-22　Treating internal hemorrhoids by loop ligation and drug injection

⑤后期内痔或伴直肠黏膜脱垂。

⑤The later internal hemorrhoids and rectal mucosal prolapse.

第 1 步,插入肛门镜,先用负压吸力式弯头套扎枪,先将痔核上方的直肠黏膜脱垂吸入枪口内套扎,并于胶圈的上方注入 1ml 消痔灵液致黏膜层隆起(图 6-23)。

The first step, the doctor inserts an anoscope, takes the muzzle to loop rectal mucosa above hemorrhoid, and breathes in it into the bore of the gun, and ligates it, and then injects 1ml Xiao ZhiLing above the rubber circle to enlarge the mucosa(Fig. 6-23).

附:Nivatvongs 介绍美国 Minnesta 大学附属医院用胶圈套扎疗法,不套扎痔体,而是借助 Hinkel-James 肛门镜在痔体上方只套扎正常直肠黏膜(图 6-24)。其优点是保存肛垫,阻止下垂;可间接治疗痔体。由于套扎地点在齿线以上,所以不痛。

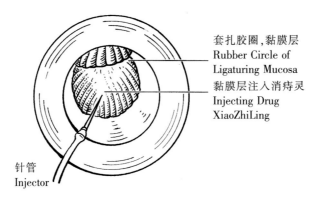

图 6 - 23　直肠黏膜层套扎

Figure 6 - 23　Loop ligation of rectal mucosal layer

Nivatvongs introduced that doctors took rubber loops to ligate the normal mucosa above hemorrhoids but not hemorrhoids by Hinkel-James' anoscopy in Affiliated Hospital of Minnesta University, US. The advantage of the technique is that it preserves anal cushions to prevent it from falling, so the technique can treat hemorrhoids indirectly. The patients don't feel pain after being treated by this therapy because the ligation is above the dental line(Fig. 6 - 24).

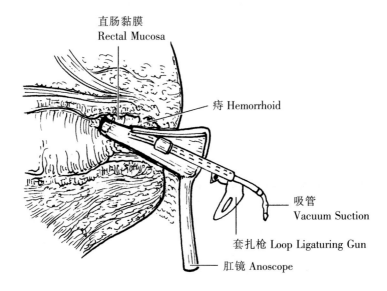

图 6 - 24　美国 Minnesta 大学附属医院胶圈套扎疗法

Figure 6 - 24　The technique of rubber loop circle ligation from
the Affiliated Hospital of Minnesta University US

第 2 步,在第 1 步的基础上,退出部分肛镜,再次用负压吸力式套扎枪将其痔核胶圈套扎,并于胶圈上方注入 1ml 消痔液致痔核隆起(图 6 - 25)。

The second step, basing on the first, to get back the anoscope partly, to take the gun of vacuum suction loop ligating to loop the hemorrhoid, and injects 1ml XiaoZhiLing above the rubber circle to enlarge the hemorrhoid(Fig. 6 - 25).

(7)非负压吸力式弯头套扎枪治疗内痔

(7) Angle head loop ligating gun treating internal hemorrhoids

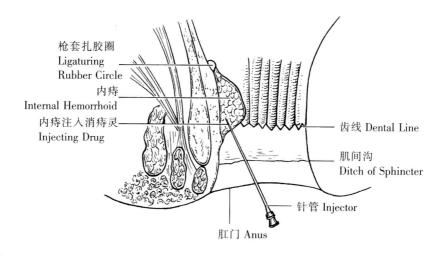

枪套扎胶圈
Ligaturing
Rubber Circle
内痔
Internal Hemorrhoid
内痔注入消痔灵
Injecting Drug

齿线 Dental Line

肌间沟
Ditch of Sphincter

针管 Injector

肛门 Anus

图 6 - 25　痔套扎

Figure 6 - 25　Loop ligaturing treating internal hemorrhoids

①适应证:内痔外脱肛门外者。

①Indication:The internal hemorrhoids prolapsing outside of anus.

②方法:将脱出肛门外的痔核,应用非负压吸引式套扎枪,于其痔核基底部套扎,并在胶圈套扎之上注入消痔灵液1ml,致痔核隆起。不必送回肛门内,仅外敷外痔贴中药膏即可(图 6 - 26)。

②Method:The hemorrhoids prolapse outside of anus. To take loop ligating gun of non negative pressure-vacuum to breathe in to loop the base of hemorrhoid and to inject 1ml XiaoZhiLing above rubber circle to enlarge the hemorrhoid(Fig. 6 - 26).

(8)小针刀配合弯头套扎枪治疗脱出痔

(8) The acupuncture scalpel cooperated with angle head loop ligating gun treating the prolapse of hemorrhoids

①适应证:脱出痔合并黏膜脱垂者。

①Indication:Prolapse of hemorrhoids with protruding mucosa.

②治疗方法:膀胱截石位,常规消毒局麻。

②Methods of treatment:　Lithotomy posture, sterilization regularly, local anesthesia.

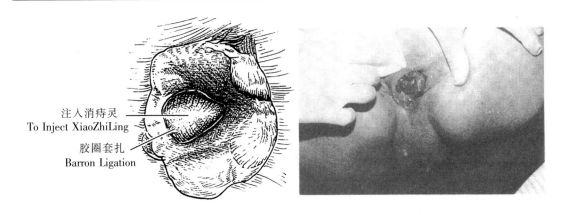

注入消痔灵
To Inject XiaoZhiLing

胶圈套扎
Barron Ligation

图6－26　内痔外脱套扎

Figure 6－26　Loop ligaturing treating internal hemorrhoids prolapsing outside of anus

第1步：小针刀将内括约肌闭合切断；左手食指伸入肛管(中)于肌肉沟上，按压固定内括约肌。然后右手持斜面小针刀于肛门(外部皮肤)3点处垂直插入到肛管内括约肌。在左手食指引导下将内括约肌纵行切断1~2cm，以松解内括约肌。拔出小针刀，针眼碘伏棉球固定即可(图6－27的3与4)。

Firstly：The acupuncture scalpel cuts the internal sphincter closely；left index finger goes into the anal canal (middle part) till the ditch of sphincters to control and fix the internal sphincter. The right hand handles the inclined plane acupuncture scalpel to insert into internal sphincter vertically from 3 o'clock position skin of outside of anus. In the introduction of left index finger to cut internal sphincter 1~2 cm vertically so as to relax muscle of internal sphincter. Then to take the scalpel out, with iodophor cotton ball pressing and sterilizing (3 and 4 from Fig. 6－27).

第2步：采用弯头负压吸入式套扎枪，先将其外脱肛外痔核(上吊)即在痔核基地部给予橡皮筋套扎，并(于套扎上部)注入1∶1的消痔灵液1ml，使其痔核于其橡皮筋前隆起(图6－27的8)。

Secondly：To take loop ligaturing gun of negative pressure-vacuum to breathe in to loop the base of hemorrhoid and to inject 1 ml 1∶1 XiaoZhiLing above the rubber circle to enlarge the hemorrhoid mass(8 from Fig. 6－27).

第3步：将其缺口电池灯肛门镜插入肛管(中)，在齿线上再用套扎枪将其相应的脱垂黏膜基底上与下部位2次套扎，上吊并于橡皮筋套扎前注入1∶1消痔灵注射。使其脱垂黏膜层隆起(图6－27的9与10)，然后肛管内注入九华膏即可。

Thirdly：The doctor inserts the incline opening optic anoscope into the anal canal (middle part), takes loop ligating gun to loop the base of mucosa of prolapse twice and to inject 1 ml 1∶1 XiaoZhi Ling above rubber circle to enlarge the mucosa(9 and 10 from Fig. 6－27), then squeezes JiuHua Gao cream into the anus at the end of the technique.

根据痔垫下移学说，将其内括约肌闭合切断，以降低直肠压力并利于痔静脉淋巴回流,使外脱痔回纳肛管内。将外脱痔核及其上部相对的松弛下垂、黏膜层纵行第 2 次分别进行套扎。起到上吊痔垫作用。注入消痔灵,使其被套扎后的痔核和黏膜均充胀隆起,其套扎橡皮筋更紧,产生药物化学,无菌纤维化,将脱垂痔垫上吊黏附直肠肌肉层。并起到防治感染和出血。

According to the anal cushions falling theory, to cut the internal sphincter closely to decrease the pressure of rectum, to help vein and lymph drainage back, so as to return external hemorrhoids to anal canal. To loop vertically relaxed falling mucosal layer above hemorrhoid twice separately, the purpose is raising anal cushions. To inject XiaoZhiLing to enlarge hemorrhoids and mucosa, the purpose is constricting rubber band tight, leaving an area of inflammation which results in fibrosis with asepsis and fixation with biologic, pharmacological and chemical changes so that the protruding mucosa raise and adhere muscular layer to prevent from infection and hemorrhage.

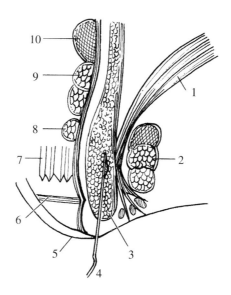

图 6 – 27　内痔上吊套扎

1 – 肛提肌;2 – 外括约肌;3 – 内括约肌;4 – 斜面小针刀;5 – 肛门;6 – 肌间沟;
7 – 齿线;8 – 套扎的内痔;9 – 下部脱垂黏膜层;10 – 上部脱垂黏膜层套扎

Figure 6 – 27　Loop ligature internal hemorrhoids

1. Levator ani muscle; 2. External sphincter; 3. Internal sphincter;
4. Inclined plane acupuncture scalpel;5. Anus; 6. Ditch of sphincter;
7. Dental line;8. Internal hemorrhoid of loop ligation;
9. Lower prolapsed mucosal layer; 10. Loop ligaturing upper prolapsed mucosal layer

（9）小针刀治疗嵌顿痔:嵌顿痔关键是以内括约肌痉挛为主,形成"狭窄环",痔核不能回纳肛门内,故采用小针刀闭合切断是治疗的重点。

（9）Acupuncture scalpel treating embedded hemorrhoids:The critical of embedded hemorrhoids is mainly spasm of internal sphincter to form "embedded circle", to prevent the hemorrhoid from getting back to inside of anus, so it is important for treatment to cut the internal sphincter by arranging acupuncture scalpel.

①麻醉,应用0.5%利多卡因8~10ml,于尾骨尖前与肛门水肿嵌顿的外缘之间给予皮肤、皮下外括约肌、内括约肌,均给予点状纵深局麻,勿污染针头。

①Anesthesia, local anesthesia:To inject 0.5% Lidocaine 8~10 ml, between anterior of coccyx tip and external edge of anus with embedded edema, into skin, external sphincter of subcutaneous muscle, internal sphincter. To take care of carrying on aseptic technique. All local anesthesia are carried on the points style local anesthesia and goes to the deep layer gradually. Don't contaminate needles.

②利用嵌顿痔暴露于肛门外的特点,要分清其解剖界线,要看准齿线和触摸内外括约肌的肌间沟,要清楚是"倒向",还是肛管呈外翻外脱状,这是治疗依据指标。

②To differentiate anatomic line, understand dental line, and feel the ditch between internal and external sphincter, that all are helpful to treat and are the aim of treatment. we must understand clearly that the anal canal model, such as it is prolapsed from the anus or others.

③首先将暴露嵌顿痔的内痔部位于齿线附近用套扎枪,先给予套扎治疗,不用负压吸,不用注药(图6-28)。

③Firstly, the doctor ligatures embedded internal hemorrhoid around dental line with loop ligating gun, but doesn't use vacuum suction, nor drug injection(Fig. 6-28).

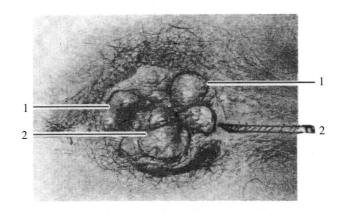

图6-28 嵌顿痔套扎与小针刀方法
1-痔套扎;2-小针刀:横行插入肛门外皮肤下层中。闭合切断外括约肌,
皮下部和内括约肌(手触及肌间沟为标记)

Figure 6-28 Loop ligation and acupuncture scalpel treating embedded hemorrhoids
1. Loop ligation; 2. To insert horizontally subcutaneous layer of outer anus to
cut closely subcutaneous muscle of external sphincter and internal sphincter
(hand touches the marker—the ditch between sphincters)

④再次应用斜面小针刀(于肛门外缘一侧的针眼插入),先将其外括约肌的皮

下部切断,肛外左手指触摸下,右手持小针刀再深入内外括约肌间沟下,将其内括约肌切割开。由于在肛门外,操作解剖界线清楚。小针刀切割线在直视下进行,故要注意防治污染,小针刀勿刺切肛管。因为内括约肌与外括约肌的皮下部被切断,立即解除了绞窄环,嵌顿痔即可回纳。治疗后将嵌顿痔回入肛管中,不要用手"送回"套扎痔,否则会脱掉。肛内注入九华膏、肛门敷消炎膏,2~3天方排便,以巩固疗效。

④Secondly, the doctor inserts inclined plane acupuncture scalpel again (from the injected point of one side of outer anal edge) to cut subcutaneous muscle of external sphincter, then along with feeling of his left hand, his right hand handles the acupuncture scalpel to insert deeply arriving at below the ditch between internal and external sphincter and cuts the internal sphincter. Because of carried on outside of anus, the anatomy is clear so that cutting courses of acupuncture scalpel cutting are seen. To take care which can't be punctured cut anal canal. Internal sphincter and subcutaneous muscle of external kphinct6i are cut, so that the narrower circle is resolved immediately no sooner than embedded hemorrhoid returns back.

4. 混合痔 采用内套外扎疗法(图6-29)。

4. Mixed Hemorrhoids carrying on interior loop and exterior ligation (Fig. 6-29).

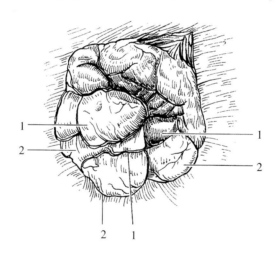

图6-29 混合痔内套外扎
1-内痔套扎;2-外痔结扎
Figure 6-29 interior loop and external ligation to treat mixed hemorrhoids
1. Loop ligation treating internal hemorrhoids;2. Thread ligation treating external hemorrhoids

(1)先用弯头负压吸力式套扎枪胶圈套扎内痔,并于胶圈上注射消痔灵液1ml,致痔核隆起。

(1)Firstly, to take rubber loop ligaturing gun of negative pressure-vacuum to breathe into loop internal hemorrhoid and to inject 1 ml XiaoZhi Ling above rubber circle to enlarge the hemorrhoid.

(2)再用粗丝线单纯结扎外痔,并于结扎丝线之上注射亚甲蓝止痛药1ml,致外痔隆起。

（2）secondly, to ligate external hemorrhoids simply with thick silk thread and to inject 1 ml methylene blue above ligating thread to enlarge the hemorrhoid for relieving pain.

（3）肛门内,挤入九华膏,肛门外敷外痔贴。

（3）Squeeze the cream of Jiuhuagao into the anus, and put the external hemorrhoid patch on the outside of the anus.

第二节　痔的伴发病症
§2　Complications of Hemorrhoids

一、痔的三联征
Ⅰ. Triad of Hemorrhoids

痔疮合并前列腺增生、阳痿称痔疮三联征。多发生于成年男性。

The triad includes hemorrhoids, hypertrophy of the prostate and impotence, often seen in adult male.

【病因病机】

【Etiology and Pathology】

肛门、肛管与泌尿生殖器官相邻,构成肛门会阴三角区。肛门直肠静脉和膀胱、前列腺和阴茎背部静脉均一同回流入髂内静脉,痔患者静脉血回流缓慢则引起肛门痔、前列腺静脉和阴茎静脉共同瘀血,血管扩张。前列腺增生压迫直肠和尿道可引起排便和排尿困难,甚至阴茎勃起障碍。

The anus and anal canal are near to urogenital organs forming the perineal triangle including anal and urogenital triangle. The veins coming from the anus, rectum, bladder, prostate and back of penis all drain into internal iliac vein. The hemorrhoidal venous drainage is slow which causes venous blood stasis and vessel spreading of anus, prostate and penis. The hypertrophy of prostate would press on the urethra and neighbor organs to cause difficult urination or defecation, even disturbance of erection.

【临床表现】

［Clinical Manifestations］

肛门会阴下坠、内痔外脱、便血伴排尿困难、滴尿、性欲减退、阴茎勃起不坚或阳痿。

The feeling of anus and even perineum falling, internal hemorrhoids protruding through the anus outside the body, defecation bleeding, urine obstruction and dripping, sexual desire decreasing, erection hindering or impotence.

【诊断】

［Diagnosis］

根据病史,有痔疮、前列腺增生和阳痿。肛指检查前列腺增生、肥大;肛门镜检查有痔疮,且阴茎勃起障碍,即可明确诊断。

According to the patient's history, who suffers from hemorrhoids, hypertrophy of prostate and impotence, it can be discovered by digital examination, hemorrhoids by anoscopy, and also disturbance of erection, so that the diagnosis is obvious.

【治疗】

［Treatment］

1.**痔治疗**　采用弯头负压吸力式套扎枪,进行内痔套扎和注射套扎的痔核治疗(见本章第一节)。

1. **Treating Hemorrhoids**　Taking rubber loop ligaturing gun of negative pressure-vacuum to breathe into loop internal hemorrhoid and to inject above rubber circle to enlarge the hemorrhoid(Refer to the first section of this chapter).

2.**肛管直肠腔减压治疗**　采用斜面小针刀针眼闭合性切断内括约肌和外括约肌皮下部治疗(见本章第一节)。

2. **Reducing Pressure of Anus and Rectum**　Taking inclined plane acupuncture scalpel to cut subcutaneous muscles of external sphincter and internal sphincter from the injected point(Refer to the first section of this chapter).

3.**前列腺增生和阳痿治疗**

3. **Treating Hypertrophy of Prostate and Impotence**

(1)采用针灸或埋羊肠线配合穴位:关元、气海、中极、命门、三阴交、足三里。

(1)Taking acupuncture points:GuanYuan, QiHai, ZhongJi, MingMen, SanYinJiao, ZuSanLi.

(2)口服中药,如健脾补肾汤。

(2)Taking herbs such as Decoction of strengthening spleen and invigorating kidney, etc.

二、痔伴便频症

Ⅱ. Hemorrhoids with Frequent Defecation

患痔疮后引起便频症,无脓血便、无腹痛,只是每日排粪便次数增加。

The hemorrhoids induce frequent defecation without pus, blood and abdominal pain, only the times of defecation increase every day.

【病因】

[Etiology]

因患痔致肛垫充血、肿胀、表面张力增大,粪便感觉器敏感,即使小量粪便刺激也会引起强烈的急迫排便,且频次多甚至排便功能紊乱。多发生在患痔初期。

Because of the hemorrhoids, the anal cushions being hyperaemia, oedema, and increasing surface tension, stimulate sensory organ of defecation that even if a little stools should cause emergency defecation so that the frequency of defecation increases, even with disordered function of defecation. All these often take place in initial stage of hemorrhoids.

【临床表现】

[Clinical Manifestations]

患痔后排大便次数增多,但不伴腹痛无脓血便。①大便常规化验无异常;②肛镜或纤维结肠镜检查见痔疮、充血水肿,无结、直肠炎表现。

The hemorrhoids induce frequent defecation without pus, blood and abdominal pain. ①The routine stool test is normal; ② The anoscopy and fibercoloscopy can discover hemorrhoids, hyperaemia, but no appearances of colitis or rectitis.

【治疗】

[Treatment]

(1)口服中药,如升举汤。

(1)Taking herbs such as Decoction of ShenJu Tang, etc.

(2)选择痔疮注射、套扎、结扎法等疗法(见本章第一节)。

(2)Treating hemorrhoids with injection, loop ligation, etc(Refer to the first section of this chapter).

三、痔伴便秘症

Ⅲ. Hemorrhoids with Constipation

患痔后引起便秘症,但没有排便困难,只是每3~4天才排便1次,粪便干燥。

The hemorrhoids induce constipation without difficult defecation, the defecation is only once every 3~4 days and of dry quality.

【病因】

[Etiology]

因患痔后期往往发生便秘,肛垫下移,直肠黏膜松弛下垂,肛管内括约肌痉挛或肥厚,引起便秘。粪便留置直肠过久,致干燥。

The hemorrhoids may result from straining to move stool, the later stage of the hemorrhoids may induce constipation, the cushions move downwards, the rectal mucosa relaxes, the sphincter of anal canal is spasm and swollen, all cause that stools stay in the rectum long time so as to form dry stools. That's called outlet obstructing constipation.

【临床表现】

[Clinical Manifestations]

患痔后期排便次数减少,每 3 ~ 4 天才排粪便 1 次,不伴排便困难。大便常规化验无异常;肛镜或纤维结肠镜检查见肛垫下移、直肠黏膜下垂,无直肠炎与狭窄;肛门指检诊断肛门内括约肌痉挛或肥厚。

The later stage of the hemorrhoids may occur times decreasing of defecation, only once every 3 ~ 4 days without difficult defecation. The routine stool rest is normal. The anoscopy and fibercoloscopy can discover that the cushions move downwards, the rectal mucosa falls, but not rectitis and narrow part; the anal digital examination shows spasm or plumping of internal anal sphincter.

【治疗】

[Treatment]

(1)口服中药,如润肠汤。

(1)Taking herbs such as Decoction of Run Chang Tang (lubricating alimentary tract).

(2)小针刀配合弯头套扎枪进行痔垫上吊法治疗(见本章第一节)。

(2)Acupuncture scalpel accompanying with angle head loop ligaturing gun to hold up cushions(Refer to the first section of this chapter).

四、痔伴贫血症
Ⅳ. Hemorrhoids Complicated with Anemia

患痔后,引起贫血症,是长期排粪便时带血或出血引起。

The most common symptom of hemorrhoids is bright red blood covering the stool or bleeding as defecation. If the symptoms last long time, then anemia will be formed.

【病因】
[Etiology]

因患痔后肛垫在长期排粪便冲击下,血管内压升高,且渐渐肿胀、充血、隆起,排粪便时,又受括约肌收缩作用,产生门槛效应,致 Treitz 肌断裂,肛垫下移,黏膜和血管破裂出血。

The cushions are stained to move stool long time, the internal vascular pressure increasing refers to a condition in which the veins are swollen leading to hyperemia, oedema, so the mucosa and their vessels break up easily to bleed as defecation.

【临床表现】
[Clinical Manifestations]

患痔后排粪便带鲜血或血凝块,甚至出血,伴全身无力,面色苍白。血常规检查见红细胞和血红蛋白明显下降;粪便隐血试验阳性;肛门镜检查见肛垫充血隆起、瘀斑;指肛、B 超、血液检查等无异常。

The symptom of hemorrhoids is bright red blood covering the stool or clot with or bleeding as defecation, if the symptom lasts long time that the patient will be weak and pale. Routine blood test shows that Hb and RBC fall obviously; Anoscopy can discover the cushions moving downwards, hyperemia, oedema; Anal digital examination, B-mode ultrasonography, and blood tests show nothing abnormal.

【治疗】
[Treatment]

（1）口服中药,如痔疮止血汤。

（1）Taking herbs such as Decoction of ZhiChuang ZhiXue Tang (hemostasis).

（2）早期治疗痔,如采用注射、套扎,或结扎法（见本章第一节）。

（2）Treating hemorrhoids with injection, loop ligation, etc (Refer to the first section of this chapter).

【点评】
[Review]

1. **钩状小针刀治疗外痔**　通过针眼,将外痔内的血栓或静脉团等钩碎而治愈。外痔是皮赘,不且切除。否则造成肛门缘缺损的溢液,瘙痒。

1. **The Hook Style Acupuncture Scalpel Treating the External Hemorrhoids**　The doctor hooks to break up the blood clot and venous bolus in the external hemorrhoids from acupuncture point.

2. 小针刀闭合性切断内外括约肌　通过左示指插入肛管内,触定肌间沟,其上为内约肌其下为外括约肌的皮下部。右手持小针刀从肛门外的针眼插入,在左示指示导下相隔肛管壁,插入内括约肌,纵行切断1cm,再切断外括约肌皮下部。以左指触及括约肌松解或凹窝为准,治疗括约肌痉挛。不宜开放切开或切除部分括约肌。否则,造成肛门缺损条沟致肛门溢液或漏气。

2. The Acupuncture Scalpel Close Cutting the Internal Sphincter　For treating spasm of sphincter along with feeling the ditch of sphincter of doctor's left index finger inserting anal canal, above the ditch is internal sphincter, below is subcutaneous muscle of external sphincter, and in the guidance of his left index finger. From acupuncture point of outside of anus his right hand handles the acupuncture scalpel to insert into internal sphincter near by the well of anal canal, and to cut vertically internal sphincter 1cm, then to cut subcutaneous muscle of external sphincter. The aim is that the left finger feels relaxation of sphincter or sunken socket.

3. 弯枪头套扎注射　将缺口电池灯肛门镜插入肛门,其脱垂黏膜和内痔则因肛门镜的缺口,而突入肛门腔,用弯枪头使气门芯可套扎于黏膜或痔核的基底。于套扎气门芯之上再注入消痔灵液于黏膜或痔核中,则会隆起胀大,致气门芯套扎更紧故干燥枯掉。不会感染,或出血。

3. Angle Head Gun Loop Ligaturing and Injection　The doctor inserts the inclined opening optical anoscope into the anus that the prolapsed mucosa and internal hemorrhoids fall into the cavity of the anoscope while the doctor makes rubber circle of angle head gun loop ligature the base of mucosa and hemorrhoids, then injects XiaoZhi Ling above ligaturing thread to enlarge them, so that the rubber circle gets strict more to do them dry up and necrosis. Don't worry about infection and bleeding because they won't occur.

第三节　肛门直肠周围脓肿
§3　Perianal and Perirectal Suppuration

中医学最早把肛门周围脓肿称为"脏毒",近代改称"肛门痈"。肛门直肠周围脓肿常见病菌为葡萄球菌、链球菌、大肠埃希菌、铜绿假单胞菌和结核杆菌等。

In the ancient days the perianal suppuration was called "dirty toxin" by traditional Chinese medicine, and in the modern time it is called anal carbuncle. The common bacteria around anus and rectum are *Staphylococcus*, *Streptococcus*, *E. coli*, *Pseudomonas aeruginosa* and *Tubercle bacillus*, etc.

按肛门直肠脓肿所在部位,可分为肛提肌上脓肿和肛提肌下脓肿。前者包括黏膜下脓肿、骨盆直肠脓肿及直肠后部脓肿;后者包括皮下脓肿及坐骨直肠窝脓肿(图6-30)。

According to the position of perianal and perirectal abscesses, they are divided into above and below of levator ani muscle abcesses, the former includes submucosal, pelvirectal, and back of rectum abscesses, while the latter includes subcutaneous and ischiorectal fossa abscesses(Fig. 6 – 30).

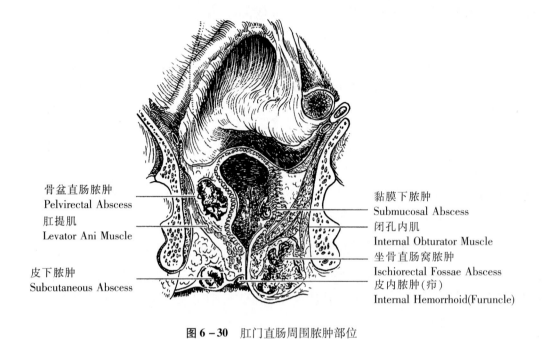

骨盆直肠脓肿
Pelvirectal Abscess
肛提肌
Levator Ani Muscle

皮下脓肿
Subcutaneous Abscess

黏膜下脓肿
Submucosal Abscess
闭孔内肌
Internal Obturator Muscle
坐骨直肠窝脓肿
Ischiorectal Fossae Abscess
皮内脓肿(疖)
Internal Hemorrhoid(Furuncle)

图 6 – 30 肛门直肠周围脓肿部位

Figure 6 – 30 Perianal and perirectal abscesses

一、皮下脓肿

I. Subcutaneous Abscess

多在肛门两侧。

The subcutaneous abscess is mainly at both sides of anus.

【临床表现】

[Clinical Manifestations]

病人先觉肛门部有跳痛,压迫时则加重,大便或行路时更甚。后在肛门周围皮下出现红肿硬块,有压痛,伴有畏寒、发热、周身不适及排尿困难等。

The throbbing pain in the perianal region is acute and aggravated by sitting, coughing, sneezing, and straining. Swelling, induration, and tenderness define the area of involvement, often with a palpable inflammatory process, and commonly with shiver, high fever, systemic uncomfortable, even difficult urination.

【诊断】

［Diagnosis］

如发现有上述全身及局部症状，即可确诊。

If those local and systemic symptom was found, the diagnosis is obvious.

【病情演变】

［Change of Disease］

此类脓肿如不早期切开，有时可引起严重的全身反应。在局部常有以下三种结局：①脓液由肛窦或肛裂流出而成内瘘；②脓液由皮肤穿出而成完全瘘；③脓液由皮下蔓延到两侧坐骨直肠窝而成蹄铁形瘘。

The abscess can change into fistula in the intersphincteric space of the anal canal, and complicated fistulas, horseshoe fistulas, etc.

【治疗】

［Treatment］

脓肿初起：应以清热解毒为主，可给予消肿止痛汤或仙方活命饮，或给予抗菌药物；另外可服缓泻药使大便稀软。局部用中药祛毒汤熏洗及热敷，并涂敷外痔贴如已化脓，宜早期用手术切开。

Initial abscess：Treatment mainly relies on clearing heat and detoxication, by taking the decoction of apocatastasis and relieving pain, or decoction of XianFangHuoMingYin, or taking antibacterial drugs, in addition to taking mild purgative medicine for making stool soft and purging free, tub baths in plain, warm water or decoction for fume and steep, application of a cream or suppository to the affected area; as festering to take incision in time.

1. 刮匙小针刀洞口单纯挂线引流　取侧卧位，常规消毒，脓肿壁点状局麻。选择肛门缘的脓肿最低位，右手持刮匙小针刀，朝向脓肿对端。先垂直刺入最低位的脓肿壁，同时旋转 1 周即完全洞式切口，边进刮匙小针刀边旋转，穿切至脓肿对端壁穿出，完成第 2 个对端脓肿壁的洞式切口。至此贯通脓腔的中心，将粗丝线挂在刮匙小针刀的刀柄前缘，原路退回并拔出刮匙小针刀，其粗丝线留挂在脓腔中，将粗丝线的两头分别由 2 个洞口牵出脓腔外再打结，形成弧形线圈，起到对口引流作用。术后敷消脓膏纱布块。待术后 1 周，脓液消失剪断引流线圈后拔去（图 6 - 31）。由于没治疗内口，故需再次行肛瘘手术。

1. Simple Hole Style Drainage by a Craping Ladle Acupuncture Scalpel and Seton　Lateral posture, sterilizing as usual, local anesthesia, choosing the lowest position of abscess, the doctor's right hand handles the curette acupuncture scalpel to insert vertically into the abscess wall from the lowest position, and spins acupuncture scalpel around so as to form hole style incision.

The doctor takes the curette acupuncture scalpel going at the same time spinning and cutting till another wall, and goes through abscess out of the wall so that these courses form 2 holes style incision on the wall of abscess. To hold up thick silk thread on the anterior of curette acupuncture scalpel, to return along the same way penetrating the abscess cavity, to put two ends of thick silk thread out of the cavity from the two holes then to tie a knot respectively, to form arc circle and to take part in open to open drainage. To apply gauze after the arrangement(Fig. 6 – 31).

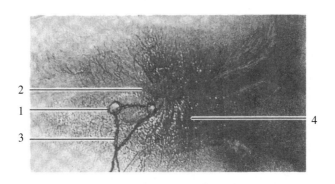

图 6 – 31　刮匙小针刀洞口挂线引流

1 – 肛门外对口挂线;2 – 肛门;3 – 丝线;4 – 阴囊肛门脓肿

Figure 6 – 31　Simple hole style drainage by a craping ladle acupuncture scalpel and seton

1. Open to open seton drainage outside of anus;2. Anus;

3. Silk thread;4. Periscrotal and perianal abscess

2. 钩刮小针刀疗法　取截石位将骶尾部托起。在局麻或骶管阻滞麻醉下,采用圆头缺口电池灯肛门镜插入肛管直肠病变一侧(图 6 – 32)。

2. Treated by the Hook and Scrape Acupuncture Scalpel　Lithotomy posture and holding up sacroiliac part, local anesthesia or sacral block anesthesia, inserting the incline opening optical anoscope into the anus. (Fig. 6 – 32).

(1)黏膜下脓肿隆起不明显,则应用钩状小针刀从脓肿上缘纵行钩割,致脓肿下缘,术毕。

(1)As submucosal abscess with indistinct projection, to hook and cut the abscess vertically from upper to bottom by carrying on hook style acupuncture scalpel.

(2)黏膜下脓肿隆起明显,则再应用刮匙小针刀,从其脓肿下缘插入脓肿腔中,并旋转一圈,拔出。脓液外溢,术毕。

(2)As submucosal abscess with distinct projection, to insert into the abscess from bottom, and to spin around by carrying on curette acupuncture scalpel, and then to take it out, the outflow of pus can be seen.

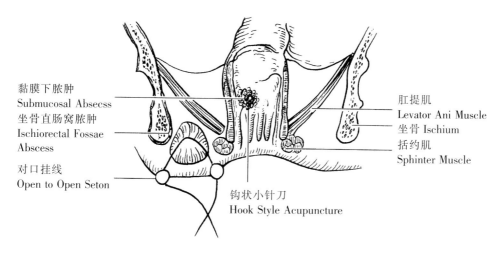

黏膜下脓肿
Submucosal Absecss
坐骨直肠窝脓肿
Ischiorectal Fossae
Abscess
对口挂线
Open to Open Seton

肛提肌
Levator Ani Muscle
坐骨 Ischium
括约肌
Sphinter Muscle

钩状小针刀
Hook Style Acupuncture

图 6 - 32　肛周脓肿的治疗

Figure 6 - 32　Treating perianal and perirectal abscesses

（3）肛门挤入九华膏。

（3）Squeezing cream of herbs.

3. 探针小弯刀一期切开挂双线治疗坐骨直肠窝脓肿　取截石位,在局麻或骶裂孔阻滞麻醉下。

3. Incision and Two Setons Drainage Treating Ischiorectal Fossa Abscess by Small Curving Probing Scalpel One Time.　Lithotomy posture, local anesthesia or sacral hiatus block anesthesia.

第 1 步,在肛门脓肿时,距肛门缘近端做第 1 个洞式切口(图 6 - 32),然后再一手示指伸入肛管,一手持探针、小弯刀从洞口探入,通过脓腔走向寻找内口。探针从内口引出,折弯拉出肛门外。再顺探针走行,其后段弯刀口切开皮肤至齿线。然后将其消毒的带橡皮筋的丝线一端系在探针球头处,拉出探针,使橡皮筋的一端由内口拉出,勒紧橡皮筋回送 3cm 后再用丝线将橡皮筋结扎固定。肛门直肠环括约肌的挂线周围同时应用亚甲蓝 1ml 和 1% 普鲁卡因 5ml 浸润注射,起长效止痛作用(图 6 - 33)。

The first step, to take a hole style incision in the near end from the fringe of anus (Fig. 6 - 32), the index finger inserted into the anal canal, the other hand handles small anus curving probing scalpel to insert from the hole, probing the track through the cavity of abscess to look for internal opening. The anterior probe is drained from internal opening, curved and put out anus. Along the track, posterior curving scalpel cuts the skin till dentate line, then ties the end of thread, of sterilized owning rubber band, with the top ball end of probe, puts the probe to make the end of rubber band draw out internal opening, hauls the rubber band tight to return 3cm, ties the silk thread to fix rubber band. A seton of anorectal ring is placed around the sphincter muscle as a marker(Fig. 6 - 33).

第2步:距肛门缘远端的脓肿,做第2个洞式切口,并探入第1个洞式切口再用第2根丝线将两个洞口贯穿成线圈,引流外部脓腔脓液,外敷消脓膏(图6-33)。

The second step, the abscess of distance from the anal fringe, to take the second hole style incision to probe the first, and to use the second silk thread through the two holes to tie a thread ring, to drain the pus from external abscess (Fig. 6-33).

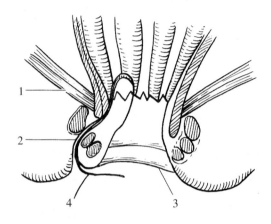

图6-33　肛管直肠环挂线

1-肛提肌;2-直肠环挂线;3-肛门;4-挂线

Figure 6-33　Use of seton in rectal ring

1. Levator ani muscle; 2. Seton in rectal ring; 3. Anus; 4. Seton

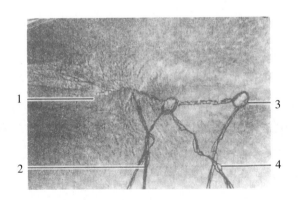

图6-34　肛门外脓肿洞口挂线

1-肛门;2-肛门内挂线;3-第2个洞口;4-第2根线

Figure 6-34　Hole style seton

1. Anus; 2. Use of seton in anus; 3. The second hole; 4. The second thread

长期以来,治疗肛周脓肿多采用脓肿切开引流,待脓腔缩小形成肛瘘后,再行第2次手术。这不但给病人增加痛苦,还使疗程延长。我们采用切开挂双线术结合中药坐浴,既可治疗肛周脓肿,又预防了肛瘘。实践证明,此法痛苦小,疗程短,可一次根治,易为患者接受。

For a long time, the common treatment of perianal and perirectal suppuration is incision and drainage. Sometimes the patient needs to suffer second operation to cure the fistula which not only increases pain but also prolongs treating course. Now we make incision and two setons integrated tub bath of warm decoction, the method not only treats perianal abscesses but also prevents from fistulae.

4. 探针小弯刀一期对口引流治疗骨盆直肠窝脓肿　采用腰俞麻醉,常规消毒皮肤,尾骨尖前肛旁在脓肿波动最明显处尽力选择近肛门缘做洞式切口,脓液流出后;右手持即将探针小弯刀前段的探针插入脓肿腔中直肠环上寻找其内口。此时左手食指伸人肛管中,与其探针自然无阻力,相触即为内口。然后将其探针,要顺其折弯而拉出肛管外,将其齿线以下脓肿壁利用探针后段小弯刀切割开。而超过括约肌直肠环部的内口给予挂橡皮筋回退 3cm 再结扎紧。其两侧的脓肿,再单纯给予挂橡皮筋,只是对口引流;但挂其橡皮筋勿结扎紧,只是起引流作用。因其主瘘脓肿来自同一个内口,当第 1 个挂紧的橡皮筋脱掉后,其分支第 2 个和第 3 个引流橡皮筋才再依次分别剪断加压法,消脓膏纱布条引流外敷(图 6 - 35)。

4. **An Open to Open Drainage Treating Ischiorectal Fossa Abscess by Small Curving Probing Scalpel Once**　Lumbar anesthesia, sterilizing the skin as usual, the hole incision and drainage in the evident fluctuation near the fringe of anus in the front of tip of coccyx; after the pus draining out. The right hand handles the front probe of the curette acupuncture scalpel to insert into the cavity of abscess and to look for internal opening in the anorectal ring, for the guidance the left index finger inserts anal canal to touch probe under nature without obstruction, it's an internal opening, then folds curving the probe, and puts the probe out the anus along the track and the curving of probe, cuts the wall of abscess below the dentate line behind the probe. If the fistula is high in relation to the rectal sphincter ring, a rubber band is placed loosely 3cm around the sphincter muscle at the two sides of abscess which is simply placed loosely for open to open drainage(Fig. 6 - 35).

二、坐骨直肠窝脓肿

Ⅱ. Ischiorectal Fossa Abscess

这类脓肿发生在坐骨直肠窝内,较皮下脓肿大且深,是一种常见的肛门直肠脓肿。

The kind of abscess takes place in the ischiorectal fossae, and is a common perianorectal abscess, which is deeper and bigger than the subcutaneous abscess.

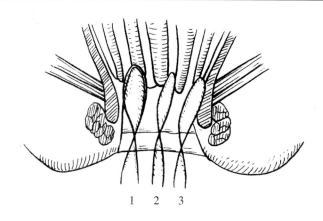

图 6 - 35　骨盆直肠窝脓肿 3 根线挂线疗法

Figure 6 - 35　Three setons treating ischiorectal fossae abscess

【临床表现】

[Clinical Manifestations]

先觉肛门部不适或微痛,并可出现头痛、寒战、发热、脉搏加速、食欲缺乏等;渐渐局部疼痛加重,肛门内觉灼痛或刺跳痛,大便时疼痛加剧,坐卧不安,排尿困难,常有尿闭发生。肛门旁皮肤肿胀、变硬、色红紫,感觉敏锐,有压痛,如脓浅时触之有波动感。

In the initial stage, the ischiorectal fossa abscess causes an infrequent aching pain in the rectum rather than in the perianal region, but excessive tenderness frequently precludes adequate examination, gradually the throbbing pain in the perianal region occurs with headache, shiver, fever, rapid pulse, jaded appetite, etc. more pain as defecation, being unable to sit down or sleep at ease, even difficult urination or aurinia. Swelling, induratrion, mass and tenderness define the perianal area. There is fluctuation as the abscess is severe.

【诊断】

[Diagnosis]

依照前述之症状,检查如肛门旁皮肤有红肿变硬,指检时可摸到肛管内一侧或两侧肿起,压之疼痛或有波动,即可诊断为坐骨直肠窝脓肿。

With manifestations mentioned above and examination shown, there are swelling and induration of the perianal skin, excessive tenderness frequently precludes digital examination in a side of anal canal or two sides, then diagnosis of ischiorectal fossa abscess can be made.

【鉴别诊断】

[Differention Diagnosis]

1. 黏膜下脓肿　其特征是生在直肠黏膜下,外部无病变,指检时在直肠壁上可摸到圆形隆起,触之疼痛或有波动感,黏膜表面常有脓苔。

1. **Submucosal Abscess**　It is below rectal mucosa, no swelling nor induration of the perianal skin. Digital rectal examination may reveal tenderness, feeling a bump and fluctuation, and pus on the surface.

2. **直肠后部脓肿**　其特征是肛门外无特殊变化,指检可在直肠后部摸到肿物且有波动感,按压肛门及尾骨中间时有痛感。

2. **Posterior anal Abscess**　There is no change around perianal region. Digital rectal examination may reveal tenderness between the anus and coccyx, feeling a bump and fluctuation.

3. **骨盆直肠间隙脓肿**　其特征是脓肿生在直肠上部肠壁之外,骨盆腔内的两侧。指诊时按压之有压痛及波动感。如在初期很难与坐骨直肠脓肿鉴别。

3. **Pelvirectal Space Abscess**　The abscess is at the outside of superior rectum, and two sides of pelvis. Digital rectal examination may reveal tenderness and fluctuation. It is difficult to diagnose differentially with ischiorectal fossa abscess in the initial stage.

【病情演变】

[Developmental Changes of Disease]

如不早期切开引流,除出现严重的全身性反应外,脓液常由内、外括约肌之间穿入肛内,或由肛门部皮肤穿出体外,形成高位坐骨直肠瘘;或经过肛门后部围绕括约肌蔓延,而传到对侧坐骨直肠窝内,形成蹄铁形复杂瘘;或骨盆直肠窝脓肿向上经肛提肌而穿入盆腔,造成盆腔内脓肿,这种脓肿往往形成复杂性肛瘘。

Besides severe systemic reactions, if there is no incision and drainage the pus goes into anus through the intersphincteric muscles, or going out anal skin to form high position fistula from ischiorectal fossae and pelvirectal space; or spreading to another side of ischiorectal fossae through by posterior midline anal gland around sphincteric muscle to form a horseshoe complicated fistula; or going upwards into pelvis through levator anal muscle to form pelvic cavity's abscess and to cause commonly complicated fistula.

【治疗】

[Treatment]

详见"皮下脓肿治疗"。

Refer to "the treatment of the subcutaneous abscess".

三、骨盆直肠窝脓肿
Ⅲ. Pelvirectal Fossa Abscess

【临床表现】

[Clinical Manifestations]

病人深部肛门胀痛,伴畏寒高热。

In deep part of anus, there is distending pain with shiver and high fever.

【诊断】

[Diagnosis]

如发现有上述表现,指检在直肠上部肠壁之外的骨盆腔间隙窝按压,压痛或波动感即可诊断。或肛门B超或穿刺。

According to manifestations mentioned above, the digital rectal examination may reveal tenderness and fluctuation, the pain is at outside of superior rectum, and space fossae of both sides of pelvis. B ultrasonic examination or puncture aspiration are helpful for the diagnosis.

【病情演变】

[Changes of Disease]

见前述。

Following as above manifestations.

【治疗】

[Treatment]

详见"皮下脓肿"治疗(在直肠盆脓肿治疗节中)。

Refer to the treatment of the subcutaneous abscess.

四、结核性脓肿
Ⅳ. Tuberculosis Abscess

原发性结核性肛门直肠周围脓肿甚少,多继发于身体其他部位的结核性病灶,而在肛门部形成脓肿。

The primary tuberculosis perianal and perirectal abscesses are seldom, secondary to perianal and perirectal abscesses from tuberculosis lesions in other parts of body.

【临床表现】

[Clinical Manifestations]

结核性肛门周围脓肿之症状,与非结核性脓肿相似。不过结核性脓肿发病缓慢,疼痛轻微或不觉疼痛;自溃或被切开后形成瘘管。另外,一般可能有身体瘦弱、食欲缺乏,午后轻度发热、盗汗,或有咳嗽、咯血等症状。

The symptoms of tuberculosis perianal and perirectal abscesses are similar to those of abscesses. The tuberculosis abscess takes place slowly and causes an infrequent aching pain in the rectum; breaking up by self and drainage by incision forming fistula easily. In addition, systemic symptoms appear, such as weak, jaded appetite, mild fever in the afternoon, night sweat, cough and hemoptysis, etc.

【诊断】

[Diagnosis]

结核性肛门周围脓肿初起缓慢,在无混合感染的情况下,不会发生急性炎症现象。肛门旁虽有肿物,压之有波动感,但无明显压痛。用空针穿刺可抽出稀薄似米泔汁样的脓液,带有微臭。

The initial tuberculosis perianal abscesses takes place slowly, acute inflammation rarely occurs without mixed infection. The abscess causes an infrequent aching pain in the anal region although a mass with fluctuation is felt. An empty injector puncturing can drain pus like thin porridge with a little foul smell.

【病情深变】

[Changes of Disease]

结核性肛门周围脓肿破溃后,将形成结核性瘘管。

The tuberculosis perianal abscesses will form tuberculosis fistula after the abscess breaks up.

【治疗】

[Treatment]

可治疗:①结核性皮下脓肿;②结核性坐骨直肠窝脓肿;③结核性骨盆直肠窝脓肿(酌病情选择前述治疗方法)。

According to above methods, we can treat: ①tuberculosis subcutaneous abscess; ②tuberculosis ischiorectal fossa abscess; ③tuberculosis pelvirectal fossa abscess.

第四节 肛 瘘
§4 Anal Fistula

肛瘘主要发生在肛门附近及直肠下部，一端进入直肠或肛管，另一端开口于肛门周围的皮外或其他邻近的器官，常由于肛门旁脓肿演变而成。

Anal fistula is an inflammatory track with a secondary opening (external opening) in the perianal skin or other organs and a primary opening (internal opening) in the anal canal or rectum. The fistula usually originates from a perianal abscess.

【病因病理】

[Etiology and Pathology]

肛瘘的发病原因，除少数患者由于穿刺性外伤等所致外，绝大部分继发于肛门脓肿溃破以后，伤口久治不愈而成。因此，凡是引起肛门旁脓肿的原因，都可成为肛瘘的病因。肛瘘是肛门旁脓肿演变的结果。

Besides a few penetrable injuries from outside of the body, most patients present with previous history of anorectal abscess associated with intermittent drainage. Recurrence of a perianal abscess suggests the presence of an anal fistula. The external opening is usually visible as a red elevation of granulation tissue with purulent or setosanguineous drainage on compression.

中医认为，肛瘘与痔的发病机制基本一致，不外乎内伤七情，外感六淫，以及饮食不节（过食辛辣、生冷、油腻等食物），或禀赋素虚，久病失养等引起机体阴阳平衡失调，障碍气血运行，致使湿热之邪乘虚流注下焦（肛门直肠部），郁久化热，溃腐成痈，穿肠窜臀，逐形成所谓"脏毒"（即肛门旁脓肿），溃后伤口不敛，最后成为肛瘘。虽然现代病理生理还不能解释"湿热"的真实意义，但是，中医对其病因的认识，既强调整体又考虑局部的观点是科学的。

In traditional Chinese medicine, it is believed that the mechanism of producing disease is similar between anal fistula and hemorrhoids, nothing more than emotion, external cause and improper diet (over eating, pungent, raw, cold food and greasy, etc), deficiency, weak, etc.. which cause imbalance of Yin and Yang, obstruct movement of Qi and blood, leading to damp heat going down into anorectal region, so long time stasis causes heat, sore causes carbuncle, gradually forming perianal abscess, and the abscess breaks up to form fistula. So the recognization of etiology from traditional Chinese medicine is both systemic and local.

肛瘘除与痔疮的发病机制有着很多相似之处外，生物因子如细菌参与也是重要因素。细菌正是在机体失常的情况下，使肛门周围出现发炎、化脓、破溃、窦道形成等一系列的病理变化。具体来说，肛门和直肠交界处（齿线上）有许多肛窦，其口向上,基底在下,并有肛门瓣围拢于其下缘,因此又增加了肛窦的深度。当粪便等异物进入肛窦内就不易排出,终会发酶分解,给细菌造成繁殖的良好场所。从而使肛窦内的分泌物增加,肛窦内压逐渐升高,其所容之物含有大量细菌脓性分泌物,即沿着所属淋巴管道进入肌肉间隙、渗流到肛门周围的软组织中,逐步形成肛门直肠周围脓肿(图 6 – 36)。

Besides many similar mechanism of producing disease between anal fistula and hemorrhoids, biological factors are also the important causes. For example, bacteria cause inflammation in anal region when the body is abnormal, make anal region a series of pathological changes, such as inflammation, suppuration, fester, etc. The pathophysiology likely relates to abscess formation in the anal glands. From this region, the function may spread downward, upward, circumferentially, or laterally to involve the various perianal and perirectal spaces. At times, other causes of infectious processes are identifiable. Those conditions include pilonidal abscess, suppurative hidradenitis, infected sebaceous cyst, folliculitis, and periprostatic abscess. Specifically, there are many crypts being the juncture of anal canal and rectum (the dentate line), are vertical with upward openings and downward bases, with anal valves around the bases, thus increasing the depth of crypts. The stools can't drain easily from anal crypts after they went there; and can take easily decomposition, making position for bacteria propagation, and then the secretion increases, the internal pressure in anal crypts heightened. A large number of bacterial secretion in anal crypts spread along lymphatic duct into intersphincteric space. From this origin, the infection may spread to involve various perianal and perirectal spaces, to form perianal and perirectal suppurations (Fig. 6 – 36).

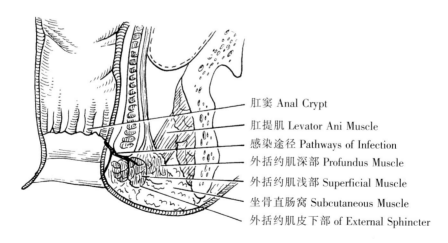

肛窦 Anal Crypt
肛提肌 Levator Ani Muscle
感染途径 Pathways of Infection
外括约肌深部 Profundus Muscle
外括约肌浅部 Superficial Muscle
坐骨直肠窝 Subcutaneous Muscle
外括约肌皮下部 of External Sphincter

图 6 – 36　肛门直肠感染蔓延方向
Figure 6 – 36　Pathways of infection in anal and rectal region

在肛门出现红、肿、热、痛,小便困难,并出现发冷发热及全身不适等。如失治或误治,脓肿可逐渐扩大,最后自行溃破或手术切开。除少数患者能自行愈合外,绝大部分将演变成肛瘘。

The systemic symptoms are shiver, fever and weak, and the local ones are red, swelling mass, hot, pain and difficult urination. The abscess can enlarge gradually if it isn't well treated or being falsely treated. The abscess can break up by itself or be cut. Some abscesses, properly drained, will heal primarily without subsequent formation of fistula, but many of these abscesses will form fistulae.

至于脓肿溃破后演变成肛瘘的原因,除了由于正气衰弱(机体抗病力低),愈合力差外,还与以下因素有关。

The abscess breaks up to form anal fistula, resulted from the condition of Qi deficiency (the body's resistance to disease reducing) and the reducing ability of healing.

(1)脓肿被切开或自行溃破,但原发部位(肛管内发炎之肛窦)仍继续有化脓性病变,并不断向下排出脓汁或粪便,影响伤口修复。

(1)Although the abscess gets being incised, or breaks up by itself, the primary inflammation (infected anal crypts)is still there and continues to drain pus downwards, which influences the healing.

(2)当排便或排尿时,肛门括约肌必然出现收缩与舒张,使患处很难得到静息生养。

(2)It's possible that the anal sphincter muscle contracts and relaxes during defecation and urination, so the healing is uneasy.

(3)肛门区血液循环较差(静脉回流迟缓),修复缓慢。

(3)The blood circulation supplying to anorectal region is slow (venous drainage is also slow), so the repair delays.

(4)破口缩小,脓肿腔道弯曲,引流不畅。

(4)The opening of breaking is small accompanying with circuitous track of fistula, so the drainage is not free.

(5)直肠腐败物质不断进入脓腔,刺激腔壁,促进结缔组织形成,尤其当瘢痕组织收缩时,可阻断新生毛细血管丛形成,终致失去愈合的可能。

(5)The material of rectal aposepsis goes into abscess, stimulates the abscess wall promoting formation of connective tissue, especially the scars contract to obstruct formation of new capillary vessels plexus, finally it's impossible to heal.

【临床表现】

[Clinical Manifestations]

肛瘘除局部表现明显外,全身也可出现各种不同的症状。

Besides local obvious symptoms, different systemic symptoms can also occur.

1. 全身症状
1. Systemic Symptoms

（1）单纯型：一般无明显全身症状。

（1）Simple stage：There aren't obvious systemic symptoms.

（2）湿热型：多表现有口苦、胃满、食欲缺乏、肢体沉重、全身无力，或有轻度畏寒发热、大便干燥或秘结、小便发黄等。

（2）Damp heat stage：Mainly showing bitter taste, abdominal distension, anorexia, heavy limb, weak, or mild shiver and fever, dry stool or constipation, deep color urine, etc.

（3）虚寒型：身体衰弱、四肢无力，劳动后有心慌气短，喜暖怕冷、食欲差、便稀、小便清白、自汗或盗汗等。

（3）Cold asthenia stage：Weak, tired, rapid heart rate, liking warm, being afraid of cold, anorexia, watery stool, light color urine, spontaneous perspiration, night sweat, etc.

（4）虚中夹实型：本属虚寒型，又加感染发炎，表现有畏寒发热，头痛身痛，口干舌燥，全身不适，并有食欲减退，或有大便干燥、排尿困难、小便色黄等。

（4）Cold sthenia stage：It belongs to cold asthenia, in case of infection, showing shiver and fever, headache, body pain, mouth parched and tongue scorched, weak, anorexia, dry stool, difficult urination, deep color urine, etc.

2. 局部症状
2. Local Symptoms

（1）流脓、流水：是肛瘘的主要症状。也有粪便及肠内气体经瘘管随脓排出。肛门内瘘的脓常与大便混合排出，有时在粪上附着几条脓血丝。外瘘脓液较少。多发性复杂瘘脓多，瘘管如与其他器官相通，则会产生相应症状，如直肠膀胱瘘，肛门可有尿流出；尿液中也可出现脓球或粪渣等。

（1）Draining pus and fluid is the main symptoms of anal fistula. There are also stools and gas draining from fistula, sometimes the stool covers some of blood streak. External fistula drains a little pus. Multiple complicated fistula drain much pus, if the fistula penetrates other organs, corresponding symptoms will occur, for example in rectum-urinary bladder fistula, the anus drain urine meanwhile urine drains pus ball and stool dregs, etc.

（2）疼痛：瘘管内有脓液积存，或内口较大，管道弯曲，粪块流入管道中。由于刺激，可以发生胀痛，尤其出现炎症反应时，可出现剧烈疼痛。单口内瘘常感觉直肠下部及肛门烧灼不适，排便时感到疼痛。

（2）Pain：There are much pus in the fistula, while the internal opening of fistula is large, the external opening is small, the tracks are curved, the stools go into track to stimulate body, so all cause the pain, especially leading to inflammation causing pain, even very painful during defecation, and to feel cauterization in the anus and the inferior of rectum.

（3）瘙痒：多因流出之分泌物刺激肛门周围皮肤，形成湿疹而致瘙痒。

（3）Pruritus：The secretion drained from fistula stimulates the skin of anal region to cause eczema leading pruritus and similar skin disease.

【诊断】

[Diagnosis]

首先询问病史。如肛门周围曾有过脓肿，经自行破溃或手术切开，其后伤口经久不愈，时常流脓、流水等，在此基础上再进行全身及局部检查。

Asking history if there were ever abscesses in the anal region, through breaking by themselves or cutting by doctors, the opening often drains pus and water, and didn't heal for a long time. On the basis of these symptoms systemic and local examinations should be made.

1. 定型诊断
1. Stage Diagnosis

（1）单纯型：脉象多为平脉，舌苔薄白或少苔。局部病变为多单纯性肛瘘较轻。

（1）Simple stage：The pulses are mainly mild, white thin or a little fur of tongue, local symptoms of fistula are also mild.

（2）湿热型：脉象多呈弦数或弦紧；舌质赤苔多黄厚而腻；局部病变多为肛瘘早期（脓肿破溃不久，分泌物较多而脓稠，或具有臭味），或单纯性肛瘘，伴有轻度感染发炎。

（2）Damp heat stage：The pulses are mainly rapid string or tense string, red tongue with yellow greasy or yellow thick even red fur; local symptoms are initial fistula (the abscess breaks up just now, the secretion is much and stiff with foul smell), or are simple fistula with mild inflammation.

（3）虚寒型：脉象多呈沉细或弦细；舌质多淡红，苔多薄白或少苔；局部病变多属病期较久的复杂性肛瘘、结核性肛瘘或一般单纯性肛瘘。因身体素虚或因其他脏腑有病而致身体衰弱。

（3）Cold asthenia stage：The pulses are mainly thin sunken or thin string, pale tongue with white thin or a little fur, local symptoms are complicated fistula with a long time, tuberculosis fistula or simple fistula. The body is weak because other organs are diseased leading to systemic weakness.

（4）虚中夹实型：脉象浮数无力或弦细而数；舌尖发红，苔黄或薄白；局部病变范围较大，多属于病期较长之肛瘘而又有严重继发感染。

（4）Asthenia in sthenia stage：The pulses are mainly rapid floating and weak or thin rapid string，pale tongue with white thin or a little fur，local symptoms are a big region and a long time fistula with secondary severe infection.

2. 分类诊断　见图 6 - 37。
2. Classification Diagnosis　See Fig. 6 - 37.

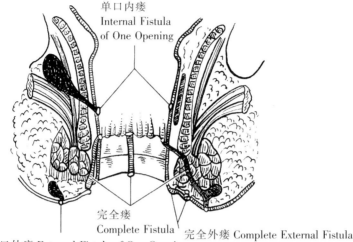

单口内瘘
Internal Fistula
of One Opening

完全瘘
Complete Fistula

完全外瘘 Complete External Fistula

单口外瘘 External Fistula of One Opening

图 6 - 37 肛门直肠瘘分类

Figure 6 - 37　Classification of anal and rectal fistulae

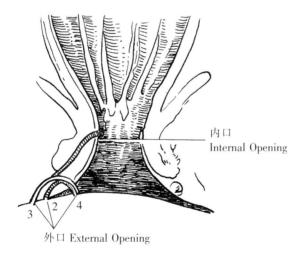

内口
Internal Opening

3　2　4

外口 External Opening

图 6 - 38 完全瘘有数个外口

Figure 6 - 38　There are some external openings in completed fistula

（1）完全瘘：外口在肛门周围皮肤上形成小的凸起，中间有瘘孔，挤压时有脓汁流出；自外口向肛内皮下可摸到一条索状物，这就是瘘管；内口大部在齿线附近，不超过

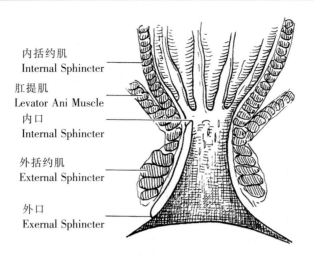

内括约肌
Internal Sphincter

肛提肌
Levator Ani Muscle

内口
Internal Sphincter

外括约肌
External Sphincter

外口
Exernal Sphincter

图 6 - 39　完全瘘管位于黏膜及括约肌之间

Figure 6 - 39　There are some completed fistula tracks between mucosa and sphincter muscle

直肠环而穿入肛管或直肠壁。有的内口虽只有一个,但外口可能有数个(图 6 - 38)。如由皮下脓肿而得的完全瘘,其内口也在齿线附近,外口多半在近于肛门附近处,瘘管则通常在皮下组织及外括约肌之间(图 6 - 39),或者在外括约肌皮下部及浅部之间(图 6 - 40)。如由坐骨直肠窝脓肿而得的完全瘘,瘘管在坐骨直肠窝内,经过外括约肌浅部及深部通入直肠(图 6 - 41)。其外口距离肛门较远,常在臀部坐骨结节附近,其内口在直肠环以下;也有的瘘管在肛门后部正中线的。

(1)Complete fistula: Around anal region the external openings form some small projections with a fistula hole in the middle point of every projection. There is pus juice draining from the holes as being pressed and squeezed, and the fistulous track can be felt and palpated as an indurated cord in subcutaneous tissue from external opening to inside of anus, the internal opening is in the anal canal near by the dentate line. Sometimes there is only an internal opening and some external openings (Fig. 6 - 38). In the simple or superficial complete fistula from subcutaneous abscess, the track can be palpated between subcutaneous tissue and external sphincteric muscle (Fig. 6 - 39), or between superficial muscle and subcutaneous muscle of external sphincter muscle (Fig. 6 - 40), the external opening in the perianal skin and the internal opening near by the dentate line either. The completed fistula from ischiorectal fossa; its track is in ischiorectal fossa going to the rectum through superficial muscle and profundus muscle of external sphincter muscle(Fig. 6 - 41); its internal opening below rectal ring; its external opening is the distance from nearby ischial tuberosity in hip. There are also fistulae in the two sides of posterior midline of anus (this kind of the fistula is rare).

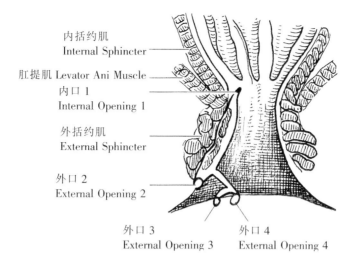

内括约肌
Internal Sphincter

肛提肌 Levator Ani Muscle

内口 1
Internal Opening 1

外括约肌
External Sphincter

外口 2
External Opening 2

外口 3
External Opening 3

外口 4
External Opening 4

图 6 - 40　完全瘘管通外括约肌皮下部及浅部之间

Figure 6 - 40　Complete fistula track between superficial and subcutaneous external sphincter

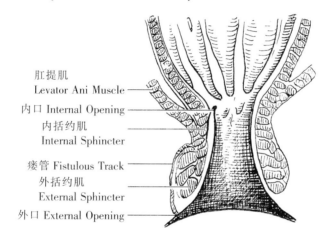

肛提肌
Levator Ani Muscle

内口 Internal Opening

内括约肌
Internal Sphincter

瘘管 Fistulous Track

外括约肌
External Sphincter

外口 External Opening

图 6 - 41　高位坐骨直肠瘘瘘管越过外括约肌浅部及深部之间

Figure 6 - 41　High positional ischiorectal fistulous track between profundus and superficial external sphincteric muscle

检查方法：先用手摸清瘘管方向、部位,将探针从外口徐徐按弯曲插入瘘管中,再以另手示指(戴指套)插入肛内寻找内口,探针自然通过或凹窝处即为内口。这类瘘管比较简单,容易治疗。

Examination：At first the hand feels clearly the direction and position of fistula track, then a hand inserts the probe into the track slowly along its curving, while the other hand inserts into anus to look for internal opening, the probe goes through the opening freely or the hand feels the sunken point, that's the internal opening. This kind of fistula is simple and can be treated easily.

(2)单纯外瘘：只有外口在肛门皮肤上,平时流脓不多,按之有少量脓液流出。这类瘘管极少见。平常所见到的多是具有内口的完全瘘,或有许多外口,但检查时未找到内口,误认为外瘘(图 6 - 40)。其实有内口,如 1 号在齿线附近,外口 2 在肛门周围,因外口 2 暂时封闭,而又由外口 3、外口 4 穿破,增加了两个外口。因此如以探针检查,可由外口 2 通到外口 4,也可由外口 3 通到外口 4,但原发内口未被发现。如图 6 - 42 未探着内口,故误认是外瘘。

(2) Simple external fistula: There is only external opening on the skin of anal region, and drainage of pus is not much, so there is a little pus drainage from the internal opening as being squeezed. This kind of fistula is rare. The complete fistula having external opening and internal opening is commonly visible. There are some external openings, but the internal opening can't be found by examination, so the complete fistula is misunderstood as simple external fistula (Fig. 6 - 40). In fact there is an internal opening nearby dentate line (No. 1 in the figure). The external opening No. 2 is near the anus. Since this opening is temporarily closed, perforations through two more openings happen. So the examination with probe goes through 2 to 4, or 3 to 4, but the internal opening can't be found; in Fig. 6 - 42 the internal opening No. 1 can't be discovered, so it is misunderstood as an external fistula.

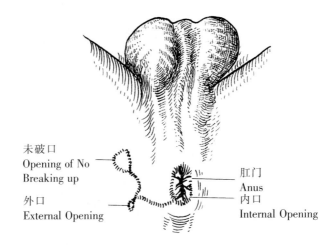

图 6 - 42　完全瘘有的外口封闭,内口也不易找到,故易误认为外瘘

Figure 6 - 42　The complete fistula is not easy to find, the internal opening is misunderstood as simple external fistula.

检查方法:用探针从外口插入(但不能通入肛内),同时在肛内指诊触不到探针顶端时,如属完全外瘘,探针顶端可从肛缘另一内口穿出;较深的外瘘也可以用色素(亚甲蓝)注射试验,或用肛钩检查肛窦,以确定诊断。

Examination: Probing the track from the external opening meanwhile digital palpation inside of anus can't touch the upper end of probe, so it is simple external fistula; if the probe goes through the internal opening, it's complete external fistula. The injection of methylene blue or checking up with hook style acupuncture scalpel may be helpful.

(3) 单纯内瘘:在肛管或直肠内,从外面看不到。这种瘘有的只有一个口,多在齿线附近,在黏膜下层有一条窦道(图 6 – 43),也有两个口均在肛管或直肠内的完全性内瘘(图 6 – 44);还有的一口开在肛管或直肠内(齿线附近为原发内口),另一口通于其他器官,如膀胱、子宫、阴道等处,这些类型极为少见。

(3)Simple internal fistula:It is not visible in the surface because it is in anal canal or rectum. It sometimes has only an internal opening usually near the dentate line, and a track in submucosa (Fig. 6 – 43). Sometimes there are two internal openings in anal canal or rectum, which is called complete internal fistula (Fig. 6 – 44); rarely it has an opening in anal canal or rectum, (primary internal opening near the dentate line), and another opening through urinary bladder, uterus, vagina, etc.

检查方法:必须用鸭嘴窥肛器扩开肛门,可见流脓的瘘口(一个或两个)。然后,再以探针插入,以了解其深度和方向,区分是单口内瘘,还是完全内瘘。

Examination:A duck mouth anoscope holds up anus:the fistula opening draining pus is visible (one or two openings), then the probe is inserted to understand its depth and direction, further to distinguish whether the one opening internal fistula or the complete internal fistula.

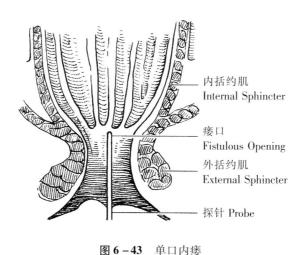

内括约肌
Internal Sphincter

瘘口
Fistulous Opening

外括约肌
External Sphincter

探针 Probe

图 6 – 43　单口内瘘

Figure 6 – 43　Internal fistula with one opening

(4)多发瘘:在肛门皮肤上有两个以上外口或瘘管,在内口仍在直肠环以下。检查方法与完全瘘相同(图 6 – 45)。

(4)Multiple fistulae:There are two or more external openings of fistulous tracks in the perianal skin and an internal opening below rectal ring. The examination is the same as that of complete fistula(Fig. 6 – 45).

(5)高位坐骨直肠瘘:外口在坐骨结节部,内口在直肠环以上或直肠环中间,是一条较长、位置又深的瘘管(图 6 – 41)。

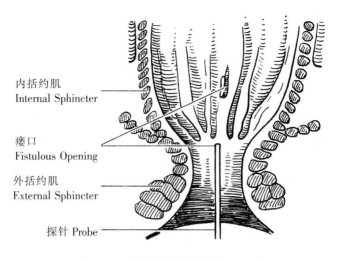

图 6 – 44　完全内瘘

Figure 6 – 44　Complete internal fistula

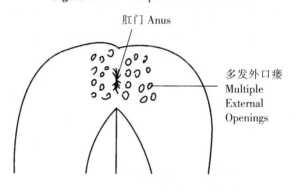

图 6 – 45　多发性复杂瘘

Figure 6 – 45　Multiple complicated fistula

(5)High positional ischiorectal fistula:There is long and deep track with the external opening in ischial tuberosity region and the internal opening above rectal ring or at this ring(Fig. 6 –41).

(6)蹄铁形肛瘘:瘘管虽不多,但管道弯曲有叉,或呈马蹄形,外口有两个,分别位于肛门两侧,内口多半有一个在前部者称为前部蹄铁形瘘(图 6 –46);在后部者称为后部蹄铁形瘘。后部蹄铁形瘘的内口,常在后部正中线上或稍偏一侧;前部蹄铁形瘘的内口则不一定在前部正中线上,而均在直肠环以上通入直肠。

(6)Horseshoe fistula:There are not a number of tracks, but the tracks are curving and biforked shape or horseshoe shape. There are two external openings in both sides of the anus. There is an internal opening. The internal opening lying on anterior is called the anterior horseshoe fistula, and its internal opening may not be locating at the anterior midline (Fig. 6 –46); the internal opening lying on posterior is called the posterior horseshoe fistula, and its internal opening locates at the posterior midline or a little inclined to one side; and their external openings locate above rectal ring going to rectum.

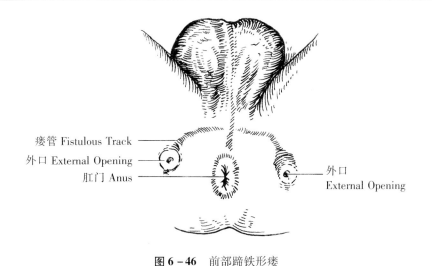

瘘管 Fistulous Track
外口 External Opening
肛门 Anus
外口
External Opening

图 6 - 46 前部蹄铁形瘘

Figure 6 - 46 Anterior horseshoe fistula

（7）多发性复杂瘘：在肛门周围皮肤上有许多外口，最多可达 30～40 个，排满两臀（图 6-45）。按之可见许多孔同时流出脓液，这些瘘口互相连通，经常发炎肿痛。外口虽多但内口一般只有一两个，在直肠环以上通入直肠。

（7）Multiple complicated fistulae：There are many external openings on the skin in the anal region, at most 30～40 external openings spreading over two hips（Fig. 6 – 45）. The pus drains in the same time from many holes as being squeezed. These tracks connect each other, and inflame frequently. There is only one or two internal openings above rectal ring into rectum although there are many external openings.

检查方法：高位坐骨直肠瘘、蹄铁形瘘和多发性复杂瘘的检查需要仔细，应用探针及肛钩检查，如查不清内口所在位置，可以做碘油造影或局部麻醉下检查。总之这些复杂性肛瘘在手术以前，必须检查清楚，否则很难治愈。

Examination：The examination should take care for high positional ischiorectal fistula, horseshoe fistula, multiple complicated fistulae, to carry on the probe and anal hook, and lipiodolography is a valuable method to identify and to manage misunderstanding the position of internal opening, or checking up in local anesthesia. In general, these complicated fistulae must be checked up clearly before operation, or they are difficult to be cured.

（8）结核性肛瘘：不论是单纯的或是复杂的，均有其大而不整的外口，边缘呈灰色，伤口肉芽水肿，缺乏弹性，摸不到索状硬条的瘘管，按之有稀薄脓液流出。对结核性肛瘘患者应做全身检查，如肺结核、骨结核，以便明确原发病灶。为了确诊，最好切除管壁送病理检查。

（8）Tuberculosis anal fistula：There is a big and disordered external opening with gray fringe, granuloma, deficient elasticity; with no feeling of fistula track with fibrous cord. There is thin pus draining out as squeezing it. The patient with tuberculosis anal fistula should carry on systemic examination, such as pulmonary tuberculosis, bone tuberculosis, so as to understand the original disease. It's better to cut off the wall of fistulous track for pathologic examination to earn a definite diagnosis.

【治疗】
[Treatment]

根据中医学"辨证论治"和"同病异治"、"异病同治"的精神,对肛瘘采用局部与整体兼治的疗法。

According to traditional Chinese medicine's "treatment based on differentiated syndrome", "the same disease treated by different methods" and "different diseases treated by the same method", an anal fistula should be treated locally meanwhile taking account of systemic treatment.

1. 整体分型治疗原则和方法
1. The Principle and Method for Treatment by Systemic Dividing Types

(1)单纯型:一般无需做全身治疗。

(1)Simple type:No need to treat systemic treatment as usual.

(2)湿热型:以清热解毒、利湿通便为原则。一般常用仙方活命饮(加减),或槐角丸、麻仁滋脾丸及其他抗生素等药物。

(2)Damp heat type:To take mainly clearing heat and relieving intoxication, infiltrating dampness and purging defecation. Taking the decoction of XianFangHuoMing Yin(add up or reduce herbs according to symptoms), or pill of scholartree pod pill of MaRenZiPi and antibiotics, etc.

(3)虚寒型:以补气养血、健脾和胃为原则。常用八珍汤(加减)或补中益气汤(丸)、十全大补丸以及维生素等药物。

(3)Cold asthenia type:To take mainly tonifying Qi and blood, invigorating spleen and stomach. Taking the BaZhen Decoction (add up or reduce herbs according to symptoms)or BuZhong YiQiTang(decoction or pill), the pill of ShiQuanDaBuWan, and vitamins, etc.

(4)虚中夹实型:以清热解毒、消肿止痛为原则。常用消肿止痛汤、仙方活命饮(加减)或用抗生素等药物。待炎症情况缓解时,再投以补养之剂。

(4)Asthenia according to sthenia type:To take mainly clearing heat and relieving intoxication, eliminating swelling and relieving pain. Taking the decoction of XiaoZhongZhiTong, XianFangHuoMingYin(add up or reduce herbs according to symptoms), or antibiotics, etc. Taking the tonifying decoctions after the inflammation being reduced.

2. 局部分类治疗原则和方法
2. The Principle and Method for Treatment by Local Dividing Stage

（1）完全瘘：不论几个瘘管，一般均可采用"简易小针刀"疗法。如因内口处有内痔（应先进行内痔注射疗法），或可采用单纯挂橡皮线挂线方法治疗。

（1）Complete fistula：To take the simple method of "acupuncture scalpel treating" no matter how many are the fistulous tracks. If there are internal hemorrhoids at the internal opening, the method is firstly to take the injection or simple rubber band seton.

（2）外瘘：用小弯刀切开方法治疗。

（2）External fistula：To take incision and drainage by the acupuncture scalpel.

（3）内瘘：用小钩刀切开瘘管后，敷外痔贴，方法治疗。

（3）Internal fistula：To take incision and drainage by the acupuncture scalpel, then apply the medicine on it.

（4）多发瘘：应采用开刀和挂线综合疗法治疗。肛外所有浅层瘘管采用"简单小针刀"方法切开，其较深部的瘘管挂线方法治疗。

（4）Multiple fistulae：To take compositing treatment by acupuncture scalpel and seton. All superficial fistulae outside of anus are given incision and drainage by "acupuncture scalpel simple treatment" while deep fistulae are treated by setons.

（5）高位坐骨直肠瘘：适用小针刀与高位挂线疗法，肛外瘘管部分只切开，从深部至通向直肠环以上内口部分，必须采用挂线（橡皮线）疗法。

（5）High positional ischiorectal fistulous track：To take treatment by acupuncture scalpel and high positional seton. The fistulae at outside of anus are taken incision and drainage while deep fistulae above the rectal ring are treated by setons（rubber band）.

（6）蹄铁形复杂瘘：用探针小弯刀切开，深部用挂橡皮筋双挂线疗法治疗。

（6）Complicated horseshoe fistula：To take incision and drainage by the small curving probing scalpel, and deep fistulae are treated by two rubber band setons.

（7）多发性复杂瘘：肛外浅部瘘管不论多少，一律采取小针刀切开法；通向直肠的瘘管，采用挂橡皮线方法治疗。

（7）Multiple complicated fistulae：To take incision and drainage by the acupuncture scalpel no matter how many shallow fistulae are outside of anus; fistulae through the rectum are treated by rubber band setons.

（8）结核性肛瘘：除瘘管部分应按以上治疗原则处理外，还应根据原发病灶情况给予适当抗结核全身治疗。

（8）Tuberculosis anal fistula：To treat the fistulous track according to above principle, meanwhile to take systemic anti-tuberculosis treatment according to the original disease.

3. 简易疗法 这种疗法可以使症状减轻,防止瘘管发炎和蔓延,但不能根除。

3. Simple Treatment The method can reduce symptoms, prevent fistula from inflaming and spreading, but can't effect a radical cure.

(1)适应证:肛瘘不宜手术者。

(1)Indication:The patients are not suitable for surgery.

(2)方法

(2)Method

①调理大便:每天多吃蔬菜,多喝白开水,定时排便。大便干燥时可吃些缓泻药(如槐角丸、五仁润肠丸、脏连丸等)。

①Regulating defecation:Take laxative drugs as there is dry stool (such as pill of Fructus Sophorae compound, WuRenRunChang, ZangLian, etc).

②保持局部清洁:每日用温开水坐浴;或用1:5000 高锰酸钾液或祛毒汤坐浴,后涂外痔贴和九华膏等,以免流出的分泌物刺激肛门周围皮肤引起湿疹。

②Keeping clear locally:Baths with warm water or 1:5000 potassium permanganate or herbal soup every day, then squeeze JiuHua cream into anus, etc. to prevent atopic eczema from sitimulation of drainage in anal region.

③消炎、止痛:肛瘘在发炎时,可用祛毒汤熏洗,或用温开水勤洗(每日 2 ~ 3 次)或坐浴,洗后敷消脓膏。还可内服清热解毒汤,每日 1 剂,分 2 次服。

③Anti-inflammatory and analgesic treatment:As inflammation with fistula QuDu decoction can be taken, tub baths in warm water, then squeeze some cream into anus, or to continue taking the decoction of QingReJieDuTang, two times per day.

4. 探针小弯刀疗法
4. Small Curving Probing Scalpel Treatment

(1)适应证:内口在直肠环以下者。

(1)Indication:The internal opening below the rectal ring.

(2)操作方法:嘱患者侧卧,屈膝向上,露出肛门(图6-47),剃去肛门周围之阴毛,对局部皮肤进行常规消毒,于瘘管及切开线处注射1%普鲁卡因溶液(内加1:1000 肾上腺素溶液数滴)4 ~ 10ml。将探针小弯刀从瘘管外口徐徐插入,并以另手示指(带指套)插入肛门内寻找内口(图6-48),以示指触到探针自然通过之口,即为内口。再将探针小弯刀前段之探针部分折弯牵出肛外(图6-49),循瘘管向上锯开(即扩开瘘管)。伤口敷外痔贴。

(2)Treatment method:The patient lies on the side, and bends his knees showing the anus

（Fig. 6 –47）. The doctor shaves his pubes around anus, sterilizes local skin as usual, injects 1% procaine（add 1 ：1000 adrenaline a few drops）4 ~ 10ml. One hand handles the curving probe acupuncture scalpel to insert slowly from fistulous external opening, While the other hand's index finger inserts into anus to look for internal opening（Fig. 6 –48）. The index finger feels the probe going through the opening freely, the opening is internal opening, and the right hand handles the front probe of the curette acupuncture scalpel to take fold curving, puts the probe out of the anus along the track and cuts the wall of fistula to enlarge the fistulous track（Fig. 6 –49）.

5. 探针挂线疗法

5. Seton on Probe Treating

（1）适应证：肛门复杂瘘，内口在或超过直肠环者。

（1）Indication：Complicated anal fistulae, internal opening is on rectal ring or above it.

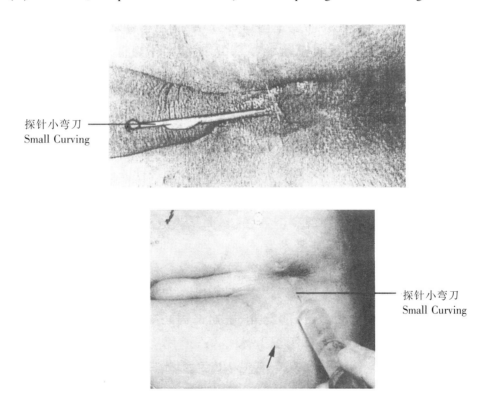

探针小弯刀
Small Curving

探针小弯刀
Small Curving

图 6 –47　侧卧后，露出肛门，探针小弯刀从瘘管外口插入

Figure 6 –47　To lie on side, show anus, insert a small curving probing scalpel into external opening of fistula

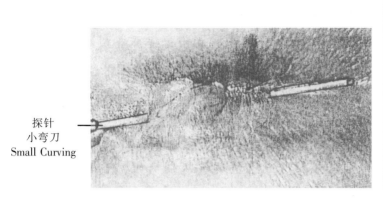
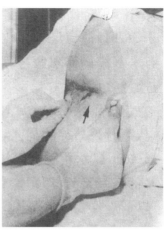

探针
小弯刀
Small Curving

图 6 - 48 另手示指由肛门插入寻找内口,将探针部分自内口牵出肛外

Figure 6 - 48 Index finger insert into anus to look for internal opening
and draws the part of probe out the internal opening

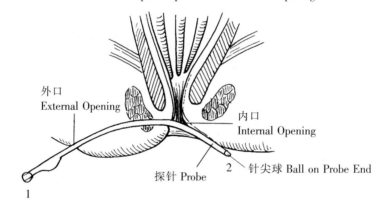

外口
External Opening

内口
Internal Opening

2 针尖球 Ball on Probe End

探针 Probe

1

图 6 - 49 探针小弯刀探出内外口

1 - 探针小弯刀;2 - 将探针牵出肛外

Figure 6 - 49 Curving probe acupuncture scalpel going through internal and external opening

1. Curving probe acupuncture scalpel;2. Carrying the probe out of the anus

　　(2)操作方法:采用挂橡皮线法。麻醉后,以探针从瘘管外口徐徐探入,同时以另手示指插入肛管内寻找内口(图 6 - 50),内口一般多在肛窦附近。若手触着探针,即为内口所在,需要慢慢上下探找,至自然通过(注意不要强力探入,以免造成人为内口,如直针不能顺利探入时,可将探针屈成弯形,以便寻找内口)即为内口。将探针从内口折弯牵出肛门后,于探针尖球部系上丝线,线上再缚上橡皮圈(图 6 - 51)。

　　(2)The method of carrying on:Seton of rubber band. After anesthesia, handles the probe to insert into slowly from fistulous external opening, meanwhile the other hand's index finger inserts

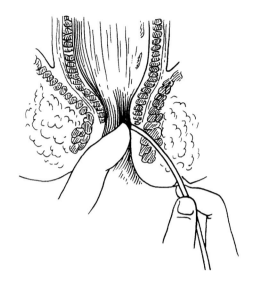

图 6 - 50　手指插入肛管内寻找内口

Figure 6 - 50　Finger inserting into anus to look for internal opening

into anal canal to look for internal opening（Fig. 6 - 50）upwards and downwards slowly, index finger feeling probe going through the opening freely, the opening is internal opening, （laterogenic track created by injudicious probing of the anal fistula）. The right hand handles the front probe of the curette acupuncture scalpel to take fold curving, and puts the probe out the anus along the track and ties the silk thread on the ball of top end of the probe wall, then ties the rubber band on the thread of fistula to enlarge the fistulous track（Fig. 6 - 51）.

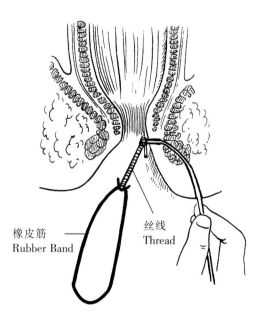

橡皮筋　丝线
Rubber Band　Thread

图 6 - 51　线上缚以橡皮圈

Figure 6 - 51　Tie the rubber band on the thread

随后将探针慢慢由原路后退,把橡皮线由瘘管内口向外口拉出(图 6 - 52)。这时橡皮圈的一端露在瘘管外口,一端从内口经肛管露出,把橡皮圈由内口拉出端合并拉紧(使其保持一定弹力),然后在近皮肤处用丝线结扎牢实(图 6 - 53)。为了减少患者痛苦,可将表面皮肤处切开至外括约肌部,填上痔瘘粉后用纱布敷盖包扎。挂线后,每日或隔日复查 1 次,如线松可再缚紧,8 ~ 9 天可脱线。

The doctor pulls back the probe slowly along the same way, and then puts thread with rubber band out of external opening through internal opening (Fig. 6 - 52). Putting rubber band out of external opening through internal opening, so that the end of rubber band shows at the external opening of fistula, and the other end shows in anal canal through internal opening, then both ends connect together and hauls tight the rubber band (keeping some tension), ties the silk thread to fix the rubber band (Fig. 6 - 53). To apply gauze after the arrangement.

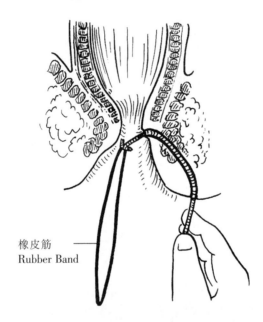

橡皮筋
Rubber Band

图 6 - 52　把橡皮圈由内口拉出

Figure 6 - 52　Puting rubber band out of external opening through internal opening

6. **小针挂药线疗法**　适应证和探针使用等与挂橡皮线疗法相同。在挂药线时,是将内口之探针牵出肛门外,在探针球部系上丝线,线上再缚上药线(图 6 - 54)。然后将探针慢慢自内口退出肛外,将药线带于管道中(图 6 - 55),并将一端割断,使两端交错接合,呈环形绕于管道(图 6 - 56)。最后将剩下的两端线拉紧,打结固定(图 6 - 57),用纱布敷盖包扎。

6. **The Method of Acupuncture Scalpel Tying Medical Thread**　The indication and the method of using probe are the same as the method of tying rubber band. The method is putting the probe out of anus from internal opening tying the silk thread at the ball of probe, taking the medicine on the thread (Fig. 6 - 54), then pulling back the probe to the outside of anus from internal

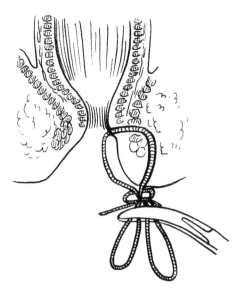

图 6 - 53 在近皮肤处用丝线结扎牢实

Figure 6 - 53 Silk thread tying near by skin

opening so as to bring the medical thread into the track（Fig. 6 - 55）, and cutting the end, making the two ends interlaced connecting to form the ring around the fistulous track（Fig. 6 - 56）, then tying two ends（Fig. 6 - 57）, at last covering the wound with gauze.

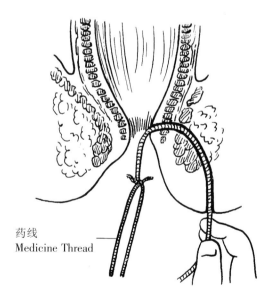

药线
Medicine Thread

图 6 - 54 丝线上缚以药线

Figure 6 - 54 Medicine thread tied on silk thread

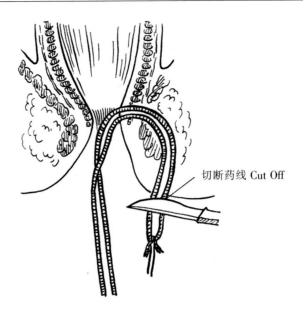

切断药线 Cut Off

图 6 -55　把药线带进管道

Figure 6 -55　Bringing medicine thread into the track

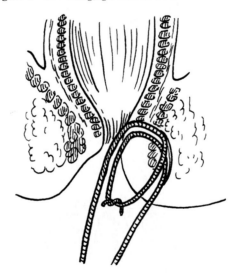

图 6 -56　药线两端交错接合,呈环形绕于管道

Figure 6 -56　Two ends of medicine thread interlaced connecting
to form the ring around the fistulous track

7. 小针刀切开高位挂线疗法

7. **To Take Acupuncture Scalpel Incision in High Position and Drainage Cutting**

(1)适应证:凡内口位于直肠环以上的复杂性肛瘘(高位坐骨直肠瘘、蹄铁形瘘、多发性复杂瘘),内口在肛门直肠环以上瘘管挂线,而齿线以下肛瘘切开。

(1)Indication:The complicated anal fistula with its internal opening above rectal ring (high

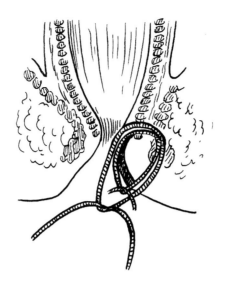

图 6 – 57 将药线拉紧打结固定

Figure 6 – 57 Tying two rests of the ends of medicine

position ischiorectal fistula, horseshoe fistula, multiple complicated fistulae), seton for the fistula with its internal opening above rectal ring, incision for the fistula with its internal opening below rectal ring.

（2）操作方法：取截石或侧卧位，肛门常规消毒后，先探查瘘管走行方向及内口所在位置。然后从瘘管外口顺瘘管切开到齿线，并将所有分支切开，最后必然找到一条总管通向内口方向（此时如发现较大之血管给以结扎止血）。切开到外括约肌浅部时，可以摸到直肠环边缘，发现腐肉处即为通入内口之瘘管。此时用探针小弯刀，自瘘管道向内徐徐插入，术者以另手示指插入肛管内寻找内口，在内口瘢痕硬结处可触到探针顶端，从此穿出，再牵出肛外。在探针球部系上丝线，线上再缚上橡皮圈，随后将探针慢慢退回，将橡皮线一端通过内口拉出至外口，另一端从内口（直肠环上）经肛管内露出肛门外。两端合并拉紧，在近直肠环处用双丝线结扎牢实（图 6 – 58）。肛门外的橡皮圈应放在纱条上面，而与创面隔开，再以纱布压迫包扎，用丁形带勒紧固定。

（2）Method：Lithotomy posture or lie on the side, sterilizing local skin as usual. At first explore the direction of fistulous track and internal opening, then cut all the offshoot of track from the fistulous external opening to dentate line finally, to find out a general track going to internal opening（at the time if the doctor finds a big blood vessel, he should ligate it tightly）. The doctor can feel the fringe of rectal ring when he cuts to the superficial external sphincter muscle；that's the fistulous track through internal opening when he finds the slough. The doctor handles the small curving probing acupuncture scalpel to insert slowly from fistulous external opening, meanwhile the other hand index finger inserting into anal canal to look for internal opening, index finger feels the top of probe going through opening acompanying with scar and hard node freely, the opening is internal opening, and then puts the probe out of the anus along the track. He ties the end of thread on top ball end of probe and ties the rubber band, then pulls back slowly the probe to the outside of anus from internal opening so as to bring the end of rubber thread into the track through internal opening to external opening, the other end putting out the anus along the track from internal opening (above rectal ring). He makes the two ends interlaced connecting to form the ring around the fistulous track then firmly ties two ends near the rectal ring (Fig. 6 – 58), at last covers the wound with gauze.

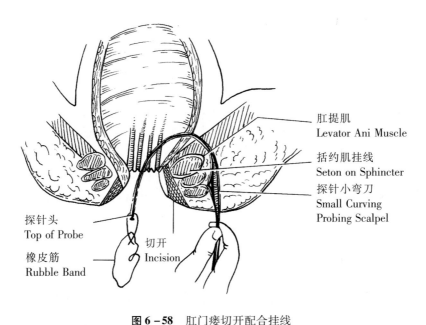

图 6 – 58　肛门瘘切开配合挂线

Figure 6 – 58　Anal fistulous incision and seton treatment

8. 探针小弯刀挂双线疗法

8. Small Curving Probing Scalpel Hanging Two Setons

(1)适应证:适宜肛门括约肌浅薄的复杂性瘘患者。

(1)Indication:Complicated anal fistula with shallow sphincter muscle.

(2)操作方法:局麻或腰俞麻醉,肛门常规消毒。右手持探针小弯刀从肛瘘的外口按其肛瘘走行徐徐插入,左手示指伸入肛门内导引并寻找肛瘘的内口;当左示指尖端触到探针头又可以自然通过之口即为内口。其内口往往通过或超过肛门直肠环深部括约肌即为复杂瘘,再将探针小弯刀前段探针部分给予从内口经肛门内折弯后牵出肛门外。用探针头挂2根粗丝线和橡皮筋备用,继用探针小弯刀后段刀锋锯开肛门直肠环以下的瘘管。但包括内口在内的肛门直肠环深部括约肌均不能锯开,以免造成肛门失禁;需采用前述挂双线治疗。然后再徐徐退回探针小弯刀,其双线即挂在包括内口在内的肛门直肠环深部括约肌上。但只将第 1 个单线挂的粗丝线给予一次性勒紧结扎,第 2 个单线橡皮筋暂不要结扎紧,容其宽松引流。当第 1 个粗丝线术后 5～6 天松弛时,才将第 2 个单线皮筋勒紧结扎,再于 9～10 天即与丝线一同自行脱掉。然后,将肛瘘敞开的外口修整成 V 形,瘘管及瘢痕均不剪除,引流通畅即可。用痔瘘粉纱布条敷盖(图 6－59)。

（2）Method ：The doctor gives local or lumbar anesthesia, and sterilizes local perianal skin as usual. The right hand handles the small curving probing acupuncture scalpel to insert slowly from fistulous external opening along the track, meanwhile the other hand index finger inserts into anal canal to look for internal opening, and index finger feels the top of probe going through the opening freely, the opening is internal opening, and then puts the anterior probe of the small curving probing acupuncture scalpel out the anus after curing along the track. The doctor ties two thick threads and the rubber band on top of probe for preparing, then cuts the fistulous track below anorectal ring by the posterior knife of the small curving probing acupuncture scalpel. Be sure that the deep sphincter muscle including internal opening should not be cut, being afraid of incontinence, it needs to be treated by hanging two setons. Then the doctor pulls back slowly the small curving probing acupuncture scalpel to the outside of anus from internal opening so as to bring the end of thread into the track through internal opening to external opening, and to hang the two threads on the deep sphincter muscle including an internal opening. The doctor ties the first thick silk thread of single thread hanging ligation, temporarily doesn't tie the second rubber band of single thread hanging ligation so as to drain freely(Fig. 6 －59) .

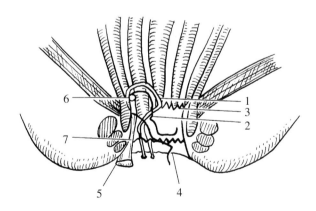

图 6 –59　复杂肛瘘探针小弯刀挂双线疗法
1 –橡皮筋;2 –丝线;3 –齿线;4 –肛门;5 –外口;6 –内口;7 –肛瘘

Figure 6 –59　Small curving probing scalpel hanging two setons treating complicated anal fistulae
1. Rubber Band; 2. Silk Thread; 3. Dentate Line; 4. Anus;
5. External Opening; 6. Internal Opening; 7. Anal Fistula

9. 小针刀挂线引流加压疗法
9. Seton Drainage and Pressure by Acupuncture Scalpel

(1)适应证:有蹄铁形肛瘘的支瘘管或多发支瘘管者。

(1)Indication:Horseshoe fistulous branch track and multiple fistulous branch track.

(2)操作方法:主瘘管治疗按常规手术进行。支瘘管采用本法治疗。以后方蹄铁形瘘为例,先插入直肠镜寻找瘘管内口,然后将探针小弯刀自一侧外口插入,由内口穿出。探明主瘘管后,于其内口相对应的肛门外缘,再以此为人造新瘘管外口。重新由新外口插入探针,再由内口穿出,并于肛门后方顺瘘管走行切开皮肤,按常规方法治疗肛门瘘主瘘管。其两侧肛瘘的支瘘管采用只挂线引流外口,并加压疗法,即将上述人造新外口及支管远端的原有瘘 2 个外口处增殖肉芽组织刮去,或内翻的皮肤边缘剪平,用刮匙小针刀清除支管壁内腐败组织。此支管不要切除,也不要切开,只将一根粗丝线从瘘管中穿过,并将线引出支瘘管外,不缚紧,松松打成一个丝线圈套即可以引流,对侧肛门蹄形支管采用同法,然后用敷料加压包扎。术后每日换药,待主瘘管的伤口将近愈合时,再去剪掉 2 个支瘘管挂的引流线。其2 个支瘘管腔因敷料外加压而粘连闭合治愈(图 6 - 60)。

(2)Method:Treating main fistulous track as usual, treating branch of track according to this method. For posterior horseshoe fistula, at first the doctor inserts rectoscope to look for internal opening of fistulous track, then inserts the small curving probing acupuncture scalpel into one side external opening, and puts out the opening. Having found the main fistulous track, the doctor takes the outer anal skin corresponding main fistulous internal opening as a new artificial fistulous external opening. Again the doctor insets the probe into new external opening and going out from old internal opening, and cuts skin along the fistulous track in posterior to the anus, to treat main fistulous track as usual. The two sides of fistulous branch track are carried on only by seton drainage and pressure. The doctor shaves out hyperplasia of granulation, and takes curette acupuncture scalpel to clear away rotten tissues in the branch of track. The same method treats the other side horseshoe fistulous branch. Then the doctor presses to bind up the wound with gauzes, and changes gauzes every day(Fig. 6 - 60).

由于本方法对支瘘管既不切除,也不切开,只是将支瘘管引流后加压,使其支瘘管前壁粘连后壁而愈合,故手术后肛门伤口小,愈合快,术后瘢痕小。

Because this method needs neither resection nor openness of the branch fistulous track, just make pressure on it following the drainage, to heal by adhesion of front wall and back wall, the anus thus has small cuts, quick union and small scars after the surgery.

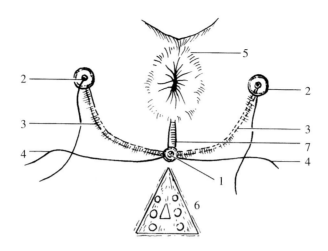

图 6－60　蹄铁形肛瘘支瘘管挂线疗法
1－主瘘管人造外口;2－外口;3－支瘘管;4－引流挂线;5－肛门;6－骶尾骨;7－主瘘管

Figure 6－60　Ligation therapy to horseshoe fistulous branch track

1. Artificial external of main fistulous track;2. External;3. Branch fistulous track;

4. Seton of drainage;5. Anus;6. Sacrococcyx;7. Main fistulous track

【点评】

[Review]

1. **探针挂线疗法**　治疗肛瘘的有效疗法之一。无论什么线,主要是利用其机械作用及药物腐蚀作用;剖开瘘管,使其引流通畅,再加换药使伤口愈合。其最大优点是对深长瘘管(内口在直肠环以上者)也不会发生后遗症,解决了手术最担心的问题。肛门括约肌一旦失禁治疗时间较长。因此目前有些瘘管(如完全瘘),均可以简易小针刀疗法代替单纯挂线疗法。但是仍然还有不少肛瘘,如复杂瘘、不适合于开刀的完全瘘,还是以此法治疗为好。

1. **The Method of Probe Hanging Thread**　It is one of effective methods in treating anal fistula. Every kind of thread makes mainly use of mechanism and medicine corroding, incision, drainage and changing gauzes to heal the wound. The most special feature and advance is there will not be any residual problem for deep and long fistulous track (the internal opening above rectal ring). Once incontinence happens, the time of treatment would be very long. The method of simply acupuncture scalpel can take place of only seton to treat some fistulae (such as complete fistula) in present time.

2. **切开配合挂线疗法**　内口位于直肠环以上的复杂性肛瘘,由于手术不慎,易造成大便失禁的后遗症。可采用切开配合高位挂线疗法。其机制:肛门直肠瘘的治疗基本原则,是通过内外口切开瘘管达到敞开引流的目的,使肉芽组织顺利生长,最后达到愈合;对直肠环以上的复杂性肛瘘,也是如此。但由于位置较高,须切断直肠环,因此在处理这个关键性问题方面有所不同。西医采取的治疗方法是分期手术,以避免造成肛门括约肌失禁,中医单纯采用挂线疗法,则痛苦多、疗程长,所以也存在一定缺点。探针小弯刀采用切开配合高位挂线的治疗方法,不必分期手术,疗程短,给予长效止痛。开刀配合高位挂线疗法,是目前治疗高位复杂性肛瘘的一种较好的方法。本法是将内口位于直肠环以下的肛瘘将其所有瘘管均行切开。(不切除)内口位于直肠环以上的肛瘘要挂橡皮线。借橡皮线之弹性回缩作用,勒于深在(通越直肠环)之内口及瘘管,由于其不断地持续地收紧而产生的压迫作用,使接触处之组织发生缺血性坏死,而逐渐将内口全部组织(包括直肠环)勒开。组织被扩开的同时,后边肉芽组织即逐渐新生而粘连愈合,不致使直肠环同时割断而失去括约的作用(由于橡皮圈对局部组织之刺激作用而产生纤维性粘连,使勒开之肌纤维仍留于原来位置,不致收回,故不易造成肛门失禁的危险)。其掉线时间以人为拉紧橡皮筋松紧为度,拉象皮筋过紧的则掉下快(3~5天),也易损伤肛门括约肌。拉橡皮筋再回送3cm再结扎,让其稍松,勒割掉下则慢些,8~10天,这是正常的,才不会损伤括约肌。

2. **The Method of Incision and Seton** The complicated anal fistula, of internal opening being above rectal ring easily causes residual syndrome of incontinence. The mechanism of the method meets a basic principle and criterion to treat anorectal fistula through incision and drainage of internal opening, external opening and fistulous track, improving granulation to arrive at aim of healing. According to this method to treat complicated anal fistula above rectal ring: if the fistula is high in relation to the anorectal ring, the rectal ring should be cut, this is an important problem. The modern medicine carries on that a two-stage procedure may be indicated for preventing anal sphincteric incontinence. This book carries on the method is that incision and setons drain through by small curving probing scalpel in the high position, the course of treatment by the method of small scalpel is short time. At present the method is a better treating high positional complicated anal fistula, all fistulous tracks which internal opening is below rectal ring should be cut. The fistulous track which internal opening is above rectal ring should be taken rubber band seton (can't be cut out). A seton of a rubber band is placed around the sphincter muscle through its elastic construction stimulates fibrosis adjacent to the sphincter muscle, the rubber band tightens into deep internal opening and track (through rectal ring). The rubber band makes the touching tissues produce ischemic necrosis so that it takes all tissues of internal opening and track (including rectal ring) unroofing gradually, because the rubber band continues to tighten to form the pressure reaction. When anterior tissues are opened, the posterior tissues having been opened forming new granulation tissues to adhere and heal gradually. These won't lead to cut off the rectal ring so that the sphincters still keep their function. (The rubber band stimulates local tissues to produce adjacent fibrosis, the muscle having been opened keeps still the original position, does not lose its reaction, so all won't lead to the risk of incontinence and won't injure the anal sphincter muscles). Use of seton in high fistula, a seton of rubber band is inserted into the fistulous track and tied loosely over the sphincter to create fibrosis. The fistulous track will be laid open in the second stage 6 to 8 weeks later.

3. **挂双线**　即将橡皮筋和丝线同时挂线。丝线松弛时,则再结扎紧橡皮筋,待一同脱掉。免去再次麻醉结扎或切断丝线。

3. **Two Setons**　The rubber band and silk thread take setons at the same time, helping each other.

4. **探针小弯刀疗法**　可将探查切开和挂线,同步完成,即将直肠环以下的肛瘘用小弯刀切开,而直肠环以上的肛瘘内口,用探针头,挂橡皮圈。故伤口愈合快,因瘘管不切除、不缝合。只将瘘管前壁切开,其瘘管后壁,则会演变肉芽组织,往上生长而愈合。无并发症,无肛门瘢痕沟,无肛门溢液。

4. **Treating Method With Small Curving Probing Scalpel**　To take the synchronous accomplishment with probing, incision and seton, these are that the small curving scalpel cuts unroofing the anal fistulous track below rectal ring, the top end of probe handing rubber band treats the anal fistulous internal opening above rectal ring. The method will not cause complications such as incontinence, stricture of anus and draining liquid.

5. **挂线疗法的发展**　挂线疗法治疗肛瘘。经过 2 次改动,第 1 次是将药线或丝线改为有弹力的橡皮筋,而解决了频繁紧线,并使挂线时间变得可以随意控制;第 2 次是采用低位切开、高位挂线的中西医结合方法,可以缩短疗程,减轻患者痛苦。

5. **Development of Seton**　The treatment of anal fistula has been changed twice. The first is that medical thread or silk thread being changed to elastic rubber band to resolve tightening the thread frequently. The second is that the method of integrated traditional Chinese medicine and modern medicine takes incision for low position anal fistula, seton for high position. The course of treatment by this method is short time.

随着医学发展,尤其西医学解剖学、生理学与中医学的结合,切开与挂线部位有了定位,即肛门复杂瘘的肛门直肠环以下,给予切开,不会造成大便失禁。其挂线只挂在肛门直肠环上或其深部肛门括约肌。这样不但减轻痛苦,缩短疗程,也提高中西医结合的疗效。

According to the development of medicine, especially integrated modern anatomy, physiology and traditional Chinese medicine, there is a distinct position for the method of incision and seton, that is taking incision to treat the complicated anal fistula below anorectal ring, seton treating above anorectal ring or deep sphincter muscles, won't cause anal incontinence. The course of treatment by this method not only reduces pain and shortens time but also improves curative effect.

第五节　肛　裂
§ 5　Anal Fissure

肛裂,如《医宗金鉴》所载:"肛门围绕,折纹破裂,便结者火燥也,初服止痛如神渴消解之。"即指肛裂是由于某些原因造成肛管皮肤损伤而形成的溃疡(图 6 - 61)。在内括约肌紧缩状态下,此溃疡呈裂隙状,排便时肛管扩张,则呈椭圆形创面,故久不愈合。

Anal fissure, such as speaking from < YiZongJinJian > : "The dermatologic break up around the anus, the patients with constipation are observed commonly. The initial disease can be treated by taking analgesic drug." Anal fissure is a tear of the skin-lined part of the anal canal to form inflammation and ulcer. A tight anal sphincter observed in this patient to make the fissure is also ellipse as defecation, so it's difficult to heal(Fig. 6 - 61).

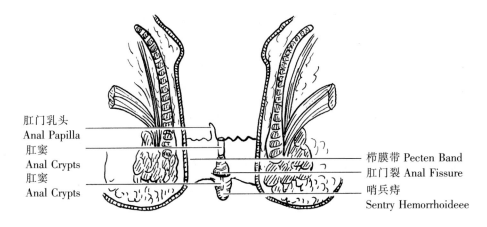

肛门乳头 Anal Papilla
肛窦 Anal Crypts
肛窦 Anal Crypts
栉膜带 Pecten Band
肛门裂 Anal Fissure
哨兵痔 Sentry Hemorrhoideee

图 6 - 61　肛门裂

Figure 6 - 61　Anal Fissure

【病因病机】

[Etiology and Pathology]

中医认为肛裂发生的原因和病机,是由于外感六淫,内伤七情,饮食不节等引起便燥火结(大便干燥或秘结);又因局部解剖的某些缺陷,致使肛管皮肤遭受损伤,形成溃疡。

In traditional Chinese medicine it is explained that etiology and pathology of anal fissure result from six kinds of bad external causes, seven kinds of internal feeling, eating and drinking without temperance, etc., to cause dry stool or constipation; another reason is some local anatomical defect so to injure the skin of anal canal easily to form ulcer.

1. **局部解剖缺陷**　肛门外括约肌从尾骨起向下至肛门后部开始分为两部分,沿肛门两则向前围绕肛门,到肛门前方连在一起(图 6 - 62)。因此,在肛门前后各留有三角空隙,同时肛门两侧有提肛门肌附着,因而肛门前后不如两侧坚固,一旦损伤,容易引起裂口感染。

1. **Local Anatomical Defect**　External anal sphincter muscle has circular and ellipse fascicles

from the tip of the coccyx towards anterior and inferior, then inserts into the posterior of anal canal, and divides into two parts, looping around the lower part of the anal canal on two sides, arrives at the anterior of the anus and syncretism forming one (Fig. 6 – 62). So there is a triangle gap in anterior and posterior of anus separately while there are levator ani muscles in the two sides of anus, so the anterior and posterior parts are not stronger than two sides, and they are easy to induce infection in the gap once being injured.

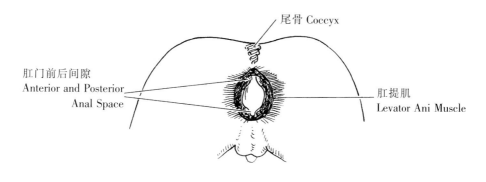

图 6 – 62　外括约肌

Figure 6 – 62　External sphincter

2. 肛管直肠位置的影响　肛管向下向后,与直肠形成一个角度,排便时,肛门后部受粪便压力较重,加之肛管后部血运较差,弹力较小,容易引起创伤,且不易愈合。

2. Positional Influence of Anal Canal and Rectum　Anal canal goes downwards and backwards to form an angle with the rectum. The relatively immobile skin overlying the posterior area and the angulation of the anal canal cause the stool to traumatize the fissure-bearing area.

3. 便秘　由于里热炽盛,排出的粪块又粗又硬,可反复损伤肛管皮肤,以致长期不能愈合。

3. Constipation　Hard and thick stool stimulates the skin on anal canal frequently. Fissure is the result of repeated trauma to the fissure-bearing area. Anal pressure studies have provided conflicting findings. A tight anal sphincter observed in these patients makes it logical to assume that defecation stimulates the sensitive fissure and causes severe reflex spasm. This would draw the anal canal cephalad during anal contraction, and the stool traumatizes the fissure repeatedly.

4. 其他疾病的影响　如妇女生产多、白带刺激过多,以及肛门狭窄、肛门乳头炎、肛窦炎、直肠炎、梅毒等,也易引起肛管损伤,形成肛裂。异物刺伤也能引起肛裂。

4. Other Diseases　Labor or having given birth more times, leukorrhea multiple stimulation, anal stricture, inflammation of anal papillae, anal sinusitis, rectitis, syphilis, and foreign body, etc. all traumatizes anal canal to form fissure.

5. 栉膜带影响　因为肛窦、乳头经常发炎充血,极易引起纤维组织增生,在肛管内形成栉膜带的纤维化。栉膜带位于黏膜下层内、齿线与白线之间,宽 0.8 ~ 1.2cm,覆被有移行上皮,缺乏弹力,使肛管经常保持紧缩状态,妨碍括约肌的松弛。

5. Pecten Band Anal crypts and papillae often cause inflammation and congestion so as to fiber, hyperplasia, and to make fibers of pecten band. It is between dentate line above and white line below, about 0.8 ~ 1.2cm gray white round band. It's covered with transitional epithelium, and connected closely to deep tissues. This area is not supplied by nerves, and no stretch, but it often keeps constriction, so it interferes with relaxation of sphincter muscles, that's why the anal fissure is not easily healed.

【临床表现】

[Clinical Manifestations]

1.疼痛 疼痛轻重和时间长短,因体质强弱及裂口大小、病期久暂、创口深浅而不同。疼痛多为阵发性,常因解大便而引起。在排便时(尤其是大便干燥时候),裂口内的感觉神经纤维被刺激而引起疼痛,持续数分钟至半小时后疼痛即可缓解,此后进入疼痛间歇期(图 6-63)。约半小时后,因肛门内括约肌痉挛收缩,遂又出现更为强烈的疼痛,常持续半小时至 10 余小时,以致坐卧不安,十分痛苦,直到括约肌因疲劳而弛缓(痉挛停止),疼痛始逐渐减轻。但在疼痛末期仍觉肛门部酸痛,此后疼痛才逐渐停止。病情严重者,在咳嗽、打喷嚏或排尿时,也会引起疼痛。疼痛有时可向骨盆及下肢等处放射。

1. Pain When the symptom is showing knife cut appearance to ache or burn defecate hind arrives several minutes later can be reduced more sorely or disappeared. Subsequently because anal constrictor is durative convulsion with acute ache, often can be alleviated continuously hours later (Fig. 6-63).

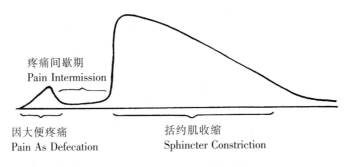

疼痛间歇期
Pain Intermission

因大便疼痛
Pain As Defecation

括约肌收缩
Sphincter Constriction

图 6-63 肛门裂疼痛间歇期图解

Figure 6-63 Diagram of intermission of anus fissure and pain

2.大便秘结 除机体内热炽盛引起便燥外,常因惧怕疼痛,想尽一切办法控制排便,如少吃饭或吃渣滓少的食物(如鸡蛋、肉类等),或有意控制便意,久之定会加重大便秘结的程度,使病情加重。

2. Constipation In traditional Chinese medicine it was thought that inner heat causes constipation. In addition, the patient may be afraid of pain, so thinks a lot to control defecation, for example to eat a little food or eat a little dross food (such as eggs, meat, etc.)or try to get the constipation passing long so with worse symptoms.

3. 出血 大量出血很少见。平时常见在大便后有几滴鲜血流出,或附于粪便上,或染红便纸;有时与黏液混合在一起排出。其原因是由于粪便损伤裂口底部的肉芽创面所致。

3. Bleeding The hemorrhage is a bleeding of little quantity or adhering to the surface of excrement, bright red color, with the result of stool traumatizing granulation wound below the anal fissure.

4. 肛门瘙痒 有时由裂口内流出分泌物(脓水)刺激肛门皮肤引起瘙痒,或由于长期刺激引起肛门周围湿疹。

4. Pruritus Ani The excrement (put with liquid) drained from anal fissure stimulates the skin of anus to cause pruritus, or eczema around the anus because of long time stimulation, and eczema exaggerates pruritus.

5. 并发肛瘘 裂口处感染,使前哨痔形成脓肿,溃破后可以成为肛瘘。其瘘管比较浅,治疗肛裂时可以一并切除。

5. Complicating Anal Fistula Inflammation of split makes the sentry hemorrhoid forming abscess, which breaks up to form anal fistula. The fistulous track is shallow, and can be cut off with anal fissure in operation.

【诊断】

[Diagnosis]

1. 定型诊断

1. Types

(1)燥火型:脉象多为弦紧或弦数;舌苔黄薄,舌边发赤;局部多为单纯肛裂或复杂肛裂,没有炎症。

(1) Dryness: Pulses are mainly rapid or string; tongue fur is yellow thin, the edge of the tongue is red. The type is simple or complicated anal fissure without inflammation.

(2)热毒型:脉象多为洪数或弦数;舌苔黄厚,舌质发赤;局部多为肛裂并有较重感染,或因前哨痔发炎及脓肿形成。

(2) Pyretic toxicity: Pulses are mainly bounding or string; red tongue with yellow thick fur; it is anal fissure with severe infection, or inflammation of sentry hemorrhoid and abscess.

2.分类诊断

2. Categorization

(1)单纯肛裂:肛外没有前哨痔,裂口(溃疡),其边软,底浅(图6-64)。

(1)Simple anal fissure:There isn't sentry hemorrhoid, split (ulcer); the edge is soft, and the bottom shallow(Fig. 6-64).

(2)复杂肛裂:溃疡深大,底部呈灰白色,周围有炎性浸润哨痔出现(图6-65)。

(2)Complicated anal fissure:The ulcer is deep and big; the bottom is gray colored; there is inflamed infiltrating sentry hemorrhoid(Fig. 6-65).

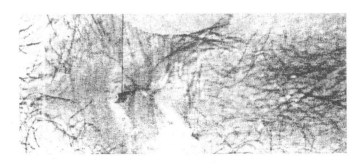

图6-64 单纯肛裂

Figure 6-64 Simple anal fissure

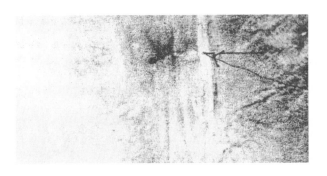

图6-65 复杂肛裂

Figure 6-65 Complicated anal fissure

【治疗】

[Treatment]

1.整体治疗原则

1. Systemic Treatment

(1)燥火型:以清热润便为主,常用脏连丸、麻仁滋脾丸。

(1)Dryness:Clear heat and lubricate stool mainly, take common pills of ZangLianWan and pills of MaRenZiPiWan.

（2）热毒型：以清热解毒为主，常用仙方活命饮、消肿止痛汤等药物。

（2）Pyretic toxicity：Clear heat and relieve toxin mainly，take common decoction of XianFang-HuoMingYin and decoction of XiaoZhongZhiTongTang.

2. 局部治疗原则
2. Local Treatment

（1）单纯性肛裂：适合简易疗法，外敷痔裂膏。小针刀钩切法、局部封闭疗法（以 1% 普鲁卡因与亚甲蓝液 5～10ml 注入裂口基底周围）。

（1）Simple anal fissure：For simple treating，put cream on the wound. Hooking and cutting by acupuncture scalpel，with local anesthesia（1% procaine adding up methylene blue 5～10ml injected around the bottom of split）.

（2）复杂肛裂：小针刀挑割结扎法。

（2）Complicated anal fissure：Pricking，cutting and ligation by acupuncture scalpel.

3. 简易疗法　单纯肛裂可以临床治愈，复杂肛裂可以减轻症状。
3. Simple Treatment　The objectives of treatment are to reduce pain and associated sphincter spasm.

（1）调理大便：排便是否正常与肛裂关系十分密切，如大便干燥可使病情加重。故每天应多吃蔬菜及容易消化的食物；大便干燥时应服缓泻药润肠汤或通便粉以保持大便稀软。

（1）To regulate defecation：The defecation has a confidential relationship with anal fissure，dry stool can aggravate the disease. The treatment includes stool lubricants，bulk stool softeners，such as Psyllium seed，vegetables and increased fluid intake，etc.，taking laxative drug to correct the constipation problem.

（2）局部处理：患者自己可以用温开水或止痒汤、去肿汤、中药等熏洗肛门，每日 2 次（病轻者可每日或隔日 1 次）。熏洗后用示指（带指套或用棉球）将痔裂膏涂于肛门裂口处。

（2）Local management ：Warm baths by water or decoction for comfort twice a day（mild disease，one time per-day or two days），or smearing cream on the anal fissure（ with glove or cotton ball）.

4. 小针刀挑割结扎疗法
4. Pricking，Cutting and Ligation by Acupuncture Scalpel

（1）适应证：①复杂肛裂底深，边硬且不整齐，缺乏弹力，外有前哨痔和齿线上有发炎的乳头者;②单纯肛裂经简易疗法治疗无效者。

(1)Indication:①In complicated anal fissure, the triad consists of deep bottom, disorder edges, inelasticity, sentinel, pile, or inflamed papillae may be present;②Simple anal fissure invalidly treated by simple treatment.

(2)禁忌证:①体弱或合并有严重心脏病、高血压及其他急性传染病者;②肛门局部有明显感染及正在患腹泻或痢疾等病者,暂缓手术。

(2)Contraindication:①Weak complicating severe heart diseases, high blood pressure or acute infectious disease;②Obvious infection around anus or diarrhea, dysentery, operation should be stopped temporarily.

(3)操作方法:局部常规消毒后,于裂口周围及基底部注射1%普鲁卡因4～10ml。麻醉后扩开肛门。肛器检查裂口的大小、位置,及上方齿线处有无发炎乳头。随后用止血钳子将肛裂下端两侧合并一同提起,用小针刀沿肛裂底部将前哨痔及肛裂挑割。其上方如有肛窦、发炎乳头,也一并提起在齿线下部用丝线结扎(图6-66)。然后将裂处的栉膜带纵行切开,并切断一部分外括约肌皮下纤维,使其呈扇面形(图6-67)。最后用枣核形棉球蘸痔瘘粉填入伤口,以压迫止血,用纱布包好,用橡皮膏固定。

(3)Procedures:Sterilization as usual, to inject 1% procaine 4～10ml, enlarge anus after anesthesia. The doctor checks up the anal fissure with anoscope the shape, position, and whether inflamed papillae in the dentate line above anus or not. By hemostatic forceps he holds up the two sides of anal fissure together, pricks and cuts anal fissure and sentinel pile along the bottom of fissure by acupuncture scalpel. If there are anal sinusitis and inflamed papillae the doctor holds up together to ligate them with silk thread below dentate line (Fig. 6-66). He cuts vertically pecten band of split, and cuts off some subcutaneous fibers of external sphincter to form sector(Fig. 6-66). Finally the doctor fills a date pit shape cotton ball in the wound, with powder of medicine to press stopping hemorrhage, then binds up the wound with gauze, fixes it with sticking plaster.

5. 小针刀钩切疗法
5. Hooking and Cutting by Acupuncture Scalpel

(1)适应证:单纯肛裂。

(1)Indication:Simple anal fissure.

(2)操作方法:骶裂孔阻滞麻醉或局麻。①小针刀内括约肌切断术:术者先用左手示指插入肛管内1.5cm确定括约肌间沟的位置,其上缘即为内括约肌,给予固定。右手持肛肠斜面小针刀从肛门外3点钟位或9点钟位点状局麻针眼插入,在肛管内以左手示指引导下隔着肛管左手示指尖摸到小针刀顶端,随着右手持斜面小针刀,两手指同时上下配合纵行切开内括约肌1.5～2cm,切勿横切,刺穿肛管腔,拔出小针刀,术毕(图6-68的1)。②小针刀肛裂钩切开术:圆头缺口电池灯肛门镜下,用钩状小针刀将肛裂上端肛窦、肛瓣纵行钩割,并下延其肛裂溃疡面下纤维化栉膜带至肛门外缘(图6-68的2和3)钩割开。并于其上伤口与周围呈扇形注入亚甲蓝长效止痛药,外敷生皮膏纱布。

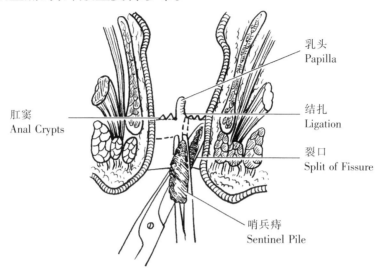

图 6-66 复杂肛裂小针刀挑割结扎疗法,将裂口、前哨痔乳头一并挑割至齿线结扎

Figure 6-66 Treating complicated anal fissure with pricking, cutting and ligation, to prick and cut anal fissure and sentinel pile together till dentate line then ligate

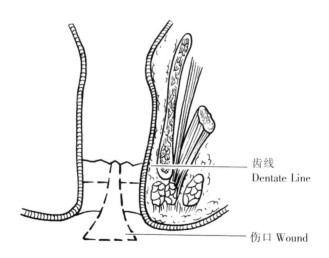

图 6-67 扇面形伤口

Figure 6-67 Fanshaped wound

(2)Procedures:To take sacral histus block anesthesia or local anesthesia. ①Cutting internal sphincter by acupuncture scalpel:The doctor's left index finger inserts into anal canal 1.5cm to define and feel the position of intersphincteric ditch, its upper fringe is the internal sphincter, and to fix the internal sphincter. His right hand handles the inclined plane acupuncture scalpel to insert into internal sphincter from local anesthetic points of outside of anus at 3 or 9 o'clock position and with the guidance of his left index finger tip touching the top of acupuncture scalpel, then his right hand handles the inclined plane acupuncture scalpel to insert into internal sphincter, and cuts vertically internal sphincter 1.5 ~ 2cm. Don't cut it horizontally. The acupuncture scalpel punctures anal canal and then the doctor pulls the acupuncture scalpel out, this operation ends (1 of Fig. 6 – 68). ②Hooking and cutting anal fissure by acupuncture scalpel: In using optical anoscope the hook style acupuncture scalpel hooks and cuts anal crypts above anal fissure, anal valves vertically and downwards cutting fibrotic pecten band below ulcer of anal fissure until outer of the anus (2 and 3 of Fig. 6 – 68). The wound is then bound up with gauze.

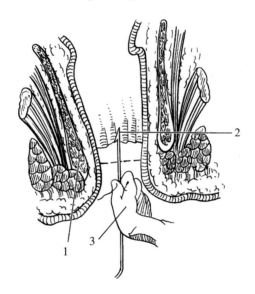

图 6 – 68　肛裂小针刀疗法
1 – 切断内括约肌;2 – 钩开肛窦;3 – 手指持钩状小针刀
Figure 6 – 68　Acupuncture scalpel treating anal fissure
1. Internal sphincterotomy;2. Hook out anal crypt;
3. Finger handles hook style acupuncture scalpel

【点评】
[Review]

1. 小针刀切断内括约肌的意义
1. Significance of Internal Sphincterotomy by Acupuncture Scalpel

(1)解除内括约肌痉挛:由于松解了肛管"外箍"紧缩,可促进肛裂溃疡面愈合。

(1) To relieve internal sphincter spasm: Relaxing outer shroud ring of anal canal to improve the healing of ulcer of anal fissure.

（2）降低肛管压力,利于肛管静脉血液、淋巴液回流通畅,减轻肛门水肿。

（2）To reduce the anal pressure:Taking helpful drainage from venous blood and lymph to decrease local edema.

（3）缓解疼痛,加速肛裂愈合。

（3）To ease pain, to accelerate healing of anal fissure.

2. 内括约肌解剖生理特点
2. Anatomical and Physical Features of Internal Sphincter

（1）内括约肌是直肠环肌层的延续,上界平肛管直肠肌环平面,下达括约肌间沟,高度为 2.32cm 左右,下端肥厚形成一条清楚的环状游离缘,居齿线以下 1.0～1.5cm。

（1）The internal sphincter is the terminal portion of the circular muscle coat of the rectum. Its upper fringe is anal canal rectal ring plane, passing downwards till ditch of intersphincter; the height is about 2.32cm; its inferior end thickens to form an obvious ring below dentate line 1.0~1.5cm.

（2）内括约肌具有消化道环肌层固有特性,属内脏神经,支配少许能量则长期易痉挛;持续性痉挛可使肌组织结构改变易致肛裂。

（2）The internal sphincter owns the inherent feature of circular muscle of alimentary tract. The anal fissure may be due to an abnormality of the internal sphincter, or sphincter spasm.

（3）内括约肌,除有机械性关闭肛门作用外,还有参与外括约肌的随意性抑制作用,故不能完全切除,只能切断内括约肌。

（3）The internal sphincter participates in optional inhibiting action of external sphincter, so it should not be cut completely.

3. 肛管内的肛裂溃疡　　其下纤维化栉膜带钩开,松解内箍。
3. Ulcer of Anal Fissure in Anal Canal　Hooking fibrotic pectin band below anal fissure open, relaxing shoulder ring.

4. 肛窦病灶　　钩开,引流后可治愈。
4. Anal Crypts Diseases　Hooking and drainage can cure the lesion.

第六节　其他肛周疾病

§6　Other Anal Diseases

一、肛窦炎

Ⅰ. Anal Sinusitis

肛管内肛窦发炎可引起肛门内疼痛,排粪便时加重。有的可伴低热。

The inflammation of anal crypts in anal channel can lead to pain, even more pain during defecation, sometimes according to low fever.

【病因病机】

[Etiology and Pathology]

肛窦炎,又称肛隐窝炎。因为肛窦位于齿线,窦口位底向下,开口呈袋状,所以易损伤,引流不畅。肛窦边缘又有游离的半月形的肛瓣,容易受到干燥的粪块擦伤或撕裂。如果腹泻频频刺激肛窦和肛瓣也容易发炎;如果粪便或异物存积肛窦,因肛窦腺分泌液引流不畅,利于病菌在肛窦繁殖引起肛窦炎。

Anal sinusitis is also called the infection of crypts. Because anal crypts are at dentate line, and vertical with upward mouths and downward bases, like bags, the contents aren't easy to be drained. In addition, there are free semilunar valves in the anal crypts, so that the valves are easy to be bruised and teared by dry stool; frequent diarrhea stimulates anal crypts and valves to cause inflammation easily; it is possible to multiply bacteria to cause the sinusitis if the stool or foreign body save in the anal crypts meanwhile the glands of anal crypts can't secrete and drain.

【临床表现】

[Clinical Manifestations]

肛窦慢性期,肛内有轻微隐痛、坠胀、不适感;急性期常伴疼痛如肛管内刺痛、撕裂痛,严重者因刺激骶神经引起臀部、会阴部放射痛。

In the chronic stage of anal sinusitis it shows mild secret anguish at the side of anus, giving a feeling of swelling and falling. In the acute stage it shows pain such as tingle, bursting pain in the anal canal; in the severe stage it stimulates sacral nerve to lead to sciatic coxal pain, radiated pain in the perineum.

【诊断】

[Diagnosis]

根据病史和临床检查。

According to history and clinical examination.

1. **肛门检查** 于齿线附近触及凹陷,硬结触痛明显。

1. **Anal Examination** To touch the crypts and hard nodes and to have obvious pain near dentate line.

2. **肛镜检查** 肛窦、肛瓣充血水肿,有脓性分泌物。

2. **Anoscopic Examination** There are congestive edema and purulent secretion in anal crypts and valves.

【鉴别诊断】

[Differential Diagnosis]

应与肛门瘘内口鉴别,如有瘘管,可沿走行触及,尤其要与瘘的内口区别,必要时用钩针探查。

The internal opening of anal fistula can feel the track along fistulous aim while can be checked up with probe.

【治疗】

[Treatment]

1. **切开引流** 肛窦一旦发炎化脓应切开,但切口不宜过大,否则易出血,愈合慢。

1. **Incision and Drainage** The anal crypts should be cut once they inflames and suppurates, however the incision shouldn't be big or they aren't easy to heal.

2. **钩状小针刀疗法** 在圆头缺口电池肛门镜下,应用0.5%利多卡因加亚甲蓝液1支,肛窦周围,即齿线下组织局部注射。然后,右手持钩状小针刀,将肛窦及炎性肛瓣呈爪形钩割开,创口敷痔瘘粉,棉球压敷后拔出肛门小针刀及肛门镜即可。术后肛门内注入九华膏,口服甲硝唑,并照常吃饭排便。

2. **Hook Style Acupuncture Scalpel Treatment** With the optical anoscope the doctor injects 0.5% lidocaine and methylene blue into perianal crypts (below dentate line). The right hand handles the hook style acupuncture scalpel to hook and cut anal crypts and inflamed anal valves to change unguiform, then pulls out acupuncture scalpel and anoscope after the doctor presses cotton ball, and squeezes the drug's cream into anus. The patient takes metronidazole, eating, drinking and defecation as usual after operation.

二、肛门潮湿综合征

Ⅱ. Anal Moist Syndrome

以肛门潮湿、肛门周围皮肤瘙痒为主要表现。

Main symptoms are anal moisture and pruritus.

【病因病机】

[Etiology and Pathology]

肛门内肛窦炎或肛管内瘘炎症分泌物外溢,引起肛门潮湿和瘙痒。

Secretion coming from drainage of anal sinusitis or fistula leads to anal moisture and pruritus.

【临床表现】

[Clinical Manifestations]

肛门周围皮肤潮湿、瘙痒;伴发炎症则疼痛。从肛门内溢出黏液或炎性分泌物,常有排便不畅或排便不尽感。

The moist and pruritic skin around anal region, and the patient feels pain accompanying with inflammation. The inflamed secretion and mucus in the anus make incomplete defecation frequently.

【诊断】

[Diagnosis]

根据肛门潮湿、瘙痒病史,肛指检查:肛窦或肛管内有瘘口,有硬结或内陷。肛门镜检查见肛管齿线、肛窦红肿,或肛瘘内口有分泌物外溢。

Diagnosis can be made according to history of anal moisture and pruritus and clinical examination. As anal digital examination, the doctor can touch the crypts and hard nodes and fistulous track and internal opening. As anoscopy checking up, the doctor can see inflamed anal crypts, the secretion from fistulous internal opening near by dentate line.

【治疗】

[Treatment]

(1)口服中药和熏洗肛门,如口服利湿止痒汤,另用止痒汤外洗(详见相关内容)。

(1)Taking herbs and fuming and bathing in plain warm herbs' water, such as taking the decoction of LiShiZhiYangTang (relieving, infiltrating mositure, and stopping itching) and bathing in warm herbs' water of stopping itching (Refer to Chapter 14).

（2）钩状小针刀疗法（详见"肛窦炎"）。

（2）Methods hook style acupuncture scalpel treatment（Refer to "anal sinusitis"）.

三、肛门瘙痒症
Ⅲ. Pruritus Ani

【病因病机】

［Etiology and Pathology］

肛门周围皮下神经末梢受到刺激，肛门出现刺痒，肛门瘙痒症十分顽固，不易治愈。体力活动较少者居多。其发病原因复杂，常不易找到确切的致病因素。中医认为，由风邪引起；现代医学认为，发病原因有以下几种。

Pruritus ani is a common problem occuring in persons lack of physical exercise, but a difficult one to solve. The perianal area is sensitive, and condition causing soiling or moisture to stimulate nerve endings of the area can induce itching. The cause is complex, no precise ones are found, and can be very difficultly treated. In traditional Chinese medicine it is believed that the wind leads to the disease, while the modern medicine thinks that there are some causes as follows.

1. **分泌物刺激**　多数因患肛瘘、痔疮、肛裂、肛窦炎等，使肛门周围经常受到分泌物的刺激而引起。

1. **Stimulation of Secretion**　Thc surgically correctable conditions contributing to this condition are anal fistula, hemorrhoids, anal fissure, anal sinusitis, etc.. They make anal region be stimulated by secretion frequently, so all cause the disease.

2. **寄生虫**　如蛲虫、阴虱等寄生虫在局部引起瘙痒。

2. **Pinworm**　Enterobius vermicularis(in children) and crab louse are the common causes to lead to local pruritus.

3. **皮肤病**　如湿疹、毛囊炎、湿疣等。

3. **Dermatosis**　eczema, folliculitis, condyloma, etc.

4. **便纸太硬、局部不洁、经常摩擦（内衣太紧）等**　均可以引起肛门瘙痒。一般由于寄生虫或真菌寄生所引起的瘙痒虽不多见，但比较顽固，治愈比较困难。

4. **Toilet Paper Being Hard**, **Local Uncleanness**, **Frequent Local Friction**（**Underclothes Being Too Tight**）, **etc.**　All factors can cause pruritus ani. The cause resulting from pinworm or epiphyte is a not common, but a difficult problem to cure.

【临床表现】

[Clinical Manifestations]

主要是肛门周围瘙痒,有的长期瘙痒,不间歇;有的时好时坏,或轻或重,非常苦恼。一般多是日轻夜重,故影响睡眠和休息。严重者因瘙痒不止,以致坐卧不宁,精神紧张。日久,可使身体衰弱。初起不久,局部可有红色斑点或丘疹,或始终无明显改变。但时间较久,皮肤多增厚变硬,呈灰白色。有的肛门两侧有丘疹,触之即可诱发瘙痒加剧。有的患者瘙痒可由局部蔓延至会阴及前阴部。

The main symptom is pruritus, sometimes long time, sometimes short, sometimes mild, sometimes severe, so it is afflicting to the patient. Pruritus may be mild in day and severe at night, influencing sleep and rest. Severe pruritus may lead to restlessness and psychosis. The patient will be weak if the pruritus lasts a long time. At the initial stage of the pruritus, the skin shows red spots or pimples, or no obvious changes. With the time flies, the skin changes thick, hard and off white. Touching the pimple can induce pruritus very much. Some pruritus can spread over to perineum.

【诊断】

[Diagnosis]

根据症状和局部情况,可以做出诊断。临床常见的瘙痒多继发于肛瘘、肛裂或肛门周围皮肤发炎,由刺激引起。

According to symptoms and local signs, the doctor can make a diagnosis. The common clinical pruritus is mainly secondary conditions, such as anal fistula, fissure and inflammation of skin.

【治疗】

[Treatment]

1. **一般治疗**　局部保持清洁,大便后用温开水及肥皂水洗净肛门,或用热水坐浴,或用中药止痒汤熏洗,每日 2 次。洗后局部涂用甲紫、痔裂膏或收湿膏,然后包扎。同时内服利湿止痒汤,每日 1 剂。另外,衣裤不要太紧;忌食有刺激性食物,如辣椒、芥末等,最好不吃鱼、蟹、虾等海味;应停止吸烟、饮酒,每日多喝开水;神经过敏者可服用镇静药。

1. **General Method**　The patient should keep clean locally. After defecation, he should rinse and wash the anal region with warm water or soap, or tub bathing in warm water, or fuming in herbal decoction of stopping itching, twice every day. One may smear drug after cleaning, meanwhile to take the decoction of LiShiZhiYangTang (relieving, infiltrating moisture, and stopping itching), a dose every day. In addition, the patient should not wear very tight clothes, forbidden eating stimulating food, such as chili, mustard, etc.; don't eat marine food products, such as fish, crab, prawn, etc.; stop smoking and drinking. The patients can drink more boiled water ev-

ery day; take sedative as neurotic.

2. 斜面小针刀悬浮疗法
2. Suspended Method with Inclined Plane Acupuncture Scalpel Treating

（1）采用长效麻药肛门周围局部浸润麻醉,再用小针刀做肛门周围皮下切割。

（1）Carrying on local infiltration anesthesia in anal region, then acupuncture scalpel cut subcutaneous tissue around anus.

（2）用甲紫将肛门瘙痒区域或范围画出。右侧卧位,常规消毒。选择尾骨尖至肛门瘙痒区之间的中点进针。将0.5%利多卡因18ml加亚甲蓝液2ml,滴入肾上腺素2滴摇匀后,进行肛门周围皮肤下浸润麻醉。右手持小针刀仍从麻醉进针处刺入皮肤,深达皮下组织。勿深入脂肪层。在肛外左示指触摸引导下,小针刀先向肛门左上侧倾斜,并潜行性缓慢切割肛周皮下组织呈扇形面,向外超过瘙痒区2cm,向内达肛门缘,向前达会阴部。切勿穿破肛周皮肤及肛管。退回小针刀,并将刀锋改为反向而紧贴肛周皮肤的内面,边搔刮边退出小针刀进针处、退出体外。同法治疗肛门右下侧,倾斜切割,并于会阴部会合,完成肛周皮肤及皮下组织的游离术（图6-69）。

（2）Drawing the region of pruritus, with the patient lying on the side, sterilizing as usual. In the middle point between the tip of coccyx and the fringe of anal pruritus, the doctor takes local infiltration anesthesia with 0.5% lidocaine 18ml with methylene blue 2 ml and dripping epinephrine 2 drops shaking up. His right hand handles the acupuncture scalpel to insert into skin and subcutaneous tissue from local anesthetic points, not to reach the fat layer. With the guidance of his left index finger touching the top of acupuncture scalpel, then his right hand handles the acupuncture scalpel to insert and to sneak into subcutaneous tissue slowly, and cut the tissue around anus to form sector from beginning at upper left inclined position to outside over the region of pruritus 2cm, to inner part reaching at anal fringe, to inferior part reaching at perineum, not to penetrate perianal skin and anal canal. And then the doctor pulls back the acupuncture scalpel, lets the edge of scalpel to cling the inner plane of perianal skin, takes acupuncture scalpel shaving at the same time going out from the position of going in. The same method treats anal inferior right region, inclines to cut till meeting at perineum, and to complete dissociation operation(Fig. 6 - 49).

【点评】
[Review]

（1）肛门瘙痒症,有长效亚甲蓝液封闭麻醉,因亚甲蓝可亲和神经细胞,麻痹神经末梢,而止痒。

（1）The subcutaneous injection of anesthetic treats pruritus ani.

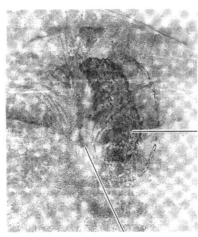

斜面小针刀呈
扇形皮下切割
Inclined Plane
Acupuncture Scalpel
Sectorial Cutting
in Subcutanea

肛门 Anus

图 6 – 69　肛门瘙痒症斜面小针刀疗法

Figure 6 – 69　Inclined plane acupuncture scalpel treating pruritus ani

（2）小针刀闭合切断瘙痒区皮下神经,而止痒。

（2）Acupuncture scalpel cuts off subcutaneous nerves of pruritus region closely so as to stop pruritus.

（3）小针刀是闭合治疗,是针眼手术,故可以多次治疗,无后遗症,无伴发症。

（3）Acupuncture scalpel is closed treatment and needle eye surgery, so it can be done many times with no sequelae or complications.

四、肛周大汗腺病

Ⅳ. Perianal Large Sudoriferous Gland Disease

肛周汗腺感染可反复发作、蔓延,呈慢性炎症,甚至形成小脓肿腔、窦道或瘘管,经久不愈,并有可能恶变。Jackman 报道发生率为 3.2%。

The infection of perianal large sudoriferous gland can take place repeatedly, spreading and forming chronic inflammation, even forming a small abscess or fistula. It's a difficult disease to cure, and easy to form cancer, with a rate of 3.2% according to Jackman's report.

【病因病机】

[Etiology and Pathology]

病因复杂,与激素代谢异常有关。肛周汗腺、皮脂腺均开口于毛囊,一旦毛囊汗腺感染则蔓延扩散,形成脓腔、窦道、瘘管,或相互沟通反复感染,或波及臀部和会阴,破溃为穿掘性化脓,形成瘢痕。病原菌多为金黄色葡萄球菌和厌氧菌。

The etiology is complicated, somewhat related to metabolic disorder of hormone. All the sudoriferous and sebaceous gland around anal region open in hair follicles, once they are infected, they spread to form abscesses and fistulas, and communicate each other, being infected repeatedly. The infection can influence the hips and perineum; the abscesses can be broken up to drain pus; they can take place frequently to form scar. The main pathogenic bacteria are staphylococcus aureus and anaerobic bacteria.

【临床表现】

[Clinical Manifestations]

发热。肛周肿痛,汗腺毛囊红肿、硬结、破溃、流脓。

Fever, swelling pain in the perianal region, red and swelling in sudoriferous gland and hair follicles, hard nodes, breaking up, draining pus.

【诊断】

[Diagnosis]

肛周皮肤汗腺、毛囊反复发炎、溃烂,呈结节、条索状,形成瘢痕、皮下脓肿、窦道或瘘管,但肛管直肠内无病变,也无肛瘘内口。碘油造影可发生肛周皮下多发性、广泛性、慢性瘘管,但应与肛周疖肿、淋巴结或肛瘘等鉴别。

Repeated infection of perianal skin sudoriferous gland and hair follicles, and their breaking up, nodes, trabs, scar, subcutaneous abscesses, fistulas, no pathological changes at internal opening of fistula inside of anus and rectum. Iodide radiography can cause many complete chronic fistulous tracks in the perianal subcutaneous tissue but need to be differentiated from perianal furuncle, lymph nodes or anal fistula, etc.

【治疗】

[Treatment]

1. 全身治疗原则

1. Systemic Treatment

(1)抗感染:首选青霉素类。

(1) Anti-infection:The first chose is Penicillins.

(2)肾上腺皮质激素类治疗。

(2) Corticoids.

(3)抗雄性激素类:如环丙氯地孕酮。

(3) Antiandrogens:Such as Cyproterone acetate, etc.

(4)口服中药清热解毒汤。

(4)Taking the decoction of clearing heat and relieving toxin.

2. 中药外用　如中药祛毒汤熏洗,或中药消脓膏外敷。

2. Herbs for External Use　Such as fuming and steeping with decoction of QuDuTang, taking inunctum cream of XiaoNongGao.

3. 小针刀治疗　骶裂孔阻滞麻醉,碘伏消毒(图6-70)。

3. Acupuncture Scalpel Treatment

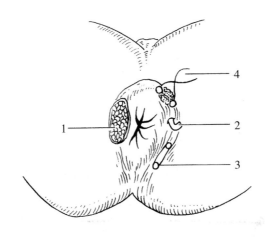

图6-70　肛周汗腺病小针刀疗法

1-斜面小针刀切割,变硬皮下组织;2-刮匙小针刀,搔刮窦道;

3-探针小弯刀,切开皮下瘘管;4-脓肿空腔,挂线引流过氧化氢冲洗空腔,外

敷消脓膏药

Figure 6-70　Acupuncture scalpel treating perianal sudoriferous gland disease

1. Inclined plane acupuncture scalpel cutting sclerosing subcutaneous tissue;

2. Curette acupuncture scalpel shaving the fistulous track;

3. Small curving probing scalpel cutting subcutaneous fistulous track;

4. Seton and drainage of the cavity of abscess

(1)探及瘘管:用探针小弯刀从前瘘口深入,在从后瘘口探出,顺之用弯刀割切开瘘管,敞开瘘管,外敷痔瘘粉中药和换药。

(1)Probing fistulas:The doctor handles small curving probing scalpel to insert from anterior fistulous opening, and to pull out from posterior fistulous opening, along the track to cut openly fistulous track by curving scalpel, then uses cream for external application.

(2)探及窦道:用刮匙小针刀将窦道搔刮,再用钩状小针刀将窦道钩割开。

(2)Probing fistulous track:The doctor handles curette acupuncture scalpel to shave the fistulous track, carries on hook style acupuncture scalpel to cut open the fistulous track.

(3)探及脓肿空腔:采用挂线探针从空腔底往顶端探出,即剪成人造2个洞口,然后挂粗丝线,从原路拔出,粗丝线置空腔中做引流丝圈。用过氧化氢冲洗空腔,外敷消脓膏药。

(3) Probing the cavity of abscess: The doctor takes the probe with thread to probe in from the bottom of the cavity and to pull out from its top, cuts to form two artificial holes, then hang seton of thick silk thread, pull back from original track with the thick silk thread using for seton drainage. Peroxide is made use of rinsing and washing the cavity, then cream is used.

(4)再于变硬的皮肤外缘的正常皮肤边缘插进斜面小针刀,将变硬的皮下组织,即达脂肪层前,潜行边切边搔刮组织至渗性出血,伤口只用消脓膏纱布敷上,痔瘘粉中药外敷即可。术后照常饮食,每天排大便后去肿汤,坐浴。外敷消脓膏纱布。

(4) The doctor handles small curving probing scalpel to insert from the fringe of normal skin near the fringe of changing hard skin into subcutaneous tissues above fat layer, to sneak in subcutaneous tissues associated with cutting and shaving to the place of oozing blood, then cover the wound with gauze or cream. After operation the patient eats as usual every day, take tub baths with QuZhongTang Decoction every day after defecation, then cover the wound with gauze or cream.

【点评】
[Review]

肛周化脓性汗腺炎,是由于肛周皮肤内汗腺感染所致,可反复发作转为慢性炎症,广泛蔓延,形成皮下脓腔、窦道或瘘管,经久不愈。采用脓肿腔挂线引流,促脓肿腔愈合后则可剪掉引流线圈;窦道采用搔刮割切开;瘘管采用割切开引流;变硬皮肤采用斜面小针刀皮下搔刮用过氧化氢冲洗,外敷痔瘘粉,消脓膏而治愈。首创小针刀疗法不损伤肛周皮肤。

Perianal suppurative hidradenitis results from infection of perianal skin sudoriferous gland, repeatedly taking place can lead to chronic inflammation. It spreads extensive wide range to form subcutaneous abscesses and fistulas, which are difficult to cure. The abscesses can be treated by seton drainage; the tracks can be opened by shaving and cutting; the fistula can be treated by incision and drainage; skinny scleroses can be treated by inclined plane acupuncture scalpel cutting and shaving sclerosmg subcutaneous tissue, then rinsing and washing with peroxide; then cover the wound with gauze or cream.

第七节 肛肠病激光小针刀疗法

§7 Using Laser Acupuncture Scalpel in Proctology

一、治疗机制

I . Mechanism of Treatment

激光探头制成的小针刀,是将激光光纤制成套管空心,然后与小针刀结合为载体,将光纤输入端准确深达。肛门内括约肌或病灶,使激光对其深部组织直接照射起到双重效果。即小针刀闭合切开深部病灶,探头可挂线,同时又可使激光对切开组织产生"凝固"止血、消炎作用,防治再"粘连";还可通过控制小针刀的进针方向,使光纤、光束顺利达到深部组织,避免激光传输过程中造成周围组织损害。

The acupuncture scalpel made of laser probe is that the laser optical fiber is made to form a tube, then combining with the acupuncture scalpel to lead the end of optical fiber to reach the exact position where the disease can be treated. The disease of anal internal sphincter can be directly shined and reach the deep tissue. It's that the acupuncture scalpel cuts deep focus, the probe hangs the thread meanwhile the laser carries on the tissue of incision to take part in "coagulation" and diminishing inflammation, to prevent "adhesion" again; the laser can control the direction of the acupuncture scalpel, making beam of optical fiber get to deep tissue lest surrounding tissues being traumatized in the course of laser communication.

采用不同激光聚光束功率密度,则可选用对组织的"汽化"切割或"碳化凝固作用"。

To carry on laser convergent pencil of rays with different power densities, to select and put to use "laser-coagulation and carbonification", tissue can be cut with "gasification".

1. CO_2 激光器　根据病理检查,采用不同量的激光,使距离、照射时间与被照射部位产生不同的效果。中、低度 CO_2 激光功率调至 $8 \sim 10W$,对组织可产生轻度碳化,至形成黄焦色的凝固膜为妥。

1. CO_2 Laser Optical Maser　According to pathological examination, the different laser doses, shiny distances and times, can make the different shiny effect for the same shiny position. CO_2 laser optical maser with middle and low power, with power regulated in $8 \sim 10W$, makes the tissue mild carbonificated, forming brown coagulation membrane.

2. **机械套管空心小针刀**　长 $5 \sim 6cm$,为激光束与组织的距离。激光探头与激光导线接头连接。

2. **Mechanical Bushing Cannula Acupuncture Scalpel**　Its length is 5 ~ 6cm, and the top of laser connects the wire.

3. **操作方法**　激光器开关采用脚踏式。脚踏开关即可发出激光束,并立即(如同电烧器一样)将深部病灶组织碳化为黄色凝固膜,穿透深度为 0.1 ~ 0.2mm,以小针刀切开与激光凝固同步完成为好。因疾病不同,要求激光作用的强度也不同。

3. **Method**　The power switch carries on foot-operated power switch. As stepping the switch, laser at once making the deep tissue carbonificated form brown coagulation membrane. Penetrable depth is 0.1 ~ 0.2mm. Incision with the scalpel and coagulation with laser should be synchronous. Different diseases need to have different laser power.

二、常见肛门直肠疾病的治疗
Ⅱ. Common Treatment of Anal and Rectal Diseases

1. **内痔**　CO_2 激光调至 8 ~ 10W。激光小针刀对准内痔,采用点状或扇形照射,至内痔表面呈焦黄色凝固斑膜,深达 0.1 ~ 0.2mm,使内痔血管蛋白变性、萎缩,达到碳化凝固、止血、消炎作用。

1. **Internal Hemorrhoids**　CO_2 laser power is regulated in 8 ~ 10W, the laser acupuncture scalpel carries on points and sectory shines to make internal hemorrhoidal surface form brown coagulation membrane, the depth is 0.1 ~ 0.2 mm, to make internal hemorrhoidal vessels and protein denaturation and shrinking to get the aim of carbonification, coagulation and diminishing inflammation.

2. **肛门内括约肌狭窄**　CO_2 激光调至 8W,应用激光小针刀从肛门外,在示指(肛内)导引下闭合插入内括约肌,边切开边给激光照射,使内括约肌切开同时切缘发生凝固、止血,防止再粘连,并有消炎作用。

2. **Narrow Anal Internal Sphincter**　CO_2 laser power is regulated in 8W, the laser acupuncture scalpel is inserted into internal sphincter from anus, in the guidance of the index finger (in side of anus) to cut internal sphincter meanwhile the laser shine to form coagulation of cut fringe and diminishing inflammation, preventing adhesion again in the incision.

3. **痉挛**　耻骨直肠肌激光小针刀治疗,同肛门内括约肌狭窄疗法。其激光小针刀切断耻骨直肠肌痉挛狭窄部(参见第 7 章第七节),勿损伤肛门直肠环肌。

3. **Spasm**　The method that laser acupuncture scalpel treats puborectalis muscle is the same as the one of treating narrow anal internal sphincter. Laser acupuncture scalpel cuts off the part of narrow spasm of puborectalis muscle (see chapter 7, §7), not to traumatize the anorectal ring.

4. **单线肛瘘**　自肛瘘外口插入激光小针刀,顺瘘管边切开边照射,使瘘管前壁敞开,伤口边缘凝固,同时清除瘘管内的坏死组织。复杂瘘应加用挂线疗法。

4. **Simple Fistula**　The laser acupuncture scalpel is inserted into fistula along its track from external opening, to cut open the frint wall of fistulous track, to coagulate fringe of wound, at the same time to eliminate necrotic tissues. Adding up seton for treating complicated fistulas.

5. **肛裂**　将肛裂上端的肛窦,中段的肛裂溃疡,下端的哨兵痔,由上至下纵行边切开边激光照射,使切口碳化凝固、止血、消炎。

5. **Anal Fissure**　The laser acupuncture scalpel cuts anal crypts above anal fissure, ulcer in middle part of anal fissure, sentinel pile from upper to inferior, cutting at the same time shining, to make the incision carbonification, coagulation and diminishing inflammation.

6. **肛旁脓肿**　自肛旁脓肿最下缘,用激光小针刀边切开边照射,使脓肿前壁敞开至内口。如内口超过直肠环,则配合挂线疗法。

6. **Perianal Abscess**　The laser acupuncture scalpel cuts and shines the sbscess from the most inferior fringe to make incision from frint wall to internal opening. Adding up seton for treating abscess above rectal ring.

7. 外痔
7. External Hemorrhoids

(1)小外痔:2cm 内者,可利用激光小针刀边切除边照射,使伤口创面凝固、止血、消炎。

(1)Small external hemorrhoid < 2cm:The laser acupuncture scalpel cuts and shines to make the incision carbonification, coagulation and diminishing inflammation.

(2)大外痔:超过 2cm 者,利用激光小针刀先散焦照射,使瘤体血管凝聚,包膜皱缩,再用激光汽化切割。

(2)Large external hemorrhoids >2cm:At first the laser acupuncture scalpel shines focus out to make the vessels coagulation, the envelope shinking, then cutting and gasification by the laser.

8. **直肠癌**　配合用激光小针刀,从肿瘤边缘边切开边汽化,深达肿瘤底部及周围使之凝固、止血。

8. **Rectal Cancer**　The laser acupuncture scalpel cuts and gasificates around cancer from the fringe to the bottom to make blood coagulation.

9. **直肠硬结症**　常因内痔注射所致,可在肛门镜下用激光小针刀边切边凝固、止血、消炎。

9. **Rectal Sclerosis**　Caused by injection treating internal hemorrhoids, the laser acupuncture

scalpel cuts, coagulates inflammation through anoscopy.

10.**肛门瘙痒症**　用激光小针刀于皮下边切边凝固、止血、消炎,破坏引起瘙痒的神经末梢。

10. **Pruritns Ani**　The laser acupuncture scalpel cuts, coagulates and diminishes inflammation to destroy nerve endings.

三、肛门尖锐湿疣的配合治疗
Ⅲ. Supportive Treatment for Condyloma Acuminatum

【病因病机】

［Etiology and Pathology］

尖锐湿疣是由 Papova 病毒的亚类——人乳头瘤病毒(HPV)引起的一种良性表皮肿瘤。据报道,HPV 病毒尚未能在体外培养成功,故人类是其唯一宿主。本病在国外的发病率较高,尤其是在欧美国家。我国近年来的发病率亦有明显增加,并已上升为国内性病的第 2 位,仅次于淋病,必须引起人们的重视。

Anal condyloma acuminatum is caused by human papilloma virus (HPV)— subtype of Papova virus. They are kinds of cuticular benign tumors. As a report that HPV has not yet been cultured outside of body, the human being is the only host. Incidence of the disease is high abroad, especially in Europe and America. In recent years the domestic incidence of the disease is increasing obviously, has risen to the second among domestic venereal diseases, only lower than the first of gonorrhea. So people must make much account of the disease.

中医学认为,本病由于房事不节,感受秽浊,房劳伤精、秽浊病毒乘虚侵入,下注阴器,浊毒而发。浊毒与痰湿蕴积,故见疣状增生;湿、毒、热互结,表面溃烂、流水、流脓,甚则出血。肛门尖锐湿疣多发生在肛管黏膜内、肛门周围皮肤等处。临床上以凸凹不平呈菜花样增生为主要特征。国内外有关资料表明,癌变率较高。近年来,病例明显增多。采用二氧化碳激光小针刀和抗病毒药物局部注射,结合中药外洗的综合疗法治疗肛门尖锐湿疣,效果显著,明显优于其他疗法。介绍如下。

In traditional Chinese medicine it is known that the disease results from sexual intercourse. Condyloma occurs in the perianal area or the squamous epithelium of the anal canal. Occasionally, the mucosa of the upper part of anal canal or the lower part of the rectum is involved. The sign of the disease varies from a few small warts to an extensive mass, occluding the anal canal. Bleeding, itching, and irritation are common symptoms; irregularity and cauliflower-like hyperplasia are main features. The abroad and domestic data stated that canceration rate was high. In recent years such cases increase obviously. The method of treating condyloma acuminatum owns good effect by using

CO_2 laser acupuncture scalpel and local injection of anti-virus medicine combined with herbs, warm baths, overmatching other therapies.

【诊断】
[Diagnosis]

根据皮疹特点、发生部位、发展情况、结合询问接触史，一般诊断不难。

The diagnosis is based on the characteristically soil papillary appearance, position, developing and sexual contact, so the diagnosis is not difficult.

【鉴别诊断】
[Differential Diagnosis]

1.**扁平湿疣**　为表面扁平的潮湿的丘疹，基底下窄，可找到梅毒螺旋体、梅毒血清学阳性。

1. **Condyloma Latum**　The surfaces are flat and wet papulae, the microspironema pallidum can be found, positive tests for syphilis.

2.**皮脂腺异位症**　丘疹在黏膜内，无重叠生长，多为淡黄色。

2. **Ectopic Sebaceous Gland**　Papulae are in mucosa, light yellow color.

3.**皮脂腺增生**　淡黄色丘疹，无蒂、无棘刺、无重叠、无融合。

3. **Hyperplasia of Sebaceous Gland**　Light yellow papulae, no stem, no spines.

4.**传染性软疣**　单个不融合的皮色半球形丘疹，周围光滑，中央有脐凹，可挤出软疣小体。

4. **Molluscum Gontagiosum**　The single lesion does not mix with other lesions, skinny color, semiglobular papula, smooth fringe, hilar depression in the middle, molluscrous bodies may be squeezed from hilar depression.

5.**阴茎珍珠丘疹病**　多见于青壮年，为冠状沟部珍珠状半透明丘疹，白色、黄色或红色，呈圆锥状、球状或不规则状，无明显自觉症状。

5. **Pearl Papules of Penis**　The disease is seen commonly in young adults, white, yellow or red, conoid, ball or disordered semitransparent pearl papules in coronary sulcus, most cases are transmitted by sexual contact, other coexisting venereal diseases, especially syphilis. The patient has no obvious independent symptom.

6.**系带旁腺增生**　包皮系带两侧成对排列的淡红色丘疹。基底不窄，栗粒或针头大，无明显自觉症状。

6. **Para-Vinculum Gland Hyperplasia**　They are light red papulae, occurring symmetrically

on the two sides of frenula praeputii, pin point shape. The patient has no obvious independent symptom.

7. 鲍温样丘疹病 皮疹常由多个色素性丘疹组成,也可单个出现,散有分布或有群集倾向,排列成线状或环形,严重可融合成斑块,发展缓慢(数月或数年)。本病为原位鳞癌,可由尖锐湿疣发展而来。本病女性稍多,主要分布在大小阴唇、肛周。

7. Bowenoid papulosis Papulosis commonly consists of a number of pigmentum papulae or only one, keeping sporadic papule, ranging on line or ring shape, the severe ones mix together to form plaque, developing slowly (for some months or some years). The disease results from developing condyloma acuminatum, easy to form squamous cell carcinoma in situ. The disease is seen more commonly in female, mainly distributed on the labia majora, labia minora and perianus.

8. 假性湿疣 又称女阴尖锐湿疣样丘疹。多见于青壮年。皮疹位于两侧小阴唇内侧面,表面为群集不融合的鱼籽状或息肉状小丘疹,触之有颗粒感或柔软感,淡红色,较潮湿。一般无自觉症状,有的有轻度痒感。

8. Pseudocondyloma It's also called female condyloma acuminatum style papula. The disease is seen commonly in young adults. Erythema are situated inner side of two sides of labia minora. The surfaces are papulae of Cluster, but don't mix like a little polypa or tobacco, a feeling of soft grain, light red, wetness. Many patients haven't obvious independent symptoms except itch.

9. 龟头炎 初起包皮肿胀、潮湿、发红,继而在龟头和包皮内发生渗液、糜烂和溃疡,其上覆盖少许淡黄色脓性分泌物。

9. Balanitis The initial symptoms are swelling, wet, red in the prepuce, gradually producing effusion, erosion and ulcer with a little covering of yellow pus secretion.

10. 肛门梅毒 肛周有扁平疣瘩隆起,亦有乳白色或灰白色奇臭滋水流出,根据其梅毒史、化验反应强阳性分泌物。

10. Anal Syphilis There are knots and some drainage with erosion or grayish white, with smelling niff. The patient has history of syphilis, and blood or secretion test positively.

11. 阴茎梅毒 肿物长大时亦步亦趋可有溃疡、奇臭的分泌物,肿块质地坚硬,呈菜花样增生,触之易出血,呈浸润性生长。初发症状类似尖锐湿疣。如诊断有困难时,可行病理组织活检,以资区别。

11. Penis Syphilis There are ulcers, niff smelling. The tumor shows infiltration proliferation, easily breeding as being touched. Initially it looks like condyloma acuminatum. Pathological examination is essential in diagnosis.

【治疗】

[Treatment]

1. **全身治疗**　加强机体免疫力,提高身体素质。选用聚肌胞 2mg,隔日一次肌内注射(也可局部注射),或病毒唑 100mg,每日 1 次肌内注射;口服病毒灵 0.5g,左旋咪唑 100mg,每日 3 次,饭后服。7 ~ 10 天为一疗程。

1. **Systemic Treatment**　The role of immune mehanisms in recurrent wart formation is yet to be determined to increase immune mechanisms, and to improve in all respects. The patients are injected Poly IC 2mg intramuscularly once every two days (or local injection), or ribavirin 100mg once every day; take Moroxydine 0.5g, Vamisole l00mg, three times every day, post meal, 7 ~ 10d is a treating course.

2. **激光小针刀治疗**　取截石位或左侧卧位,常规消毒、局麻;先用 0.9% 生理盐水湿赘尖锐湿疣,再用激光小针刀探头对尖锐湿疣逐一碳化,碳化至略低于皮肤为准;外涂甲紫药水或氟尿嘧啶软膏,纱布包扎固定。

2. **Laser Acupuncture Scalpel Treating**　Lithotomy position or lying on right side, sterilizing as usual, local anesthesia, at first the doctor takes the anal condyloma acuminatum wet with 0.9% physiological saline, puts to use " laser-coagulation and carbonification" to cut tissue with " gasification".

第7章　肛肠出口排便障碍性疾病
Chapter 7　Difficult Defecation in Anal Outlet

第一节　肛门直肠脱垂
§1　Prolapse of the Anorectum

中医有关肛门直肠脱垂症记载很多,如《医学入门》中载有"脱肛全是气下陷"。

There are many records about prolapse of the anorectum, as is said in ＜ Elementary Medicine ＞: "procidentia is Qi sinking".

【病因病机】

[Etiology and Pathology]

肛门直肠脱垂,俗称脱肛,是肛门和直肠或黏膜因某种原因失去支持遂向下移位。脱出肛外的叫外脱垂;脱垂部分仍在肛管内,外面不能看见的叫内脱垂。依照脱出程度可分为三级。

Prolapse of the anorectum (procidentia) is an uncommon condition in which full thickness of the rectal wall turns inside out, into or through the anal canal. Typically, the extruded rectum is seen as concentric rings of mucosa extruding out of the anus. The other type of rectal mucosal prolapse is in which the radial folds of mucosa inside the anus. According to the degree of procidentia, it is divided into three grades.

第1级:仅是肛管或直肠的黏膜与肌层分离,向下移位。若仅是肛管皮肤脱出的称为脱肛,或叫肛管黏膜脱出;若只是直肠黏膜脱出的称为直肠脱垂,或叫直肠黏膜脱出。

The first grade:Only the mucosa of anal canal or rectum separates from muscle layer, and goes downwards. If only the skin of anal canal prolapses, it is called anal prolapse, or called mucous prolapse of anal canal; if only the rectal mucosa prolapses, it's called the rectal prolapse, or called rectal mucous prolapse.

第2级:是指肛门直肠各层全部向下移位,有时上部直肠可脱入到直肠壶腹,叫直肠套叠。

The second grade:Every layer of anus and rectum goes downwards from normal position, sometimes the upper part of rectum can prolapse into rectal ampullae, it's called rectal intussusception.

第 3 级:是盆结肠向下移位,称为盆结肠套叠,可脱出肛门外很长,甚至可达 30cm 以上。

The third grade:The colon goes downwards to form colonic intussusception. It can prolapse out of anus for long distance, even over 30cm.

中医学认为,由于气虚(中气下陷),以致升提无力而形成直肠脱出。现代医学则认为是由于解剖上发育缺陷,如骶骨弯曲度小,直肠失去其有效的支持,或直肠前陷凹腹膜反折处过低,当腹腔内压力增高时,均可使直肠被直接向下推移。另外,由于支持直肠的组织软弱,如坐骨直肠窝脂肪被吸收,失去支持直肠的作用;也可因为神经系统疾病引起提肛门肌及括约肌松弛或瘫痪;或由于腹腔内压力经常增高,促使直肠向外脱出。最常见的肛管黏膜脱出,则多由于较大的内痔反复脱出,使黏膜与肌层间组织松脱,与内痔一并脱出。

In traditional Chinese medicine it is believed that Qi asthesia causes little power raising to form rectal prolapse. The modern medicine shows that developmental defect in human body anatomy, such as small degree of sacral curvature, rectum losing effective support, very low peritoneal reflection in front of sunken rectum, causes rectum going down as the inner pressure of abdominal cavity increasing. In addition, because the supporting tissues of rectum become soft, for example the fat is absorbed in the ischiorectal fossa, the action of supposing rectum decreases in the course of the disease; another reason is pathological changes of nerve system lead to levator ani muscles and sphincter relaxation and paralysis. The high inner pressure of abdominal cavity induces the rectum prolapse outside. The most common mucous prolapse of anal canal results from repeated prolapse of big internal hemorroids leading to loose tissues between mucosa and muscle. This kind of prolapse gets together with internal hemorrhoids.

【临床表现】
[Clinical Manifestations]

初起大便时有黏膜自肛门脱出,便后自然缩回。这是因为直肠环还有紧张力的关系,以后由于反复脱出,直肠环渐渐松弛,脱出的黏膜则不能自然复回,必须用手推回肛内,并常有少许黏液由肛门流出。如果长久反复脱出,在打喷嚏、咳嗽、行走稍久时,均可脱出。这是因为直肠环过于松弛。因为黏膜常受刺激而糜烂,所以大便有时有少量出血。常自觉肛门部坠胀、酸痛。内脱垂一般坠胀较明显,常自觉大便未排净,常有血和黏液排出。

Initially the mucosa prolapses during defecation, and retracts back after defecation, because the rectum still keeps its tense power in this period. Later repeated prolapsis make rectal ring relax, the mucosa cannot get back naturally, and needs to be pushed into the anus by hand, usually a little mucus drains out of anus. Long time later, the prolapse occurs repeatedly, so the prolapse can take place in sneeze, cough and walking. Sometimes stool is covered by a little blood, due to mucous projection being stimulated repeatedly to cause mucous erosion. The patient often feels anal falling and distension, sore pain, incomplete defecation, with some blood or mucus in the stool.

【诊断】
[Diagnosis]

第 1 级脱垂：大便后可见黏膜脱出，便后自然缩回。在脱出时可见红色环形肿物，长数厘米，自肛管中央向周围有放射状纵沟。指诊可摸出两层折叠黏膜，没有弹性（不同于内痔）；在突出黏膜外侧与肛管之间，可摸到一沟，即直肠脱垂或称直肠内黏膜脱出（图 7-1）。如无此沟就证明是肛管黏膜也随着脱下。如果黏膜未脱出肛外，指诊时在直肠上部可摸到折叠的黏膜，质柔软，上下可移动。用窥肛器检查可见直肠黏膜折叠，有时也可能有部分黏膜脱出。

The first grade: The mucosa projects after defecation, then retracts naturally. The red ring shape mass can be seen as projecting. The intussusception begins circumferentially at 6 to 7cm from the anal verge. The redness of the rectal mucosa, especially anteriorly at the 6~7cm level, gives a clue to the diagnosis(Fig. 7-1). When the prolapse remains in the upper anal canal, the radial folds of mucosa extrude from the centre of anal canal to around through the anus that the finger can find two folds of mucosa, no flexibility (different from internal hemorrhoids).

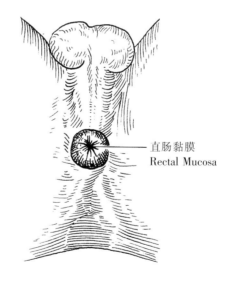

图 7-1　直肠脱垂（肛管中央有向外放射状纵沟）

Figure 7-1　Prolapse of the anorectum(radial folds of mucosa extrude from the centre of anal canal)

第 2、3 级脱垂：是直肠及盆结肠各层完全脱出肛外，脱出部分如螺旋形环状皱襞，且较第 1 级长，有时可达 30cm 以上。有时稍微弯腰、略一用劲即可脱出。如未脱出肛外，在直肠内可摸到脱出部分为一硬块，光滑、活动；手指可摸到脱下部分与肠壁之间有一环状沟;用窥肛器检查可见脱出部分塞满肠腔,黏膜充血(图7-2)。

The second and third grade:Every layer of anus, rectum and colon goes downwards from normal position, with spiral ring shaped folds of mucosa prolapse. It is longer than the first grade, even over 30cm. If it does not prolapse out of the anus, it can be felt in the rectum as a hard mass, smooth and movable, together with a circular groove or sulcus. Anoscopy may reveal the prolapsed portion fills the rectal lumen and congested mucosa (Fig. 7-2).

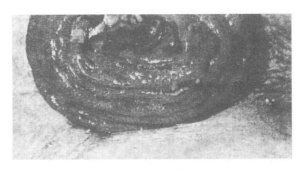

图 7-2 第 2 级直肠脱垂

Figure 7-2 The second grade prolapse of the rectum

【治疗】

[Treatment]

1. 简易疗法 调理大便如内服补中益气汤。

1. Simple Treatment To regulate stool by taking the decoction of BuZhongYiQiTang.

2. 直肠黏膜内脱垂治疗

2. Treating Hidden Prolapse： The prolapse in the upper anal canal.

(1)弯头负压吸力式套扎枪配合小针刀治疗:①小针刀治疗:采用斜面小针刀和钩状小针刀,从肛门外,点状皮肤针眼分次刺入肛门内括约肌和外括约肌皮下层。将内括约肌和外括约肌皮下层闭合性切断。②弯头负压吸力式套扎枪治疗:用圆头缺口电池灯肛门镜,分4次分别插入肛门直肠腔使脱垂黏膜层突入缺口肛门镜中,再用弯头套扎枪于截石位3点、6点、9点和12点钟位分别套扎,直肠(腔内)黏膜层的4个部位。先将3点钟位的松弛黏膜,用胶圈套扎,并于被胶圈套扎上方的黏膜层内注消痔灵液1ml以隆起为度。此后,依次分别套扎6点、9点和12点钟位松弛的黏膜层(图7-3)。

(1) Angle head loop ligaturing gun with vacuum suction combining acupuncture scalpel. ①Acupuncture scalpel treatment:Carrying on inclined plane and hook style acupuncture scalpel to insert into internal sphincter and subcutaneous layer of external sphincter from points of injection outside of anus, separately. Cut off internal sphincter and subcutaneous layer of external sphincter.

②Angle head loop ligaturing gun with vacuum suction: lithotomy position, through by 4 times, with optical anoscope the doctor inserts gun into anorectal cavity to make mucosa of prolapse fall in anoscope, then make ligatures of 3, 6, 9, 12 o'clock four positions of mucous layer separately. The projecting relaxing mucosa of 3 o'clock is ligated with rubber circle, and injected 1ml XiaoZhi Ling to enlarge the position above rubber circle. According to the technique the flabby mucosas of 9, 6, 12 o'clock positions are separately ligated (Fig. 7 – 3).

（2）多点单纯结扎配合小针刀治疗：取截石位，局麻或腰俞麻醉、扩肛后于两叶肛门镜直视下，从齿线上至直肠壶腹，用直角血管钳夹住，并提起直肠前壁松弛的黏膜，包括黏膜下层波及肌层。每点仅钳夹 1cm² 用粗丝线于基底部单纯结扎，由近至远行呈点状结扎，每点之间应留 0.3～0.5cm 黏膜桥，并避免在同一水平结扎，使结扎点纵横交错，呈均匀分布的网状结节。直肠全周黏膜内脱垂，则在直肠前与后壁及侧壁用同法处理；若合并内痔、息肉或直肠前凸也采取同法处理，但直肠前凸要以前突凹陷消失为准进行多点单纯结扎，以加强直肠前壁支撑。配合小针刀治疗：于肛管腔将肛管后侧栉膜带切断，再于后尾骨尖至肛缘肛外皮肤中点旁开 1cm 为进针点，潜行刺入小针刀，深达肛门白线，即肛门内外括约肌的分界线，下端外括约肌皮下部用小针刀闭合切断，再用小针刀将上端内括约肌潜行闭合性纵行切开 1～1.5cm，使肛管松解，术毕肛内外置干纱布（图 7 – 4）。

（2）Simple multiple points ligation combining with acupuncture scalpel treatment: using lithotomy position, local anesthesia or lumbar anesthesia, with anoscope the doctor enlarges the anus, takes right-angle vessel forceps to infibulate and holds up flabby mucosa of anterior rectal wall including submucosa and muscle layers, only 1 cm² every point, then ligate simply the bottom with thick silk thread, from near point to distant point. Every point maintains 0.3～0.5cm mucous bridge to avoid being in same level, to make crisscross ligated points form even well-distributed netty nodes. The same method was used to treat anterior, posterior and side rectal walls. In case of combined internal hemorrhoids, polypus, and anterior, posterior rectal projection on treat them in the same technique, but for anterior rectal projection treatment must be pointed to disappearance by use of simple multiple points ligation so as to increase the sustaining of anterior anal wall. Combining with acupuncture scalpel treating, the doctor cuts posterior pecten band of anal canal in the cavity of anal canal, then in sinking inserts and punctures acupuncture scalpel from 1cm skin position near the midpoint between the tip of coccyx and the fringe of anus to anal white line, that's the intermuscular sulcus between the internal sphincter muscles and external sphincter muscles, downwards cuts closely subcutaneous layer of external sphincter, then sinking upwards cuts the internal sphincter 1 – 1.5 cm vertically and closely so as to relax the anal canal. To cover with dry gauze inside and outside of anus(Fig. 7 – 4).

3. 双位注射配合小钩针点状缩肛术治疗肛门直肠脱垂

3. Two Position Injection Cooperated with Small Hook Points Style Contracting Anus to

Treating Prolapse of the Anorectum

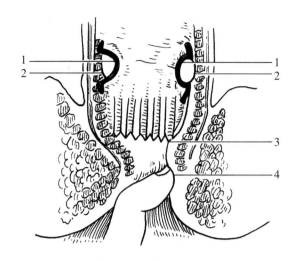

图 7 – 3　直肠黏膜内脱垂套扎枪治疗

1 – 套扎胶圈上,注入消痔灵;2 – 胶圈套扎;3 – 齿线;4 – 肌间沟

Figure 7 – 3　Loop ligaturing gun treating the prolapse of inner anorectum

1. Injected XiaoZhiLing in rubber circle of loop ligaturing;

2. Loop ligaturing of rubber circle; 3. Dentate line; 4. Internal sphincter ditch

　　肛门直肠脱垂治疗方法较多,但老年患者体弱多病,不愿接受手术治疗,因此,宜采用双位注射,配合小钩针点状缩肛术治疗。

　　There are many methods to treat prolapse of the anorectum with small hook points style contracting anus to treat prolapse of the anorectum.

　　(1)肛管镜下注射法:用肛门镜较高位插入才有利于向松弛黏膜上方注射药物。用碘伏消毒,取20ml注射器抽0.5%普鲁卡因与消痔灵液1ml。用心内注射器的长针头在3、6、9点钟位置及齿线上,最好选择在脱垂起始部,即直肠乙状结肠交界处的尖端,直肠中下段末端,于第3个直肠瓣为标界,每点注入6ml。呈扇状注射,即针头向上注射再往回吸(没回血),边退针,边注射药液至齿线止。注射总量3处共18ml。每点间隔相距1.5cm。注射后,以上3个点位置呈纵行分布于肠腔中,以注射在黏膜下层为准,勿注入过浅(黏膜层),也勿注入过深(波及直肠肛管壁的肌层),以黏膜层充盈隆起,毛细血管清晰可见为度。

　　(1)Injection through anoscopy:The doctor inserts the anoscope in high position so as to inject medicine into relaxing mucosa. After sterilization, draws 0.5% procaine and the liquid of XiaoZhiLing 1∶1 into 20ml injector, by long syringe needle of intracardial to inject, in the 3,6,9, o'clock position and above dentate line, the best position is the initial position of prolapse in which the sulcus between rectum and sigmoid colon, and the position of end part of inferior middle of rectum, takes the direction of the third rectal valve, injects 6ml in every point. Sector style injection,

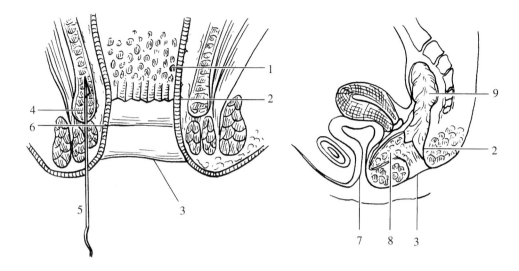

图 7 - 4　直肠黏膜内脱垂多点单纯结扎与小针刀治疗
1 - 多点结扎黏膜层;2 - 齿线;3 - 肛门;4 - 内括约肌;5 - 小针刀;
6 - 肌间沟;7 - 阴道;8 - 前凸;9 - 直肠

Figure 7 - 4　Simple multiple points ligation combining with acupuncture
scalpel treating the prolapse of inner anorectum

1. Multiple points ligation of mucosa; 2. Dentate line; 3. Anus; 4. Internal sphincter;

5. Acupuncture scalpel; 6. Internal sphincter ditch; 7. Vagina; 8. Anterior projection 9. Rectum

it's that to inject with upward syringe needle, then retract syringe needle at the same time to inject (draw back no blood) the medicine to dentate line. Total dose of injection is 18ml in 3 parts, every two points keep a distance of 1. 5cm. The positions of three points are vertically distributed in the intestinal cavity after being injected. The injection should go into the submucosa, neither inject into very shallow position (mucosa), nor over deep (involving the muscle layer of anal canal and rectum). The depth of injection should be mucosa upheaval and blood capillary be seen clearly.

（2）肛管与直肠间隙注射法:将肛周皮肤消毒,分别于截石位 3 点和 9 点钟位,肛缘外 1.5cm,选用腰麻针头接 20ml 针管,抽鱼肝油酸钠注射液 15～20ml 或 1∶1 的消痔灵液。将左手示指伸入肛管直肠腔,先触摸内外括约肌分界的肌间沟。其上为内括约肌,两侧为坐骨结节,即找到坐骨直肠窝。如为脱肛,则各注入 5ml 至两侧的坐骨直肠间隙。如为直肠脱垂,则将药注入两侧骨盆直肠窝,(也叫骨盆直肠间隙)第 2 个针头刺空感,一般在提肛肌与盆肌膜之间(图 7 - 5)。刺入并穿过提肛肌才可进入骨盆直肠窝。其针头类似刺入橡皮感觉后,再有刺空感。

（2）Injection method in anal canal and rectal spaces:The doctor sterilizes the perianal skin with the patient in lithotomy posture at 3 and 9 o'clock positions, distance from anal fringe 1. 5cm, using syringe needle for lumbar anesthesia to connect with 20ml syringe, draws 15～20ml sodium morrhuate or 1∶1 XiaoZhiLing. The left index finger goes into the anus, to touch the ditch of intermuscular sulcus between the internal sphincter muscles and external sphincter muscles, upwards from the ditch being internal sphincter, two sides being ischial tuberodties, so ischiorectal fossa is here. In case of anal prolapse, the doctor injects the two kinds of medicine, 5ml each into the two sides of ischiorectal fossa (another name is pelvirectal fossa). The second space of feeling syringe needle falling is usually between levator ani muscle and pelvic muscular membrance (Fig. 7 – 5). Only by puncturing into levator ani muscle and going through the muscle, can the injector go into the ischiorectal fossa. The feeling is that the syringe needle punctures into the rubber then falling.

4. **小钩针点状缩肛术**　消毒,取尾骨尖与肛门缘之间的皮肤行点状局麻,右手持钩状小针,从局麻针眼刺入,在左手示指伸人肛内辅助,将肛周外括约肌皮下部向尾骨方向推移,找到条状肌束,然后右手用钩状小钩针从针眼钩出肌束。最后再用细羊肠线做 2 次结扎紧缩。紧缩程度以示,中指可插入肛管,并有紧缩感为度。最后仍从原针眼处将扎紧的外括约肌皮下部推入原位针眼,用乙醇纱布块压迫即可(图 7 – 6)。

4. **Small hook points style contracting anus**　The doctor sterilizes the skin, takes local point anesthesia between the tip of coccyx and the fringe of anus, his right hand handles small hook acupuncture scalpel to insert into muscular bundle from the injected local anesthesia points, his left index finger goes into the anus for helping, to push subcutaneous muscle of external sphincter towards the coccyx, hooks out sliver of muscular bundle, then ties thin sheep bowel thread twice to ligate and contract strictly up to the condition that index and middle fingers can insert into anal canal with a feeling of strict contraction. Lastly he pushes the subcutaneous muscle of external sphincter towards primary position, covers and presses with ethyl gauze (Fig. 7 – 6).

【注意事项】

[Note]

(1)不要将药注入括约肌中;回吸无回血再注入药,以免注入血管中。

(1)Don't inject medicine into sphincter, injection made after drawing back the injector showing no blood injected into vessels.

(2)肛管与直肠间隙勿注入过深或过浅,必须在左手示指肛管直肠腔内导引下,左手示指与右手持腰麻针或心内注射长针头,两者与相离图肛管或直肠壁有一定距离,又可触及针尖,以相距 0.5 ~ 1cm 为宜。每处注药 5 ~ 6ml。

(2)Don't inject medicine into spaces of anus and anal canal too shallow or too deep. His left index finger goes into canal and rectum from the anus for introduction. There are some distances between anal canal and rectum, the tip of syringe needle can be felt. The optimal distance is 0.5 ~ 1 cm. To inject 5 ~ 6 ml of the medicine.

(3)骨盆直肠窝,注射部位一定要准确。针刺通过肛提肌,一定要体验出通过

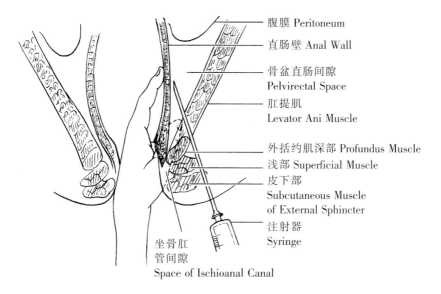

图 7 - 5 肛门直肠脱垂注射疗法

Figure 7 - 5 Injection treatment for the prolapse of the anorectum

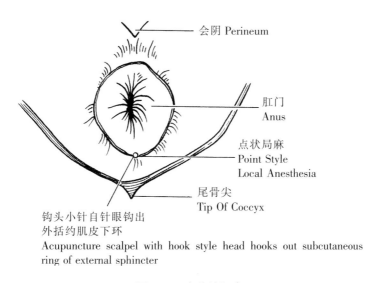

图 7 - 6 点状缩肛术

Figure 7 - 6 Points style contracting anus

类似肌性橡皮针感后针头有至明显落空感,回抽无回血再注射药。然后,再伸入示指按摩注射间隙,以避免药物过于集中。

（3）The injecting position must be exactly in ischiorectal fossa. The feeling through levator muscle is that the syringe needle punctures into the rubber then falling.

（4）黏膜下层镜下注药时,针尖勿穿破肛管直肠腔,以免引起感染或内瘘。勿注入括约肌中,尤其不可注入肛门直肠环内。

(4) As injecting medicine into submucosa through anoscopy, the syringe needle can't go through anal canal and rectum, for fear of causing infection and internal fistula. Don't go into sphincter especially the anorectal ring.

(5)肛管和直肠窝分别注射,位置要确切,针刺要有明显的刺空感,针尖上下有一定移动度,没阻力,回吸没回血才可缓慢、定向注入药物。

(5) Injection of anal canal and rectal fossa should be taken separately, the position must be exact, we should feel obvious falling as puncturing, the tip of needle can be moved up and down in the certain extension, without resistance. Injection should be carried on slowly at the correct direction.

【术后处理】

[Postoperative Care]

手术后俯卧(或侧卧),臀部垫高 10～20cm,给流质或半流质食物 3～5 天,并给鸦片酊 0.5ml 口服,每日 2～3 次,以防排泄大便。治疗后第 3 天在排泄大便之前用盐水洗肠,或服五仁润肠丸等,保持大便稀软。如排便后黏膜脱出须立即送回,否则时间长久,注射局部组织已粘连固定,即不易送回。术后经常练习收肛活动(有意识地收缩肛门)。1 周后下地活动,但大便仍应保持稀软。脱垂从此即不会再出现。

The patient should lie pronated (or on their side), being held up the hips 10～20cm. A bulk-producing compound and a lubricant are administered orally, starting on the day of operation, take liquid or semifluid food 3～5 days postoperatively, walk after one week.

【点评】

[Review]

(1)直肠脱垂的起始部在直肠与乙状结肠交界部,脱垂首先发生在黏膜松弛处,形成内脱垂性肠管上尖端脱套,远端直肠腔中进入直肠中下段,最后才经肛门脱出。因此,采用多点位黏膜下层注射硬化剂造成无菌粘连(悬吊)固定法。但勿注入直肠肌肉层,其针头似刺入橡皮感则回退。

(1) The initial site of prolapse of the rectum is the juncture of rectum and sigmoid, and relaxation of mucosa. When the prolapse remains in the upper anal canal, it's hidden prolapse. The distal intestinal canal goes into the middle inferior rectum, at last goes outside of anus. So carrying on the method of treatment, it's that sclerosing agent being injected into submucosa by the multiple point style to cause sterile adhesion and location (hanging). But don't inject into rectal muscular layer. The syringe needle should be retracted when the doctor feels it punctures into the rubber.

(2)盆底肌群和肛管松弛,失去支持作用和承托作用,排便腹压增高时,尤其在原有直肠黏膜内脱垂的基础上,可迫使全直肠和黏膜层组织外脱出。肛管和直肠间隙注入消痔灵等可起粘连、固定、承托作用,使肛管、直肠与周围组织粘连固定,恢复生理状态。

(2)Because the tissues of supporting rectum become soft, the muscles relax in pelvic bottom and anal canal, all these cause rectum going down as the inner pressure of abdominal cavity increases. Especially on the base of hidden prolapse, high inner pressure of abdominal cavity induces the rectum prolapse out. Injecting XiaoZhiLing into the space of anal canal and rectum can take use of adhesion, location and support to cause environmental tissues adhesion with anal canal and rectum, to recover the physical state.

(3)由于单纯双位注射法不能使已松弛的肛门缩小到理想程度,所以采用钩状小钩针将外括约肌皮环钩出至肛外,用羊肠线结扎紧缩再送回肛内。羊肠线为异体蛋白,易与肌组织粘连、纤维化,起到缩肛及固定双重作用。

(3)Simple two positions injection can't make relaxed anus contract to an ideal degree, so the author takes small hook acupuncture scalpel to hook subcutaneous ring of external sphincter out of the anus, and ties it tightly with thread, then makes it return to inside of the anus to take the action of contracting and locating the anus.

第二节 直肠前凸与便秘

§2 Rectocele and Constipation

【病因症状】

[Etiology and Symptoms]

直肠前凸又称阴道后壁膨出,主要是阴道损伤造成直肠阴道壁薄弱而形成,大部分患者与便秘无关。肛管因括约肌痉挛使排便受阻,粪便挤入薄弱的直肠前凸而加重。常需用手指插入阴道,挤回前凸以协助排便。

Rectocele is also called posterior vaginal prolapse, mainly as a result of vaginal trauma causing thin rectovaginal septum. The spasm of anal canal sphincter suffocates defecation, and the stool is squeezed toward anterior thin rectovaginal septum, making more serious rectocele. Commonly the patient has to insert a finger into vagina to push and squeeze the rectocele for defecation.

【临床表现】

[Clinical Manifestations]

阴道后壁膨出导致出口梗阻,引起便秘。但手术后约一半病人虽然前凸消失,但便秘症状仍不缓解或缓解后再复发,其原因与女性盆腔解剖生理特点有关。直肠前凸程度有轻、中、重之分。

Prolapse of posterior vaginal causes constipation by outlet obstruction. Although about a half of patients who received operation had resolved rectocele, the constipation might not be relieved or has postoperative recrudescence. The cause has something to do with female pelvic features in anatomy and physiology. Rectocele can be divided into three degrees:mild, middle and severe.

【诊断】

[Diagnosis]

1. **轻度前凸**　直肠前凸囊袋深 2cm,如果肠壁张力较大,也属不正常,称为直肠前壁薄弱。

1. **Mild Rectocele**　The thin rectovaginal septum is similar to sack which projects toward anterior about 2cm, or the tension of intestinal wall has kept high.

2. **中度前凸**　直肠前凸囊袋深超过 2~3cm,前壁复原缓慢,不能复原。

2. **Middle Rectocele**　The forward septum is deep over 2~3cm, or the septum restores slowly even difficult reversion.

3. **重度前凸**　直肠前凸囊袋有的深达4~5cm。肛指检查直肠前凸不但要明确直肠前凹深度,更要了解直肠前凸的肠壁张力。

3. **Severe Rectocele**　The forward septum is deep over 4~5cm. By digital examination not only the deepness of rectocele, but also the tension of intestinal wall of rectocele should be understood.

【治疗】

[Treatment]

采用小针刀配合套扎枪双向治疗。

Loop ligation gun combining with acupuncture scalpel double action treatment.

(1)点状局麻,从肛门外3点或9点钟位侧面插入斜面小针刀,在左手示指肛管内导引下将内括约肌和外括约肌皮下部闭合性切断,以解除肛管压力,利于排便(图7-4)。

(1) Points style local anesthesia, from the 3 o'clock or 9 o'clock outside of anus the doctor's right hand handles the inclined plane acupuncture scalpel to insert into sphincter and to cut closely internal sphincter and subcutaneous portion of external sphincter in order to resolve pressure of anal canal, to help defecation(Fig. 7-4).

(2)从肛门插入圆头缺口电池灯肛门镜,应用弯头套扎枪将直肠阴道前凸的黏膜层及下层一同多点套扎,直至直肠前凸消失,以变平坦为度。然后在阴道口应用套扎枪同法将阴道后壁,即直肠前凸的囊袋全套扎或用丝线单纯多点结扎。直至直肠阴道后壁变平直(图 7 - 14)。将九华膏挤入肛门。

(2) With optical anoscopy, the doctor carries on the angle head loop ligation gun to loop many points of ligation in mucosa and submucosa of rectovaginal septum till the rectocele disappears and the septum becomes flat. Then in the vagina he carries on the loop ligation gun to loop ligation, or uses silk thread to tie many points with simple ligation, of sack of rectocele in posterior vaginal wall until the wall becomes straight (Fig. 7 - 14). Then squeeze the Jiuhuagao to the anus.

(3)从阴道插入窥器,用弯血管钳,钳夹其阴道后壁的突凸(束袋)用丝线,多点单纯结扎(勿缝扎)至阴道后壁平坦(图 7 - 14)置入阴道栓药剂。

(3) With vaginoscopy, the doctor takes curved hemostatic forceps to clip up projective posterior vaginal wall (sack of rectocele), then uses silk thread to tie many points with simple ligation until the wall changes to a plane (Fig. 7 - 4). Then squeeze the cream to the vagina.

【点评】
[Review]

1. 从肛门直肠与阴道的双向结扎治疗,直肠前凸,方法简单,效果好。

1. The double action treatment of ligation between anus and vagina to treat rectocele is simple method with good effect.

2. 因采用单纯结扎致"前凸"平直,没有缝合的针眼,故不会发生感染引起直肠阴道漏,也没有后遗症。

2. Because the author carries on simple ligation to cause "rectocele" plane and straight, so rectovaginal fistula won't occur.

第三节　直肠瓣增生与便秘
§ 3　The Hyperplasia of Rectal Valves and Constipation

病因不清,长期便秘腹胀,需服用泻药。

There are no obvious causes of disease with long time constipation, so laxative has to be taken.

【诊断】
[Diagnosis]

肛指检查可触及直肠瓣增生,呈半月形。肛门镜检查直肠瓣隔板样增生,将直肠横行阻断,直肠上方扩张,有粪便堆积。

In digital rectal examination, the finger touches the rectum disc hyperplasia, with the shape of crescent. Anoscope shows that the diaphragm hyperplasia of rectum valve blocks the rectum in transverse section, and the upper part of the rectum expands with fetus accumulation.

【治疗】
[Treatment]

采用钩状小针刀治疗。

Carrying on hook style acupuncture scalpel.

洗肠,肌内注射地西泮 1 支。取膀胱截石位,骶尾部托升。左手示指伸入肛管扩肛。在圆头缺口电池灯肛门镜下,用钩状小针刀沿肛门直肠瓣正中线及左侧右侧纵行钩断成 3 处纵沟。敞开隔板状增生直肠瓣,用痔瘘粉纱布条上敷即可(图 7 - 7)。

Lithotomy position, holding up sacrococcygeal region, the doctor's left index finger goes into the anal canal to enlarge the anus. In the optical anoscope the hook style acupuncture scalpel hooks and cuts anorectal valves vertically forming 3 vertical ditches in middle line, left side and right side to open rectal valves of clapboard style hyperplasia, then the wound is covered by gauze with medicine (Fig. 7 - 7).

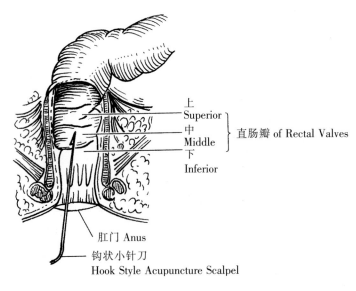

图 7 - 7　直肠增生
Figure 7 - 7　Hyperplasia of rectal valves

【点评】
[Review]

直肠瓣由霍斯顿 1830 年首先叙述,一般为 3 个横行皱襞。直肠瓣的功能是支撑粪便,减慢排入直肠肛管。但增生成隔板状则会引起便秘。采用小针刀纵行钩断敞开即可使排便通畅。该方法简单,没有后遗症和并发症。

Rectal valves were described first by Houston in 1830, usually there are three horizontal folds. Their purpose seems to serve as steps or spiral supports to modify the flow of the feces as they descend into the lower rectum, but clapboard style hyperplasia can induce the constipation. Acupuncture scalpel hooks off and cuts open anorectal valves vertically so as to defecate stool freely. The method is simple, won't leave sequel and complication.

第四节 内括约肌失弛缓与便秘

§ 4 Nonrelaxing Internal Sphincter and Constipation

【病因病机】

[Etiology and Pathology]

患者无痛性粪便排出困难。其诱发因素有长期抑制便意;精神负担过重致自主神经功能紊乱;心理压力过大,使内括约肌紧张度增生,舒缩功能紊乱。

The patient suffers from difficult defecation painlessly. The predisposing factors are long time inhibiting desire to defecate, dysautonomia and mental over-pressure. All these causes increase tensity of internal sphincter and functional disturbances of contraction and relaxation.

【临床表现】

[Clinical Manifestations]

患者无痛性排便困难,且排便多次仍感排出困难,有一半患者大便干结。

The patient suffers from difficult defecation painlessly. Although he defecates many times, he still feels difficult defecation. About a half of the patients defecate dry stool.

【诊断】

[Diagnosis]

内括约肌失弛缓症者直肠指检可摸及内括约肌增厚、弹性增强、肛管压力增高。内括约肌肌电图放电频率均超过9.4周/分,肛管压力测定静息压和直肠最大耐受量 MTV 均高于正常。

Digital examination can show thicker internal sphincter, with elasticity increasing and pressure of anal canal rising. Internal sphincter electromyogram shows discharge frequency of internal sphincter over 9.4 cycles per minute. Pressure monitor of anal canal shows resting pressure of anal canal and maximum rectal tolerance are over normal.

【治疗】
[Treatment]

取侧卧位,消毒,局麻。术者先用左手示指插入肛管内约1.5cm,确定括约肌间沟的位置,其上缘即为内括约肌,可按压固定。右手持肛肠斜面小针刀从肛门处3点钟位点状局麻针眼插入。在肛管内的左手示指引导下,隔着肛管左手示指尖摸到小针刀顶端,随着右手持斜面小针刀,两手指同时上下配合小针刀纵行切开内括约肌1.5~2cm。禁忌横切,切勿刺穿肛管腔。拔出小针刀,术毕(图7-8)。

With patient lying on side, sterilizing and local anesthesia, the doctor's left index finger inserts into anal canal 1.5cm to define and feel the position of intersphincteric ditch, the upper fringe is the internal sphincter, and to fix the internal sphincter. His right hand handles the inclined plane acupuncture scalpel to insert into internal sphincter from local anesthetic points outside of anus at 3 o'clock position, and in the guidance of his left index finger tip touching the top of acupuncture scalpel through anal canal, then his right hand handles the inclined plane acupuncture scalpel to insert into internal sphincter, and cuts vertically the internal sphincter 1.5~2cm, but not cut horizontally. The acupuncture scalpel should not puncture anal canal and then the doctor puts the acupuncture scalpel out (Fig. 7-8).

【点评】
[Review]

肛管内括约肌失弛缓性便秘常为顽固性便秘,女性多于男性,病因不清。内括约肌是参与排便的重要肌束,它处于生理状态,是排便不可缺少的重要条件。如肛管内括约肌舒缩功能紊乱,出现失弛缓,采用内括约肌切断术即可治愈。

Constipation suffering from nonrelaxing internal sphincter of anal canal is usually intractable constipation. This disease is more in female than in male, and is agnogenic. Internal sphincter is the important muscle to participate in defecation, indispensable condition for normal defecation. If the internal sphincter dysfunction causes nonrelaxing, cutting off internal sphincter can cure the disease.

第五节　肛门直肠狭窄
§5　Anorectal Stricture

肛门直肠狭窄可分为单纯肛门狭窄、单纯直肠狭窄和肛门直肠联合狭窄。后者是前二者的结合,因此,其病因、临床表现、诊断基本上也是前二者的综合,其治疗也更相复杂。

Anorectal stricture can be divided into simple anal stricture, simple rectal stricture and anorec-

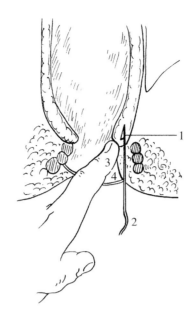

图 7 - 8　内括约肌失弛缓小针刀治疗
1 - 内括约肌;2 - 斜面小针刀;3 - 指尖;4 - 肛门
Figure 7 - 8　Acupuncture scalpel treating nonrelaxing internal sphincter
1. Internal Sphincter; 2. Inclined Plane Acupuncture Scalpel; 3. Top of Finger; 4. Anus

tal stricture. The latter is syntheses of the former two, so the etiology, clinical manifestations and diagnosis are the syntheses of the former two, and the treatment is more complicated.

一、肛门狭窄
I. Anal Stricture

【病因】

[Etiology]

肛门或直肠发炎、糜烂,或内外痔手术切除皮肤黏膜太多,或肛门瘘手术后有较大的瘢痕形成(多见于多发性复杂肛瘘手术后),以及肛门部外伤、肿瘤等影响,都可使肛门变窄。

Anal stricture results from anal or rectal inflammation, erosion, or complication of anorectal surgery such as cutting off more skin in surgery of internal and external hemorrhoids, forming larger scar after treating anal fistula (multiple complicated anal fistula), anal trauma and tumor, etc.

【临床表现】

[Clinical Manifestations]

主要是排便困难和排便时或排便后肛门疼痛,有时为刺痛或剧烈疼痛,可持续数分钟至数小时。有的伴里急后重感。

Clinical manifestations are mainly difficult defecation, and anal pain during defecation or post-defecation, sometimes tingle or throe. The pain continues or lasts for a month and tenesmus for sometimes.

【诊断】

[Diagnosis]

根据临床表现结合病史,如已往患者肛门部有过损伤感染,或肛门部做过手术等,指检可摸及肛管缩窄,有时在齿线下触到坚硬的瘢痕组织;或呈环形狭窄,有的伴肛裂(图7-9)。

Diagnosis is based on clinical manifestations and history of anal inflammation, trauma and surgery, etc. Digital examination reveals narrowring of anal canal, sometimes touching hard scar tissues below dentate line, sometimes accompanying with fissure (Fig. 7-9).

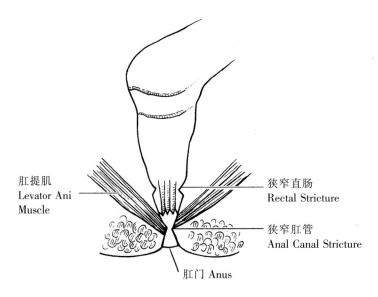

肛提肌
Levator Ani
Muscle

狭窄直肠
Rectal Stricture

狭窄肛管
Anal Canal Stricture

肛门 Anus

图7-9 直肠与肛管狭窄

Figure 7-9 Stricture in rectum and anal canal

【治疗】

[Treatment]

参考"直肠狭窄"。

Refer to "rectal stricture".

二、直肠狭窄

II. Rectal Stricture

【病因】

[Etiology]

主要是由于直肠手术后引起瘢痕收缩。如内痔手术时将直肠黏膜切除太多，或因用内痔注射疗法时，不慎波及黏膜下层肌肉形成坏死。另外，直肠损伤后(如枪弹伤、穿刺伤、烫伤等)引起感染，以及因误用过强腐蚀性药或接受放射治疗等，均可损伤直肠组织，造成瘢痕收缩，引起直肠狭窄。另外，慢性痢疾、直肠癌、腹股沟淋巴肉芽肿(女性多见)等也可引起直肠狭窄。

Rectal stricture is a main dreaded complication of rectal surgerys such as postoperative scar contraction. Cutting off more rectal mucosa in surgery of internal hemorrhoids causes stricture, improper injecting method for internal hemorrhoids may injure the muscles in submucosal layer to form necrosis. In addition, infection of the rectal trauma (gunshot wound, scald, and puncture for examination and treatment, etc.), misusing corrosive drug, and others such as postradiotherapy, chronic diarrhea, rectal cancer, inguinal lymphogranuloma (mainly female), etc., all can injure rectal tissues to form scar and stricture.

【临床表现】

[Clinical Manifestations]

初起常感肛门直肠坠胀不适，长期便秘，并日渐加重。排便后常感未排净，仍有便意，粪便形状细而扁；晚期则伴黏液、脓血便。肛门周围皮肤常因分泌物刺激形成湿疹，或出现表皮糜烂。

Initial symptoms include common falling and distension in anorectal region, constipation for a long time, gradually becoming severe, feeling of incomplete defecation, still desiring to defecate, thin and small stool; in later stage there would be some mucus, pus and blood in stool. Perianal skin frequently shows eczema or erosion of epidermis because of secretion stimulation.

【诊断】

[Diagnosis]

根据上述症状，结合专科检查结果诊断。指诊检查时，可摸及括约肌多处狭窄，多位于齿线上2.5~5cm，直肠壁变硬，弹性消失。狭窄孔大者，可将手指伸过狭窄的上方，并可摸出狭窄范围之大小；如不能通过手指，则不能勉强，否则会引起疼痛、出血，或撕破肠壁。用窥肛器检查时，可见到狭窄下端黏膜色淡。如用狭窄镜

(细形结肠镜)检查,则可见狭窄上端溃疡及肠内情况,可区别线状、片状、环形或全管状狭窄。钡剂灌肠后做 X 线检查,可确定狭窄范围和形状:直肠腔由周围向内缩小成一环形,如狭窄部分上下宽度不过 2.5cm,为环形狭窄。直肠腔由周围向内缩小,狭窄区域较长,成管状,则为管状狭窄;直肠腔部分狭窄,不波及全管周围,为线状狭窄;表面不平、坚硬,常在肠壁一侧为片状狭窄,发展快,甚至出现恶病质,多为恶性肿瘤狭窄。

Diagnosis is based on symptoms mentioned above combined with specialized examination. Digital examination can show many narrow parts, mainly above dentate line 2.5 ~ 5cm, and hard rectal wall with less elasticity. As the hole of stricture is not very small, the finger can insert into the part through it to feel the extension; squeezing through it can easily cause pain, bleeding, or tearing intestinal wall. Examination with anoscope, one can find out color changing light below narrow part; with colonscopy, one can find out ulcer and narrow degree such as linearity, patch, ring and total canal above the strictured part; with X-ray barium enema, the narrow extension and shape forming stricture of centrality can be detected. As the diameter of stricture of centrality is not over 2.5cm, it's called canal shape stricture; to form line shape, not influencing total intestinal wall, it's called linearity shape stricture; as irregular surface, hard, patch on the side of intestinal wall, rapid development, it's the stricture of malignancy.

【治疗】

[Treatment]

1. 安全套气囊扩张疗法

1. Dilatation with Condom-Balloon Therapy

(1)适应证:直肠腔内的黏膜层狭窄与直肠线状或片状狭窄。

(1)Indication:Rectal mucous layer, linearity and patch style stricture.

(2)安全套气束制造方法:见第 11 章第七节。

(2)Making method of condom-ballonet:refer to chapter 11, §7.

(3)方法:按相关章节介绍的方法制作安全套气囊。①治疗前用开塞露 3 枚灌入肛门,洗肠,使直肠内粪便排空。②先将安全套外涂九华膏润滑剂,用手指推进肛管齿线上方的直肠腔。③注入 150ml 或 250ml 空气后针头与安全套气囊连接,然后给安全套气囊充气,扩张狭窄的直肠的,并留置 1h 或 3h,等待患者不能忍耐,则可剪断塑料管,排出空气,安全套即可自行排出。④按上述方法,每天治疗 1 次,3 ~ 7 天为一疗程。

(3)Method:According to involved chapter the condom-balloon is made. The doctor takes the inunction of lubricant on the outside of condom, then inserts the condom into rectal cavity above dentate line through anal canal with his finger, then injects 150 or 250 ml air into the condom-balloon through connected injector to the narrow rectum, then keeps the condom-balloon in the rectum 1 ~ 3 hours. Treat once every day, 3 ~ 7 days is a period of treatment.

2. 探针小针刀配合挂线疗法　鞍麻或腰俞麻醉,截石位。

2. Probe Acupuncture Scalpel Coordinating with Hanging Thread Treatment　Sacral hiatus or lumbar anesthesia, lithotomy position.

（1）肛管狭窄:左手示指伸入肛管内导引,或用两叶肛镜,右手持小针刀先从肛门后侧(6 点钟位)狭窄下端下部、浅部及内括约肌下端,将小针刀刀锋对向肛管腔,边探查边切割,并穿过肛管狭窄后侧全下缘,再刺破肛管,进入肛管腔,顺小针刀锋由肛管内向肛管外弧形割开狭窄的肛管壁,并延长切口到肛缘下 1cm,即完成弧形切开术。肛管直肠指检若认为松解不理想,再选肛门两侧缘(3 点或 9 点钟位),按上法用小针刀割开,一般可以扩肛至可容 3 ~ 4 横指。

（1）Stricture of anal canal:The doctor's left index finger inserts into anal canal for introduction, or using bifoliate dilator. His right hand handles the acupuncture scalpel from posterior part of anus (6 o'clock position), of the interior part of stricture and shallow part and the interior part of internal sphincter, to take the edge of scalpel toward anal canal cavity, probing at the same time cutting and going through the posterior anal canal of stricture, then punctures and breaks anal canal, and inserting into anal canal cavity, then arch cutting narrow wall of anal canal from the inside of anal canal to the outside of anal canal along the edge of acupuncture scalpel and prolongs the incision till below the anal fringe l cm. That's all complete arch incision. If the digital examination shows that the relaxation is unsatisfactory, the doctor may cut the two sides of anus (3 or 9 o clock position), according to above method the anus can be expanded to receive 3 ~ 4 fingers.

（2）直肠狭窄:需探针小针刀配合挂线治疗。齿线以下肛管部分仍可用小针刀按上述方法进行切开。此后右手持探针小针刀继续向纵深边探查边插入,在狭窄的直肠后壁上缘绕过,再刺破直肠壁进入直肠腔。此时小针刀不能切割,需配合挂线治疗。在两叶肛门镜观察下,用左手指或血管钳协助,将小针刀前部探针拉至肛门外;在小针刀探针头系上粗丝线,再将小针刀前部探针原路退回,使粗丝线挂在直肠狭窄处(包括深部括约肌或肛门直肠环)一次性勒紧结扎。直肠指检如认为松解不满意,可选择肛门两侧缘(3 点或 9 点钟位),再按上述方法挂第 2 根或第 3 根引流丝线(不要勒紧结扎),待第 1 根线脱掉后再依次勒紧第 2 根及第 3 根挂线。以防括约肌同时受损、术后肛门内置入痔瘘粉纱布条。照常饮食排便(图 7 - 10)。

（2）Rectal stricture:Probe acupuncture scalpel coordinating with hanging thread treatment. According to the method mentioned above, the acupuncture scalpel can cut anal canal below the dental line. Then the doctor's right hand handles the acupuncture scalpel into the depth, probing at the same time inserting. Let acupuncture scalpel go around the anterior fringe of narrow posterior rectal wall, but not through it. Then puncture through the rectal wall into rectum. Now the acupuncture scalpel can't cut for hang thread. In observing with bifoliate dilator, coordinating left finger or vessel forceps, the doctor puts the anterior probe of acupuncture scalpel out of the anus, then ties the thick silk thread on the top of probe, retracts the acupuncture scalpel along the same way, makes the thick silk thread hanging the narrow part of rectum (including deep sphincter and anorectal ring) to tie tight once. If the digital examination shows that the relaxation is unsatisfactory, the doctor may hang the second or third thread on the two sides of anus (3 or 9 o'clock position), according to above method (don't tie tight) to prevent injuring the sphincter. Cover with gauze at the anal region. After the operation, the patient can eat and defecate as usual (Fig. 7 – 10).

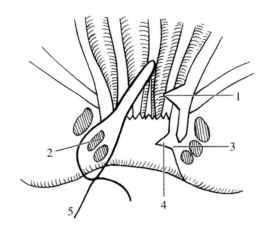

图 7 – 10　肛管直肠狭窄小针刀挂线疗法

1 – 直肠狭窄;2 – 肛门直肠环;3 – 肛管狭窄;4 – 肛管切开;5 – 肛门直肠环挂线

Figure 7 – 10　Acupuncture scalpel hanging thread treating anorectal stricture

1. Rectal stricture; 2. Anorectal ring; 3. Stricture of anal canal;

4. Cutting anal canal; 5. Seton on anorectal ring

第六节　巨直肠与便秘

§6　Megarectum and Constipation

病因不清,长期便秘,排便困难。采用人工扩肛,服泻药长期治疗后,病情反复发作。肛指检查为巨直肠,行肛管直肠压力测定、排粪造影、钡剂灌肠造影、肌电图、直肠镜检查等确诊。

The agnogenic disease manifestations include difficult defecation and long time constipation. Dilation and taking laxative have been used for many years, but this is painful and often unsuccessful. The examination can make a definite diagnosis through digital pressure monitor of anal canal, defecography, barium enema, muscle electromyogram, rectoscopy, etc.

【治疗】

[Treatment]

采用小针刀闭合切断内括约肌治疗。取侧卧位,消毒、局麻。术者先用左手示指插入肛管内约 1.5cm,确定括约肌肌间沟上缘即为内括约肌,按压固定。右手持肛肠斜面小针刀从肛门外 3 点或 9 点钟位点状局麻的针眼插入。在肛管内的左手示指引导下,隔着肛管左手示指尖摸到小针刀顶端,随着右手握持的斜面小针刀,两手指同时上下配合纵行切开内括约肌 1.5～2cm,禁忌横切,切勿刺穿肛管腔。拔出小针刀,术毕(图 7－11)。

Acupuncture scalpel is used to cut off internal sphincter. Taking lateral posture for sterilizing and local anesthesia, the doctor's left index finger inserts into anal canal 1.5cm to define and feel the position of intersphincteric ditch, its upper fringe is the internal sphincter, and to fix the internal sphincter. His right hand handles the inclined plane acupuncture scalpel to insert into internal sphincter from local anesthetic points outside of anus at 3 or 9 o'clock position, and in the guidance of his left index finger tip touching the top of acupuncture scalpel through anal canal, then his right hand handles the inclined plane acupuncture scalpel to insert into internal sphincter, and cuts vertically internal sphincter 1.5～2cm but doesn't cut horizontally. The acupuncture scalpel does not puncture the anal canal and then the doctor puts the acupuncture scalpel out (Fig. 7－11).

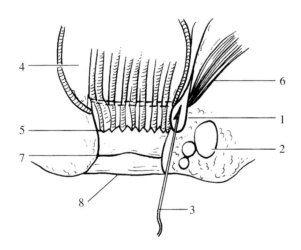

图 7－11　巨直肠便秘小针刀疗法

1－内括约肌;2－外括约肌;3－小针刀;4－巨直肠;

5－齿线;6－肛提肌;7－肌间沟;8－肛门

Figure 7－11　Acupuncture scalpel treating megarectal constipation

1. Internal Sphincter; 2. External Sphincter; 3. Acupuncture Scalpel; 4. Megarectum;

5. Dentate Line; 6. Levator Ani Muscle; 7. Intersphincteric Ditch; 8. Anus

【点评】

[Review]

特发性巨直肠的肛管长度明显高于正常人,直肠腔宽大,腔内压力低,内括约肌反射虽然存在,但排便阈值(即注入直肠气囊的空气量)高出正常人 1 倍多。指检无狭窄。可触及大量蓄积粪便。采用小针刀闭合切断内括约肌术式简单,效果好。

The length of megarectum is obviously longer than that in normal persons. The rectal cavity is large, and the pressure in the cavity is low. Although the reflection of internal sphincter exists, defecation threshold (the air dose being injected) is twice as high as that of normal person. Digital examination can show a large amount of stool. Carrying on acupuncture scalpel cutting off internal sphincter is a simple method with a good effect.

第七节　耻骨直肠肌痉挛与便秘

§7　Spasm of Puborectal Muscle and Constipation

【病因】

[Etiology]

耻骨直肠肌痉挛是一种以耻骨直肠肌肥大引起的功能性与器质性出口梗阻、排粪障碍性疾病,常与慢性炎症、滥用泻药等有关。

Puborectal muscular spasm is a kind of disease resulted from puborectal muscular hypertrophy leading to functional and organic obstruction of outlet and difficult defecation, commonly related to chronic inflammation and abusive laxative.

【临床表现】

[Clinical Manifestations]

严重的排粪条细窄,排便频繁,但仍有排粪不畅感,伴肛门或骶尾部坠胀疼痛。

Very thin stool, difficulty in initiating bowel movement, the feeling of incomplete evacuation, the pain with falling and distension in sacrococcygeal region is also common.

【诊断】

[Diagnosis]

肛门直肠指检,手指通过肛管有狭窄感,肛管明显延长,伴触痛,直肠环后部边缘锐利,直肠后方呈囊袋状,耻骨直肠呈搁板状,亦称"搁架征",即可确诊。排便造影检查 X 线片见肛直角变小,肛管延长见图 7 - 12。

Digital examination can reveal narrow and obviously long anal canal with touching pain, posterior hard fringe of rectal ring, posterior rectal wall forming sack shape, puborectal muscle changing clapboard style, it's also called "clapboard syndrome". The clapboard syndrome can make a definite diagnosis. Defecography X-ray shows the anorectal angle becoming smaller and prolongation of anal canal(Fig. 7 – 12).

【治疗】

[Treatment]

手术切断痉挛的耻骨直肠肌。过去认为,耻骨直肠是组成肛门直肠环的重要部分,其功能是控制排便,一旦切断将造成大便失禁。但耻骨直肠肌一旦发生痉挛性肥大等病理改变,其肌纤维往往呈纤维化,与周围肌组织产生粘连,因此手术切断后不会发生肛门失禁。

The spastic puborectal muscle is cut off through surgery. Puborectal muscle is an important part to form rectal ring, and its function is to control defecation. Once being cut off, incontinence will occur. But now the doctor thinks that once puborectal muscle becomes spastic hypertrophy with other pathological changes, the muscles often form fibrosis to adhere with surrounding tissues. So incontinence can't occur after it has been cut off by operation.

常规消毒,腰麻或局麻,肛门缘与尾骨尖的中点为小针刀进口。右手持钩头小针刀,于此进针点垂直刺入,左手示指先伸入肛管直肠做导诊,触及尾骨尖为耻骨直肠肌上缘标志,用左手示指伸入直肠腔向上顶起,并扣住痉挛耻骨直肠肌,右手持小针刀纵行钩割切断 1 ~ 2cm。再用左手示指触及加压,对凹陷、已被切断的耻骨直肠肌按摩,加大其间隙,以防术后肌断端肌纤维粘连,并隔着直肠后壁可钝性分离,扩大切断面。以左手示指触及并感到耻骨直肠变松弛,有凹陷感为度。如不理想可再纵行重切,但勿横切,勿刺破肠腔引起感染。以在左示指尖与右手小针刀头部相吻合、相触及为原则,确认左手示指触摸到右手小针刀头才可以钩割切断痉挛的耻骨直肠肌。切忌只使用小针刀盲目切割,以防损伤肛提肌及外括约肌深部,造成大便失禁。该法可以将以往复杂的开放性耻骨直肠肌切开缝合术变成简单的闭合微创术,手术简单,效果好,无并发症(图 7 – 12,图 7 – 13)。

Sterilization as usual and lumbar anesthesia or local anesthesia is performed. The doctor's left finger inserts into anal canal to touch the tip of coccyx. The tip of coccyx is index the mark of upper fringe of puborectal muscle. Then the left index finger inserts rectum to hold up and fix spastic puborectal muscle right. His right hand handles the acupuncture scalpel to insert into puborectal muscle from the middle point between anal fringe and the tip of coccyx, and with the guidance of his left index finger a forehand inserting into anal canal to touch the tip of coccyx, then his right hand handles the acupuncture scalpel to cut off vertically spastic puborectal muscle 1 ~ 2cm. Then again his left index finger touches and presses to massage the sunk puborectal muscle having been cut off so as to increase the space of section lest postoperative adhesion of sectional fiber. The massage can enlarge the section through posterior rectal wall. The standard of incision is that the doctor's left index finger touches relaxing and sunks in puborectal muscle. If the operation can't make relaxation, cut it vertically again. Don't cut it horizontally for fear of breaking up intestinal cavity to cause infection. The doctor confirms his left index finger tip touching the top of acupuncture scalpel, then cuts and hooks the spastic puborectal muscle. Avoiding by all means blind cutting, for fear of injuring levator ani muscle and deep part of external sphincter to cause incontinence (Fig. 7 – 12, Fig. 7 – 13).

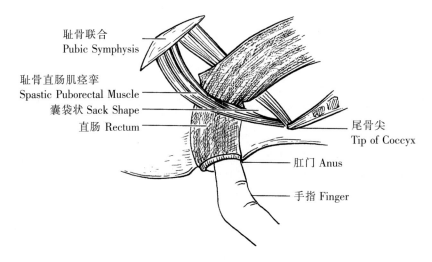

图 7 – 12 耻骨直肠肌痉挛图

Figure 7 – 12 Spastic puborectal muscle

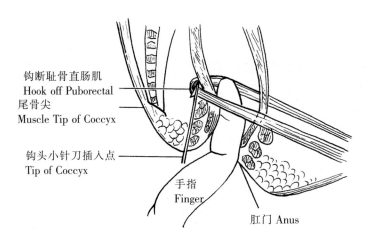

图 7 – 13 小针刀钩断耻骨直肠肌

Figure 7 – 13 Acupuncture scalpel hooking off puborectal muscle

第八节　粪便嵌塞

§8　Stool Block

粪便嵌塞是粪便梗阻于肛管、直肠中,患者无能力自行排出,须协助治疗。多见于老年人、卧床患者及长期用泻药者;多为功能性,少有器质性;可并发粪块性直肠溃疡、出血或穿孔。

Stool block means the stool blocks in anal canal and rectum. The patients may not be able to defect stool, in need of help. It is commonly seen in the persons who are old, sickbed and taking laxative for long time. It is commonly functional but not organic obstruction. It may be complicated with rectal ulcer, bleeding or perforation.

【病因病机】

[Etiology and Pathology]

中医便秘、脱肛、虚劳、肠痹,就是西医的粪便嵌塞、便秘、出口梗阻。中医称肛门为魄门、后阴、司开阖,排出糟粕,为肾所主。位于大肠之末端,其需肾气之温煦气化,肺气之宣发肃降,脾之健运,心血滋养,肝气疏泄。若饮食不节,七情失调,劳倦过度,生育过多,年老气衰,久病不愈,导致脾气失健运。其"中气受损"清阳不升,浊阴下降,脾气不能散,精于肺,而洒其六腑致大肠功能失常,肾元气亏损,不能气化温煦,心血失其滋润,肝气郁结而气机不畅,使肛门不能开阖,糟粕不能排出,致粪便嵌塞。关键是"清阳不升,浊阴不降"《内经》说"清阳出上窍,浊阴出下窍。清阳发腠理,浊阴走五脏,清阳实四肢,浊阴归六腑。"

In traditional Chinese medicine it is thought that the anus is a soul gate, it controls the excretion of waste material controlled by kidney which is end of the large intestine. The anus needs to be taken warm by the kidneys' Qi, raised and descended by the lungs' Qi, moved by the spleen, nourished by the heart, and dredged by the liver's Qi. In case of crapulent, maladjustment of emotion, very tied, over birth, old age, long time sick, that all may cause spleen deficiency. In addition, the middle Qi being hurt so that the clear Yang can't rise up; the dirty Yin can't fall down; the spleen Qi can't go normally but concentrates in lungs and spreads to six hollow organs; so the large intestine loses normal function.

【诊断】

[Diagnosis]

1. 病因诊断

1. Diagnosis of Etiology

（1）长期卧床,尤其腹部、盆部手术、骨折、妇科、泌尿科手术后,以老年人多发。

（1）Sickbed long time, especially in postoperative period of abdominal, pelvic, post-fracture, gynecologic, and urologic surgeries in old persons commonly.

（2）精神病、失眠、习惯看报排便者等。

（2）Persons with psychosis, insomnia and reading during defecation.

（3）长期习惯服泻药者或灌肠者,导致结直肠蠕动减弱,一旦停止服泻药则造成粪便嵌塞。

（3）Persons taking laxative or enema for a long time cause hypoperistalsis of intestine, once stop taking laxative, then stool block will occur.

（4）截瘫患者不仅粪便谳塞,有时还会大便失禁。

（4）Paraplegic patients may have not only stool block, but also stool incontinence sometimes.

2. 鉴别诊断

2. Differential Diagnosis

（1）先天性巨结肠病:主要是病变肠远侧节段神经节细胞缺如,导致肠无力、肠管扩张巨大。

（1）Congenital megacolon:Mainly resulted from that deficiency of nervous ganglion cells in distant pathologic colon, to cause no power of bowel movement while enlarging the cavity of colon.

（2）直肠无力:与巨结肠病的区分是,直肠无力不存在神经节细胞缺如;也有继发巨、结肠病者,其特点是直肠对粪便容量的刺激不起反应,而且肛门的括约肌明显松弛无力。

（2）No power of rectum:No power of bowel movement is different from megacolon of deficient nervous ganglion cells. Another is secondary to the disease from megacolon. The feature is that the rectum won't react for stimulation of stool volume, while anal sphincter is relaxed.

（3）肛门内括约肌痉挛:肛裂、肛窦炎、内外痔、肛瘘等致肛门内括约肌痉挛加重或纤维化变窄。因为这类患者长期惧怕排便疼痛,抑制排便或服用止痛药而加重,以至恶性循环。

（3）Anal internal sphincteric spasm:All these diseases, such as anal fissure, anal sinusitis, internal hemorrhoids, anal fistula, etc., can cause exaggeration of anal internal sphincteric spasm or narrow fibrosis. Because these patients are afraid of pain defecation so as to inhibit bowel movement, or take anodyne, thus causing a vicious circle to make the illness growing worse.

（4）直肠内异物:误吞金属异物或骨片,致嵌插直肠内壁,引起粪便嵌塞。

（4）Foreign material in the rectum:The foreign metal material or section of bone eaten inadvertently cause incarceration in the rectal wall to lead to stool block.

（5）肛门耻骨直肠肌痉挛综合征：使直肠颈牵拉、悬吊、狭窄。

（5）Syndrome of anal puborectal muscular spasm：Make the rectal neck be involved and hung up to cause stricture.

（6）直肠黏膜内脱垂：排便时直肠松弛的黏膜层阻塞肛管。

（6）Inner rectal mucous prolapse：The relaxed rectal mucosa obstructs the anal canal in bowel movement.

（7）直肠阴道前突症：排便时粪块经直肠前壁疝囊经阴道后壁凸入阴道。

（7）Rectocele toward vagina：Stools project towards posterior vaginal wall through rectovaginal septum of anterior thin sack-style rectal wall in bowel movement.

（8）肛管直肠先天或后天手术、外伤致狭窄，或病久。

（8）Congenital or acquired stricture in anal canal and rectum, the latter results from frequent operations, trauma, or prolonged sickness.

（9）肛管直肠套叠。

（9）Anal canal-rectum intussusception.

（10）肛管直肠肿瘤：如癌肿增生，狭窄。

（10）Tumor in anal canal and rectum.

粪块嵌塞，不但引起直肠腔极度扩张，并可刺激直肠黏膜引起炎症、糜烂、出血，诱发溃疡穿孔和腹膜炎。

Stool block can not only induce enlarged rectal cavity, but also stimulate rectal mucosa to cause inflammation, erosion, bleeding, ulcer, perforation and peritonitis.

【治疗】
[Treatment]

1. 针对性治疗
1. Suit the Remedy to the Case

（1）根据病因采用治疗方案、方法。

（1）To adopt treating scheme and method according to etiology.

（2）配合小针刀闭合切断：①内括约肌痉挛；②耻骨直肠肌痉挛。

（2）To cut off with the acupuncture scalpel：①Spasm of internal sphincter；②Spasm of puborectal muscle.

(3)腰俞麻醉下,用手指挖出嵌塞粪便或用圆头圈钳夹住,嵌塞粪块取出肛管外;或配合"刮匙小针刀"将嵌塞粪块化整为条,取出肛门外。

(3)To put out the obstructive material from inner anus by round-head forceps or the acupuncture scalpel in YaoShu acupoint local anesthesia.

(4)对合并直肠出血者,在圆头缺口电池灯肛门下,找到出血点,用消痔灵液封闭注射。并放置撒有痔瘘粉的止血海绵块。

(4)To treat complicated rectal bleeding, finding out the bleeding points and doing hemostasis with optical anoscopy, then covering with gauze.

(5)对并直肠穿孔者,则开腹行直肠穿孔单纯修补术及盆腔橡皮管引流术。

(5)To treat rectal perforation, using abdominal incision to repair perforation simply and to make drainage with a rubber tube.

2. 中医辨证施治
2. Differentiation Treatment by Traditional Chinese Medicine

(1)首先根据西医的正确诊断,再进行中医辨证施治,以防止误诊误治。

(1)To carry on treatment first according to correct modern medical diagnosis, then relying on traditional Chinese medical differentiating syndrome, for preventing mistakes of diagnosis and treatment.

(2)做肛门直肠动力学检查、结肠传输功能检查、肛门肌电图、排粪造影检查、光导纤维直结肠镜、肛门直肠腔内 B 超检查等,为确诊提供依据,也为缩小中医辨证范围提供依据。

(2)To take anorectal dynamical examination, functional transmission of colon, muscle electromyogram and defecography, and optical fibrous rectocolonoscopic examination, ultrasonography in lumen of anus and rectum examination, barium enema, electromyogram, rectoscopy, etc., for making a definite diagnosis, and for shrinking extent of differentiated syndrome by traditional Chinese medicine.

根据辨证,可采取依热则寒之,燥则调之,风则驱之。例如补脾健胃,口服通便汤,配合小针刀治疗等(参阅相关内容)。

According to differentiated syndrome, the doctors can carry on expelling heat with cold herbs, regulate dry disease, and repel wind toxin (Refer to related sections in this book).

第九节　盆底痉挛综合征
§9　Syndrome of Pelvic Bottom Spasm

盆底痉挛综合征,多合并耻骨直肠肌痉挛综合征或内括约肌痉挛综合征。在排便过程中,盆底和肛门不舒张,不开放,反而收缩痉挛,使肛门关闭,造成粪便滞留、便秘,引起排便困难或粪便梗阻性疾病。

The syndrome of pelvic bottom spasm complicates commonly the spasmic syndrome of puborectus muscle and internal sphincter. In the bowel movement, the pelvic bottom and anus are not dilated and open, but contract to make the anus spasm, with the stool in the intestinal lumen, thus inducing difficult defecation and constipation or stool block.

【病因病机】

[Etiology and Pathology]

根据临床和盆底肌电图等分析,多种因素牵拉或损伤盆底神经、骶神经和盆底肌肉群可引起盆底痉挛。

According to clinical analysis and pelvic muscle electromyogram, the spasm of pelvic bottom results from many factors of traction and trauma involving the pelvic bottom nerves, sacral nerve and pelvic bottom muscles.

1. **神经系统** 受损伤神经纤维缩小,传导迟缓,甚至丧失。

1. **Nervous System** Injured nervous fibers become smaller, slower transmission and even lost.

2. **肌肉群** 一组或某一囊肌肉纤维被牵拉延长、变细,甚至纤维断裂,影响肌肉功能,引起收缩痉挛,故造成盆底功能紊乱。

2. **Muscles** A sheaf of muscle or a group of muscles is prolonged with traction, becomes thin and even breaks off. These changes affect muscular function to give rise to muscular spasm and to cause pelvic bottom functional disorder.

【临床表现】

[Clinical Manifestations]

便秘 3 ~ 5d 排便 1 次。粪便干燥或球形粪块,排便困难。排便后肛门仍有下坠感,或排不尽感,伴肛门、会阴胀痛,甚至粪便阻塞。

The patient defecates once every 3 – 5 days or has constipation. His stools are dry or ball shape, with difficult defecation, the feeling of incomplete evacuation, pain with falling and distension in anal and perineal region, even stool block.

【诊断】

[Diagnosis]

根据病史、临床症状和如下检查可以明确诊断。

According to medical history, clinical symptoms and examination as follows, definite diagnosis can be made.

1. 肛指检查

1. Digital Examination

（1）合并耻骨直肠肌痉挛者。肛指检查触及尾骨尖上、直肠环后缘有囊袋、搁板征。

（1）The doctor can feel sack and "clapboard syndrome" above the tip of coccyx and posterior fringe of rectal ring in puborectal muscular spasm.

（2）合并内括约肌痉挛者。肛指检查触及肌间沟上内括约肌痉挛或肥厚。

（2）The doctor can feel spasm or hypertrophy of internal sphincter above intersphincteric ditch.

2. 排便造影　检查结直肠肛管的功能、动力和解剖结构，有无病灶。

2. Defecography　To check up the rectocolon function, dynamical force and anatomical structure.

3. 肛管直肠测压　检查肛门直肠的括约肌功能。

3. Pressure Monitor of Anal Canal and Rectum　To check up anorectal sphincteric function.

4. 盆底肌电图检查

4. Pelvic Bottom Muscular Electromyography

（1）耻骨直肠肌痉挛，肌电图静息相下紧张表现异常。

（1）Puborectal muscular spasm： Tension in resting muscular electromyography.

（2）盆底肌肉痉挛，肌电图静息相收缩，肛门相和用力排便动作相出现反常肌电表现，如呈反向收缩的异常肌电征。

（2）Pelvic bottom spasm：Resting pelvic muscle electromyogram shows contraction, anal-gram and headlong defecating movement-gram shows abnormal expressions such as reverse contraction, and abnormal features of electromyogram.

【治疗】

[Treatment]

1. 针灸或电针　大肠俞、气海俞、太溪俞、肾俞、脾俞、次谬俞。

1. Acupuncture and Electroacupuncture　To puncture points of DaChangShu (large intestine), QiHaiShu (Qi's controlling centre), TaiXiShu, ShenShu (kidney), PiShu (spleen), and CiLiaoShu.

2. 中药治疗　①通便汤,一煎,口服。②二煎,灌肠。

2. Herbal Treatment　To take the herbal decoction of TongBianTang (let the defecation free) first and then give enema with the secondary boiled decoction.

3. 钩针埋入羊肠线　穴位:长强、会阴、双侧足三里等穴。

3. Hook Style Needle Hanging Thread in Acupuncture Points　Points：ChangQiang, HuiYin(perineum), ZuSanLi of both sides, etc.

4. 穴位注入药液疗法

4. Injecting the Drugs into the Acupuncture Points

(1)用针管经腰俞穴(骶骨裂孔),注入药液,治疗骶盆、神经见(第 5 章第三节)。

(1)Injecting the drugs into the lumbar points (sacral hiatus) to treat sacral, pelvic nervous diseases (see chapter 5, § 9).

(2)药液组合:①1% 利多卡因 10ml 加入生理盐水 5ml,共 15ml。②维生素 B_1 100g,维生素 B_6 100g,维生素 B_{12} 100g;加辅酶 A 50U,肌苷 100g,山莨菪碱 10mg。③曲安奈德注射液(曲安缩松注射液)40mg。

(2)Components of drugs：①1% Lidocaine 10ml with physiological saline 5ml, totally 15ml. ②Vitamin B_1 100mg, Vitamin B_{12} 100mg, add in Coenzyme A 50U, Camine 100g, Anisodamine 100mg. ③Triamcinonlone acetonide injecta (acetospan injecta) 40mg.

注意:上述药液不能静脉注射。针头插入腰俞穴回吸无回血可吸入 20ml 针管中,改用细小短的 7 号针头,18min 一次性注入腰俞穴,每周 1 次,1 个月为一疗程。

Notice：All drugs mentioned above can't be injected into veins. To inject through by a 20ml syringe, 7# syringe needle into lumbar points as sucking in no blood, should be injected slowly in 18 minutes, once every week, one month as a treating course .

5. 小针刀手术　①合并耻骨直肠肌痉挛者采用钩头小针刀治疗;②合并内括约肌痉挛者,采用斜面小针刀治疗。

5. Acupuncture Scalpel Surgery　①The patient complicated with puborectal muscular spasm can be treated by hook style head acupuncture scalpel. ②The patient complicated with internal sphincteric muscular spasm can be treated by the inclined plane acupuncture scalpel.

第十节 其他排便障碍性疾病

§10 Other Diseases about Difficult Defecation

一、盆底失弛缓综合征

I. Nonrelaxing Pelvic Floor Syndrome

盆底肌肉和肛管内括约肌失弛缓,引起排便困难,称为盆底失弛缓综合征。

It's called nonrelaxing pelvic floor syndrome that pelvic floor muscles and internal sphincter of anal canal lose relaxed function to cause difficult defecation.

【病因病机】

[Etiology and Pathology]

盆底失弛缓综合征,是排便时盆腔底部的横纹肌,尤其是肛管内括约肌不协同松弛,使肛管不开放,粪便不能排出肛门外而引起便秘。

The nonrelaxing pelvic bottom syndrome results from striated muscles of pelvic bottom that can't coordinate relaxation with internal sphincter of anal canal to cause that anal canal can't work normally, the stool can't be defecated out, so that constipation occurs.

【临床表现】

[Clinical Manifestations]

通过盆底肌电图或肛管内括约肌的肌电图和肛管测压检查,证明主要是内括约肌持续痉挛,使肛管腔压力升高;同时盆底横纹肌细小收缩短暂,因而出现排便困难,便秘,肛门坠胀痛。

The examinations through electromyography of pelvic floor muscles and internal sphincter of anal canal, and pressure monitor of anal canal, prove mainly that lasting spasm of internal sphincter increase the pressure of anal canal lumen, together with small, thin and short contraction of pelvic floor striated muscles at the same time, so as to difficult defecation, constipation and anal pain with falling and distension.

【诊断】

[Diagnosis]

根据便秘病史,肛指检查触及肛管内括约肌痉挛和肥厚;患者做排粪便动作时,肛管不松弛反而紧缩。排粪造影呈盆底失弛缓综合征典型特征。

According to medical history of constipation, digital examination can feel spasm and hypertrophy of anal canal internal sphincter. In the bowel movement, the anal canal is not only nonrelaxing, but also contracting. Defecography shows classical features of nonrelaxing pelvic floor syndrome.

【治疗】
[Treatment]

1. 口服中药　如通便汤。
1. **Taking Herbs**　Decoction of TongBianTang (keep free bowel movement).

2. 小针刀治疗　参考"内括约肌失弛缓与便秘。"
2. **Acupuncture Scalpel Treatment**　Refer to "Nonrelaxing Internal sphincter and constipation."

二、盆底松弛综合征
II. Relaxing Pelvic Bottom Syndrome

盆底松弛综合征多合并直肠前凸或会阴下降,以女性多见,由于盆腔多个脏器或单个脏器下垂,盆底失去承托,而脱出盆底外,引起排粪便紊乱,肛门功能或器质性失控或便秘;也有出现泌尿或生殖脏器下垂或外脱者。

Relaxing pelvic bottom syndrome commonly combined with rectocele or perineum falling, is commonly seen in female, many visceroptosis or single visceroptosis go outside of pelvic bottom because the pelvic bottom loses holding function, so as to disordered defecation, functional and organic incontinence and constipation. Others may have also urinary or generative organs prolapse, even prolapse toward outside.

【病因病机】
[Etiology and Pathology]

多是综合因素作用的结果。例如妇科、泌尿科和肛肠科疾病等,引起盆底、会阴和肛门神经、肌肉、韧带损伤。

It results from composite factors commonly, for example, the diseases of gynecology, urology and proctology injury nerves, muscles and ligaments of pelvic bottom, perineum and anus.

1. 神经系统　盆底下降加重对盆底神经、阴部神经和肛门直肠神经的牵拉,神经纤维被拉牵长后失去传导功能而失控。
1. **Nervous System**　The pelvic bottom prolapse increases tractive force for nerves of pelvic bottom, perineum, anus and rectum. The nervous fibers are pulled long and lose its transmitting function so as to lose control.

2. **肌肉群**　脏器下垂可加重肌肉群牵拉,尤其长期患盆底痉挛者肌肉松弛,肌肉、韧带纤维化、变性或断裂,以至失去收缩、粘连作用。不能悬吊、固定和承托盆腔上口的脏器。

2. **Muscular Group**　The visceroptosis increases tractive force for muscular group, especially suffering from pelvic bottom spasm long, to make muscle and ligaments relaxation, fibrosis, degeneration and rupture so that muscles and ligaments won't take part in contraction and adhesion. One can't hang, locate and hold up organs in inlet of pelvic cavity.

【临床表现】
[Clinical Manifestations]

1. 排便紊乱
1. Disordered Defecation

(1)排便失控,尤其老年人,粪便液外溢,甚至大便失禁。

(1)Uncontrollable defecation, especially in old persons, even incontinence of feces.

(2)便秘,排便困难:有的需用手指插入肛门;女性用手指伸入阴道来协助排便。

(2)Difficult defecation and constipation.

2. 盆底受压
2. Pelvic Floor Being Pressed

(1)肛门、会阴下坠或坠痛,堵塞胀满感。与其体位变化有关,往往站立或坐位加重,平卧位可缓解或减轻。

(1)The falling pain of anus and perineum, and feeling of distension and obstruction, are related to changes of body posture. The illness grows worse as standing or sitting, while relieves as lying.

(2)盆底会阴下凸或会阴突出包块物。

(2)Pelvic bottom and perineum prolapse.

(3)合并盆底疝、会阴下降、肛门直肠三角下降,以致脱肛、直肠脱垂、直肠黏膜脱垂等。

(3)Combined with pelvic bottom hernia, perineum and anorectal triangle falling leading to anus, rectum and rectal mucosa prolapse, etc.

【诊断】
[Diagnosis]

根据病史、临床表现和如下检查可确诊。

According to medical history, clinical symptoms and examination are as follows, and definite diagnosis can be made.

1.肛指检查
1. Digital Rectal Examination

（1）触及肛门直肠括约肌松弛，无张力，收缩功能欠佳，甚至失禁。

（1）The doctor can feel anorectal sphincter relaxation, no strain to influence the contractive function, even to cause incontinence.

（2）会阴下降，整个盆腔、盆底，松弛下垂，臀沟变浅且外凸。

（2）The doctor can feel perineum falling, total pelvic cavity and pelvic bottom relaxing and falling to cause the ditch of hips becoming shallow.

（3）直肠突凸于阴道后壁呈囊袋状。

（3）The doctor can feel the rectum projecting towards posterior of vaginal wall to form sack shape.

（4）子宫后倾压迫直肠前壁，致肛门直肠腔窄小，甚至脱肛、直肠脱垂。

（4）Tipbacked uterus presses the anterior of rectal wall to cause the rectal cavity becoming smaller, even anal prolapse and rectal prolapse.

（5）直肠内套叠、盆底疝、会阴下降、肠疝等特征。

（5）Intussusception in rectum, pelvic bottom hernia, perineum falling, intestinal hernia, etc.

2.排便造影检查　见横结肠、乙状结肠过长，纡曲垂入盆腔。
2. Defecography　Transverse and sigmoid colon are too long, circular falling in the pelvic cavity.

3.B 超检查　可确定脏器下垂程度、性质。
3. B Style Ultrasonography　To decide the degree and characteristics of visceroptosis.

4.CT 或 MRI 检查　确定盆腔器官性质、病灶、部位、程度、脏器彼此的关系。
4. CT or MRI examination　To decide the degree, characteristics and position of normal and abnormal viscerae, and their relationship.

5.肌电图检查　了解盆底、会阴、肛门、直肠肌肉松弛表现、程度、范围等。
5. Muscular Electromyography　To understand muscular relaxing manifestation, degree and extension, etc. in pelvic bottom, perineum, anus and rectum.

【治疗】

[Treatment]

1. 针灸或电针　白环俞穴、三阴交、阴陵泉、脾俞、肾俞、足三里。

1. Acupuncture and Electroacupuncture　To puncture points of BaiHuanShu, SanYinJiao, YinLingQuan, ShenShu (kidney), PiShu (spleen), and ZuSanLi.

2. 中药治疗　口服补中益气汤。

2. Herbal Treatment　To take the decoction of BuZhongYiQiTang.

3. 封闭疗法　如在骶骨上缘腧穴封闭疗法。

3. Blocking Therapy　Point-blocking therapy above the fringe of sacrum.

(1)腧穴在解剖学上相当于骶部、会阴部的神经丛区域,是椎体旁交感神经干下端的神经分支相吻合处,对肛提肌、尾骨肌的分支感觉、运动均有重要作用。

(1) The points are placed similar to anatomical nervous plexus in sacrum and perineum region, which are the identical nervous branches lying on inferior end of sympathetic trunk in paravertebrate region, and have an important part in feeling and moving of the branch of levator ani muscles and coccygeal muscle.

(2)封闭方法用 7 号针头,以此腧穴为中心封闭 3～5cm^2。深入皮下脂肪层及骶骨前面。

(2) The method of blocking: To inject through 7# syringe needle into adipose layer and anterior of sacrum around the points 3~5cm^2.

(3)药液组合:①0.5% 利多卡因 2ml;②维生素 B$_1$ 100mg;③维生素 B$_{12}$ 100mg;④复方丹参注射液 3ml(不能静脉注射)。

(3) Components of drugs: ①0.5% Lidocaine 2ml; ②Vitamins B$_1$ 100mg; ③Vitamins B$_{12}$ 100mg; ④Compound injection of red sage root 3ml (not to inject into veins).

(4)疗程:每周封闭 1 次,4 次为一疗程。

(4) Treating course: Once every week, one month is one treating course.

4. 小针刀手术

4. Surgery

(1)盆底肌肉修补术:多用于合并妇科疾病、会阴下凸、阴道松弛下凸或外脱等,伴肛门下垂。缝合,上吊松弛的盆底,并修补阴道前壁。

(1) Repairing pelvic bottom muscles: Using the method in anal falling common complicated gynecological diseases, such as perineal falling, vaginal relaxation, falling or prolapse towards out-

side. To tie to hand up the relaxed pelvic bottom and to repair the anterior vaginal wall.

（2）子宫疾病：压迫严重,且年长者可行子宫摘除术,主韧带可缝合悬掸腹直肠后鞘,提升盆底以减轻对直肠前壁的压迫;封闭子宫与直肠陷窝,膀胱直肠间隙,以前后腹膜缝合封闭,以及行肛门坐骨间隙、骨盆直肠间隙盆底抬高缝合固定术。

（2）Treating uterine diseases：To perform uterectomy for patients whose rectum is pressed seriously and ages are big, to tie to hand up posterior rectal wall, so as to hold up pelvic bottom, and reduce the pressure to anterior rectal wall; to close cavum Douglas rectovesical pouch and anterior and posterior peritoneum; to tie, hand up and fix relaxed pelvic bottom in ischioanal space and pelvirectal space.

（3）盆腔下垂肠管手术：将下垂纡曲过长的横结肠或乙状结肠切除,缩短肠管,回位腹腔,解除对盆底的压迫。

（3）Intestinal operation in falling pelvic cavity：To cut off over long circular falling transverse or sigmoid colon make shorten intestine, retire back abdominal cavity to relieve pressure for pelvic bottom.

（4）直肠前凸治疗（图 7 - 14）,见第 7 章第二节。

（4）Treating rectocele （Fig. 7 - 14）,refer to chapter 7 § 2.

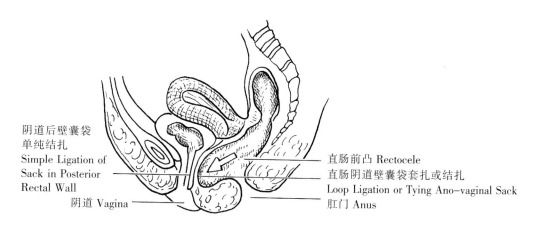

阴道后壁囊袋单纯结扎　Simple Ligation of Sack in Posterior Rectal Wall

直肠前凸 Rectocele
直肠阴道壁囊袋套扎或结扎 Loop Ligation or Tying Ano-vaginal Sack

阴道 Vagina

肛门 Anus

图 7 - 14　直肠前凸治疗
Figure 7 - 14　Treating rectocele

（5）直肠黏膜内脱垂、脱肛直肠脱垂治疗（图 7 - 15,图 7 - 16）;见第 7 章第一节。

（5）Treating mucosa prolapse in rectum, anal prolapse and rectal prolapse （Fig. 7 - 15, Fig. 7 - 16）, refer to chapter 7 § 1.

（6）肠套叠治疗：采用手指或肛管内灌中药"通便汤",送回套叠的肠管。

（6）Treating intussusception：To carry on finger-manipulative reduction or enema with the decoction of TongBianTang (let the defecation free).

（7）合并直肠子宫凹、滑动疝配合小针刀修补术。

（7）Repairing slipped hernia of cavum Douglasi with acupuncture scalpel.

（8）合并肛门括约肌松弛,甚至外溢粪液。采用钩头小针,紧缩肛门术。

（8）Contracting anus with hook style head acupuncture scalpel for treating anosphincteric relaxation.

（9）手术后仍要口服中药升举汤辅助治疗。

（9）Taking decoction of ShengJuTang for postoperative adjuvant therapy.

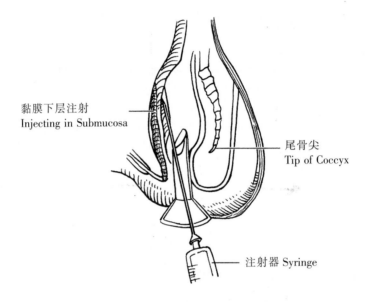

图 7 - 15　直肠黏膜内脱垂治疗

Figure 7 - 15　Treating mucosa prolapse in rectum

三、肛门三角下降综合征

III. Anal Triangle Falling Syndrome

【病因病机】

[Etiology and Pathology]

肛门和肛管位于两侧坐骨结节连线水平位置之上,骶尾骨前侧的肛门三角正中。由于长期用力排便,尤其是干燥粪块时可引起盆底肌肉和肛管直肠肌肉松弛,迫使肛门和肛管下降,甚至脱出肛门外,并引起相应的症状。

Anus and anal canal are located above an interischial line between two ischial tuberosities, at

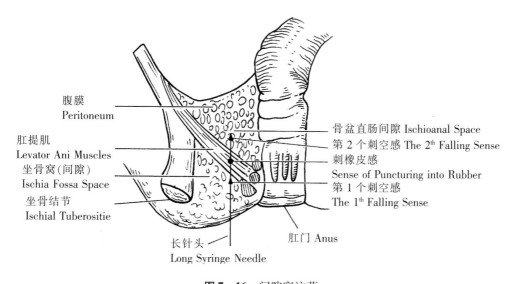

图 7 – 16　间隙窝注药

Figure 7 – 16　Injecting medicine into space and fossa

the middle position of anal triangle in anterior part of sacrum and coccyx. Because defecation strain lasts long especial dry stools can cause the muscles of pelvic bottom and anal canal relaxing to make the prolapse of anus and anal canal even prolapse out of anus with symptoms.

【临床表现】

[Clinical Manifestations]

排便困难,排粪便后肛管内感觉不通畅,或肛门三角下坠感。有的伴内痔或直肠黏膜脱垂、脱肛。老年人患肛门括约肌松弛性大便失禁。

The difficulty in initiating bowel movement, the feeling of incomplete evacuation, and the feeling with falling in anal triangle region are also common. Some patients complicated with internal hemorrhoids and prolapses of rectal mucosa and anus. The old patients are easy to have incontinence of stool due to relaxing of anal sphincter.

【诊断】

[Diagnosis]

根据排便困难的病史和症状。蹲位检查以肛门和肛管为中心的肛三角下降,并超越两侧坐骨结节连线水平之下 2～3cm。肛指检查触及,肛门内括约肌和外括约肌松弛。排便造影见肛管、直肠、肛门三角,或盆底位置下降,肛肠角加大,肛管下降超过 2～3cm。

Diagnosis relies on the medical history, clinical symptoms and examinations. In squat position examination, anal triangle relying on the center of anus and anal canal falls below the interischial line 2～3cm. In digital examination, the doctor can feel anal internal sphincter relaxation. Defecography shows the positions of anal canal, rectum, anal triangle or pelvic bottom falling, anorectal angle increasing, the falling anal canal is over 2 ~ 3cm.

【治疗】

[Treatment]

1. 一般治疗

1. General Treatment

(1)早期患者口服中药升举汤。

(1) To take the decoction of ShengJuTang in initial disease.

(2)合并直肠黏膜脱垂,或内痔患者采用弯头负压吸力式套扎枪套扎和注射治疗(详见"痔疮")。

(2) Angle head loop ligaturing with vacuum suction gun and injection treatment for those complicated with rectal mucous prolapse (see "hemorrhoids").

(3)合并脱肛患者采用两侧坐骨直肠窝注射治疗法(详见"肛门直肠脱垂")。

(3) Injecting into two sides of ischiorectal fossa treatment for those complicated with anal prolapse (see "anorectal prolapse").

(4)合并肛门松弛性大便失禁(详见"老年人肛门括约肌松弛性大便失禁")。

(4) Complicated with anal incontinence (see "old persons anal incontinence with loss of control of the anal sphincter").

2. 钩头小针,紧缩肛门术

钩头小针沿肛外针眼插入,将内括约肌和外括约肌皮下环钩出分别结扎。送回原针眼,肛门。

2. Contracting Anus with Hook Style Head Acupuncture Scalpel   The doctor inserts the hook style head acupuncture scalpel and hooks into internal sphincter and subcutaneous ring of external sphincter out of the anus, ties separately, then retires along the same road.

第8章 肛肠出口排便失控性疾病

Chapter 8 Losing Controlled Defecation

第一节 慢性溃疡性结肠直肠炎

§ 1 Chronic Ulcerative Colorectitis

慢性溃疡性结肠直肠炎是一种多种原因及不明原因的炎性肠道病,其发病率较高。溃疡性结肠炎相当于中医学泄泻与痢疾病,纵观整个病程,还是属于痢疾,以久痢为多。另外,结肠与直肠均属大肠腑范围,如痢疾入脏,可由肠胃累及脾肾或入侵营血与肝肾。

Chronic ulcerocolorectitis is a kind of inflammatory bowel disease resulting from many causes and undefined causes. The incidence of the disease is high. The disease corresponds to diarrhea and dysentery in traditional Chinese medicine of long pathologic course. In addition, colon and rectum belong to large intestine, if the dysentery goes into the viscerae, the disease invades into blood, spleen, kidney and liver from gastrointestinal tract.

【病因病机】

[Etiology and Pathology]

多与遗传因素、感染、精神、免疫及酸的学说(肠道分泌过多、溶菌酸酶、破坏黏膜,对肠壁的保护作用,引起细菌侵入,发生黏膜坏死导致溃疡形成)等有关,并发生病理改变。非特异性者多局限于结肠黏膜层、黏膜下层,严重者可侵犯肌层和浆膜。内镜下早期黏膜充血、水肿颗粒状、点状出血,渗出发展成溃疡。慢性期黏膜挛缩,纤维包围或假息肉。

The disease has something to do with inherited factor, infection, psychology, immunization and acid theory (the stimulation of the acid materials make alimentary tract secrete more enzymes of bacterioclasis, these enzymes destroy mucosa taking part in intestinal wall to induce bacteria invasion, mucosa necrosis, and ulcer formation etc.), and produce pathologic changes. Ordinarily the pathologic change mainly locates in colonic mucosa, submucosa, in severe cases can invade muscular serosa and layers. In endoscopy the disease shows initial mucous hyperemia, edema, grain or point style bleeding, with infiltration developing to form ulcer. The chronic period shows mucosa depauperating, fibers packing and pseudo-polypus.

本病有实证和虚证之分。①实证:病变机制是虚热或寒虚蕴结大肠。大肠转运功能失利,以致腑气不行,气机不利,故腹痛为主。热迫大肠故里急;邪伤肠络故耳红面赤,气血延滞,温蕴不化,故败瘀夹温;化而为脓及黏液。②虚证:病久肠肾损伤至中气虚亏,脾阳不振。再由脾胃反肾(子病累母)命火衰微,形成脾肾两虚,是痢久伤阳病机。以上为伤阳。久痢伤阴致营血耗伤,损及脾肾与肝阴,也有温热不化致寒温郁而化热,致邪热入侵营血致动风惊厥或自闭外脱。以上为伤阳伤阴、动风惊厥。

There are strong and deficient syndromes in the disease. ①Strong syndrome: Pathology is that deficient heat or deficient cold stays in large intestine. The large intestine can't move normally, visceral Qi can't move normally, either, so that causing abdominal pain. The heat invades large intestine to cause inner heat; the toxin injures intestine to induce red ears and face; the Qi and blood stasis, can't work so as to induce infection and fever; draining pus and mucus from anus. ②Deficient syndrome:Long-time disease injures kidneys function, leading to middle Qi deficiency and spleen Yang deficiency. The spleen and stomach react kidneys to cause kidneys functional deficiency, further both spleen and kidney deficiency, this is a pathology that long-time diarrhea must injure Yang. Meanwhile long-time diarrhea may also injure Yin to cause blood consuming, spleen, kidneys and liver injury. In addition that lasting fever makes cold, warm and stasis translate heat, toxic heat invades into blood to cause convulsion, to cause drainage to outside. All are injuring Yang and Yin both.

【临床表现】

[Clinical Manifestations]

1. **湿热型** 腹泻,便脓血,赤白夹杂、里急后重,腹胀、腹痛、发热身倦,口苦咽干,小便短赤,舌苔黄腻脉滑数。

1. **Damp Heat Stage** Mainly shows diarrhea, pus and blood defecation, tenesmus, abdominal pain and distension, having a fever, bitter taste, pharyngoxerosis, short and deep colored urine, yellow tongue with greasy fur, slippery and rapid pulses.

2. **肝脾不和型** 腹泻、腹痛、痛即欲泻夹黏液脓血、苔薄白,脉弦细。

2. **Liver and Spleen Discording Stage** Mainly shows diarrhea, abdominal pain, mucus, pus and blood defecation; thin and white tongue fur, thin and string pulses.

3. **脾胃气虚型** 腹痛时作时止,里急后重黏膜液血便腹胀隐痛,舌淡苔白脉细。

3. **Qi Deficiency of Spleen and Stomach Stage** Abdominal pain with secret anguish sometimes taken place, sometimes stops; tenesmus, mucus, and bloody defecation, pale tongue, white fur, thin pulses.

4. **脾肾阳虚型** 便溏胶陈夹脓血,五更泻,腹胀冷痛,舌淡苔薄白,脉沉细无力。

4. Spleen-Kidney Yang Deficiency Stage Mainly shows diarrhea with pus and blood defecation, diarrhea in the early morning; abdominal pain and distension, getting worse as meeting cold; pale tongue, white thin fur, sunken thin and feeble pulses.

5. **血瘀型**　泄泻不爽,腹痛有定处,按之痛甚,舌暗红,舌边有紫斑,脉弦小涩。

5. **Blood Stasis Stage** Diarrhea and feeling of incomplete evacuation are common. The pain has a fixed position, more pain as pressing; black red tongue, purplish red spots in the fringe of tongue, string, thin and hesitant pulses.

【诊断】

[Diagnosis]

首先通过光导纤结肠镜检查确诊,并与肠癌、菌痢、阿米巴肠炎等鉴别。中医辨证以脾、肾为主,脾肾阳虚及气滞血瘀多见。临床多表现为虚中夹实。

According to fiberoptic colonoscopic examination, definite diagnosis can be made. The differential diagnosis includes: intestinal cancer, bacillary dysentery, amebic colitis, etc. Differentiation of syndrome from traditional Chinese medicine denotes that the disease is mainly in spleen and kidneys, Yang deficiency of spleen and kidneys is common. Main clinical manifestation is strong in deficiency.

【治疗】

[Treatment]

1. 中药汤剂治疗

1. Herbal Decoction Treatment

(1)湿热型:健脾清热汤,一煎口服,二煎保留灌肠。

(1)Damp heat stage：The decoction of JianPiQingReTang (invigorating the spleen and relieving heat). To take the decoction first, and then give enema with the secondly boiled decoction.

(2)肝脾不和型:健脾疏肝汤,一煎口服,二煎保留灌肠。

(2)Liver and spleen discording stage：The decoction of JianPiShuGan Tang (invigorating the spleen and soothing the liver). To take the decoction first and then give enema with the secondly boiled decoction.

(3)脾胃气虚型:健脾和胃汤,一煎口服,二煎保留灌肠。

(3)Qi deficiency of spleen and stomach stage：The decoction of JianPiHeWeiTang (invigorating the spleen and stomach). To take the decoction first and then give enema with the secondly boiled decoction.

(4)脾肾阳虚型:健脾补肾汤,一煎口服,二煎灌肠。

(4) Spleen-kidney Yang deficiency stage：The decoction of JianPiBuShenTang (invigorating the spleen and tonifying kidneys). To take the decoction first and then give enema with the secondly boiled decoction.

（5）血瘀型：健脾化瘀汤，一煎口服，二煎灌肠。

（5）Blood stasis stage：The decoction of JianPiHuaYuTang (invigorating the spleen and dispelling stasis). To take the decoction first and then give enema with the secondly boiled decoction.

2. 钩针穴位埋线
2. Hook Style Acupuncture Hanging Thread in Acupuncture Points

（1）主穴取中脘、下脘、足三里（双）、天枢（双）、气海。有五更泄者加脊俞、关元；有脓血便者加大肠俞、胃俞、长强俞、阴陵泉；脾虚者加脾俞，肾虚者加肾俞。穴位消毒麻醉，1%利多卡因加亚甲蓝长效液点状局麻。

（1）Main points are ZhongWan, XiaWan, ZuSanLi (two sides), TianSu (two sides), QiHai (Qi's controlling centre). For diarrhea in the early morning adds up LvSu, GuanYuan; for diarrhea with pus and blod adds up DaChangSu, WeiSu(stomach), ChangQiangSu, YinLingQuan; for spleen's deficiency adds up PiSu (spleen), for kidneys deficiency, adds up ShenSu (kidney). Points are sterilized and taken anesthesia with 1% Lidocaine adding up Methylene blue in located points style.

（2）用钩针从穴位下缘刺入，从穴位上缘穿出，再将0-0羊肠线钩入双股进穴位留置，拔出钩针，并剪断羊肠线。穴位针眼用创可贴敷。

（2）The doctor handles the hook style acupuncture to insert into the point from below fringe of the point to upper fringe, then hooks two 0-0 threads into the point to stay here, puts out the acupuncture, cuts off the thread, covers with gauzes on the points.

第二节　老年人肛门括约肌松弛性大便失禁
§2　Old Person Anal Incontinence with Loss of Control of the Anal Sphincter

老年人肛门括约肌松弛、萎缩性大便失禁是指老年人机体功能减退，肛门括约肌萎缩，直肠环松弛引起肛门括约功能减弱，不能随意控制排便和排气。

Old person anal incontinence with loss of control of the anal sphincter results when the body function retires, with anal sphincter atrophy and relaxed rectal ring. Anal incontinence is soiling or passage of flatus involuntarily.

【临床表现】

[Clinical Manifestations]

咳嗽、下蹲时有粪便黏液外溢;走路时内裤有粪便溢出;不能随意控制排便排气。肛门检查见肛门闭合不严,呈椭圆形张开,肛门潮湿,肛门收缩无力。直肠检查肛门括约肌收缩无力,肛门直肠环张力差,肛管直肠测压肛管波静息压和最大缩窄压均较正常对照组差,盆底肌电图检查轻度收缩,电压降低。

There are mucus and stool drainage in cough, squat and walk with involuntary passage of formed stool and gas. Anal examinations discover anal incomplete closing and even oval opening, anal moistness and contraction with disability. Rectal examinations discover anal sphincter contraction with disability, anorectal ring lacking strain. Pressure monitor of anal canal and rectum: resting pressure of anal canal wave and the most contracted pressure are lower than in normal contrast. Pelvic bottom muscular electromyogram: mild contraction and low electropressure.

【诊断】

[Diagnosis]

主要是依据病史、肛指检查、钡灌(肠造)影测压试验。但要鉴别诊断。肛肠测压仪图像分析:肛管波静息压均在 5cmH$_2$O 以下,肛管收缩压均为 100 ~ 150cmH$_2$O 电图像分析所示:盆底肌电压均为 150 ~ 220PV,盆底肌运动单位电位均为 3 ~ 4.5ms。横纹肌电位两例均产生多相波。

Diagnosis and differential diagnosis rely on the medical history, digital examination, pressure monitor of barium enema examination, image analysis from pressure monitor of anal canal and rectum: the resting pressure of anal canal wave is below 5cm H$_2$O, the contracted pressure is 100 ~ 150cm H$_2$O. Image analysis from pelvic bottom muscular electromyogram: pelvic bottom muscular electropressure is 150 – 220 PV, electric potential of pelvic bottom muscular moved unite is 3 ~ 4.5ms. The electric potential of striated muscles produce multiple waves.

【治疗】

[Treatment]

右侧卧位,消毒铺巾,于尾骨尖与肛门缘中点进行点状局麻,左手示指深入肛管,摸到肌间沟其上缘为内括约肌,其下缘为外括约肌皮下部。右手持钩状小针,仍从点状局麻针眼插入肛管后侧。在左手示指肛管内导引下,右手持钩针先将内括约肌钩出,用弯蚊式血管钳对拢钳夹,羊肠线结扎,然后再送回针眼,再将外括约肌皮下部同法钩出结扎也送回针眼。针眼外敷创可贴即可(图 8 -1)。

Patient lying on the right side, skin sterilizing, covering with a cloth, taking points style anesthesia from the middle point between anal fringe and the tip of coccyx, the doctor's left index finger inserts into anal canal to define and feel the position of intersphincteric ditch, its upper fringe is the internal sphincter, its lower fringe is the subcutaneous portion of external sphincter. His right hand handles the hook style acupuncture scalpel to insert into posterior anal canal from local anesthetic points, in the guidance of his left index finger, his right hand handles the hook style acupuncture scalpel to hook out the internal sphincter, takes curved hemostatic forceps to jaw, ties with thread, and retires back the internal sphincter from initial points. According to the same method the doctor hooks out the subcutaneous portion of external sphincter, ties and tums back, covers with gauzes on the points(Fig. 8 – 1).

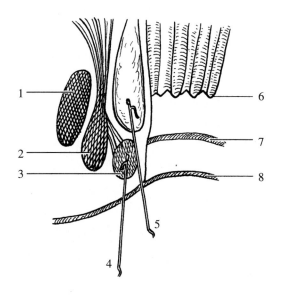

图 8 – 1 肛门括约肌松弛钩头小针紧缩术

1 – 外括约肌深部;2 – 外括约肌浅部;3 – 外括约肌皮下部;

4 – 钩头小针钩出外括约肌;5 – 钩头小针钩出内括约肌;6 – 齿线;7 – 肌间沟;8 – 肛门

Figure 8 – 1 To contract tightly relaxing anal sphincter with

hook style head acupuncture scalpel

1. Profundus Muscle of External Sphincter;2. Superficialis Muscle of External Sphincter;

3. Subcutaneous Portion of External Sphincter;

4. Hook Style Head Acupuncture Scalpel Hooking out the External Sphincter;

5. Hook Style Head Acupuncture Scalpel Hooking out the Internal Sphincter;

6. Dentate Line;7. Intersphincteric Ditch;8. Anus

第三节　肛门失禁

§3　Anal Incontinence

【病因】

[Etiology]

1.**神经源性失禁**　儿童因先天性畸形,如脊柱裂、脑脊膜膨出,或者成年人因脊髓外伤引起肛门失禁。

1．**Central Nervous System Disease Causing Incontinence**　These patients with anal incontinence are either the young children with congenital malformation as spina bifida and meningocele, or the adult with injury of spinal cord.

2．**外伤性失禁**　因肛门直肠外伤,括约肌断裂、粉碎、感染、瘢痕形成等。

2．**Damage Causing Incontinence**　Anorectal injury causes sphincter breaking up, inflammation, and the following stigmatization.

3．**医源性失禁**　因手术不当损伤肛门括约肌,分娩撕裂伤,注射药物感染,瘢痕形成等。

3．**Iatrogenic Incontinence**　Anorectal surgery, obstetrical procedures and infection of injection and scar formation.

4．**其他**　如肛门直肠先天性畸形、直肠低位癌和肛管癌、会阴人工肛门等。

4．**Others**　Other causes include inflammatory bowel disease, anorectal carcinoma, rectal prolapse, and perineal artificial anus.

【发病机制】

［Pathology］

肛门主要功能是控制排便,其机制非常复杂,至今尚了解不多。但认为括约肌功能、直肠肛门角、直肠肛门感觉、直肠抑制反射、直肠储存大便量及直肠腔的可忍受量、大便量及其稠度、直肠的推进力均参与控制排便。在肛门、直肠严重外伤,或直肠低位癌、肛管癌患者肛门、括约肌、直肠已严重损伤或整个被手术切除,需要用结肠或乙状结肠人工代替直肠、肛管、肛门。手术重建直肠肛管后,随着时间延长,直肠肛门的感觉、直肠抑制反射、直肠储存大便量等会逐渐完全或部分恢复。

Anal incontinence results when there is a loss of control of the anal sphincter. The term actually covers a broad spectrum of anal function impairment, ranging from simple involuntary passage of flatus to complete loss of sphincter tone with involuntary passage of formed stool. Total anal incontinence, with complete loss of sphincter muscle control, is due to physical loss of muscle mass, sensory innervation damage, or central nervous system diseases. Partial anal incontinence is intermittent soiling or passage of flatus involuntarily. Overflow anal incontinence is found in patients with fecal impaction or chronic constipation with prolonged laxative abuse. The sphincter muscle mechanism is intact, but the large bolus of feces distends the rectal ampulla, and is responsible for loss of defecation reflex.

【治疗】

［Treatment］

主要采用股薄肌移植术。

Tine gracilis muscle is transplanted to encircle the anus.

1. **术前准备** 一般准备 2 天,即手术前 2 天流质、洗肠。服甲硝唑 0.4g,每日 3 次;女性准备阴道。术前 1 天清洁洗肠、流质,洗刷大腿、小腿上部,用碘酒、乙醇消毒,然后用干净绷带包扎,静脉输入红霉素 0.5～1g 和甲硝唑 250ml。手术当天禁食。一般腰麻生效后,移植手术开始。

1. **Preoperative Preparation** In general preparation should be 2 days, it's that liquid food, enema, taking Metronidazole 0.4g three times a day preoperatively for 2 days. Giving enema till being clean preoperatively for one day.

2. 手术过程

2. Operation Procedure

(1)整个手术过程包括:①大腿内侧 2 个切口;②小腿胫骨粗隆处 1 个切口;③肛门处 1 个切口;④腹股沟或坐骨结节 1 个切口共 5 个切口,另有 3 个隧道:①大腿上 1/3 切口至肛门切口之间,围绕肛门隧道;②肛门切口至股薄肌止腱固定处之间的隧道;③关键在围绕肛门的隧道。隧道需呈"喇叭"状,这符合股薄肌解剖特点,股薄肌植入后易成活并起滑车作用,达到恢复肛门功能最好水平(图 8－2～图 8－13)。

(1)Total operative course includes:①Two incisions on inner sides of two thighs;②One incision on the tibial tuberosity of the leg;③One incision on anus;④One incision on groin or ischial tuberosity. There are totally 5 incisions. In addition, there are 3 tracks:①Wrapping around anal track between the incision upper 1/3 of the thigh and anal incision;②The tracks between anal incision and located position of the gracilis muscular insertion;③The tracks wrapped around anus are the pivotal. The tracks show trumpet shape fitting to the gracilis muscular anatomic feature. The gracilis muscular sling is substituted in an attempt to gain voluntary control (Fig. 8－2～Fig. 8－13).

(2)距耻骨结节下方 12cm 处,相当于大腿上 1/3 和中 1/3 之间内后侧有股薄肌血管神经束(应用探针小斜刀分离),是主要供应营养的血管及支配神经。一旦损伤,会造成股薄肌供血不足或坏死,手术失败,必须加以保护,切勿损伤。

(2)The vascular and nervous bunch of the gracilis muscle, located inner posterior between upper 1/3 and middle 1/3 of the thigh, 12cm below ischial tuberosity. It is very important (should be dissociated by small inclined probing acupuncture scalpel). Once the bunch is injured, gracilis muscular insufficiency or necrosis will occur, the operation is defeated. So it must be protected, not be injured.

(3)股薄肌移植最后肌腱固定前,另换手套,示指插入肛门肛管,测量其紧缩程度,认为越紧越好。助手牵紧股薄肌的末端,维持已确定的紧缩程度,把双腿放平,进行缝合固定。

（3）Before completion, an index finger inserts in anal canal to monitor the pressure and the degree of contraction, the tighter the better. The doctor tracts the end of the gracilis muscle to keep the degree of tight contraction, put back the patient's two legs, ties and fixes the muscle.

（4）术毕，一定把取股薄肌的大腿侧用绷带包扎压紧，目的是防大腿皮下出血。

（4）Wrapping the gauze-band tight around the legs.

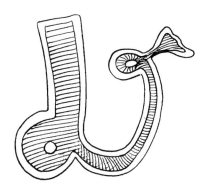

图 8 - 2　肛门移植股薄肌基本术式

Figure 8 - 2　The gracilis muscle being transferred to encircle the anus

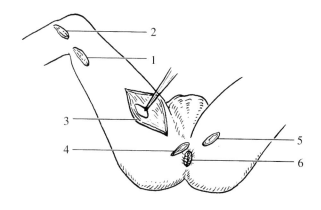

图 8 - 3　手术切口

1、2 - 股薄肌下端切口；3 - 股薄肌上端切口；

4、5 - 股薄肌围绕肛门口切口；6 - 肛门隧道切口

Figure 8 - 3　Operation of tumor in posterior rectal wall combined double plane acupuncture scalpel

1,2. Inferior incision of gracilis muscle; 3. Anterior incision of gracilis muscle;

4,5. The incision around anus; 6. The incision of anal track

3. 手术后护理　禁食 3 天，不禁水，平卧，可轻轻翻身或活动下肢。应用抗生素，以防感染。肛门部伤口以暴露为好，保持干燥、清洁，有分泌物或稀便溢出，随时清洁消毒。手术后 2 周开始轻轻做肛门收缩练习，坐马桶排便。注意动作要轻缓，3 周后逐渐加强肛门收缩练习，随时间延长长期坚持功能训练，肛门功能恢复良好。

3. Postoperative Care　Fasting 3 days, water is not fasted. Patient lying on the back, should turn around the body and move the lower limbs. Using antibiotics to prevent infection. The wound of anal region should show at best meanwhile keeping dry and clean. To take sterilization and cleanliness as soon as discharge and drainage from anus. Two weeks after operation the patient should do anal contraction exercises gradually.

4. 肛门功能评定标准
4. The Anal Functional Standard

(1)优：排便功能与正常人相同。

(1)Excellent：Normal defecation.

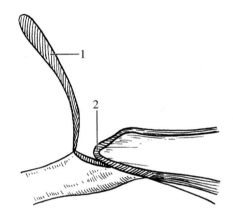

图 8 - 4　小针刀游离股薄肌

Figure 8 - 4　Acupuncture scalpel dissociating the gracilis muscle

(2)良好：能完全控制干粪,不能很好地控制稀便。有的患者有时用灌肠来调节排便,不用带垫。

(2)Good：The patient can control completely solid stool, not well for liquid.

(3)较好：因有稀便污染衣裤,需要经常带垫。

(3)Middle：The patient is instructed to keep cotton dressing in the anal area to collect liquid stool.

(4)无效：无排便感觉,完全失禁。

(4)No effect：No bowel feeling, totally incontinent.

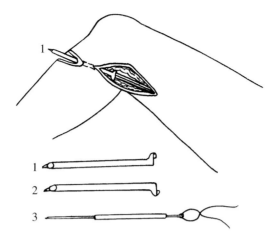

图 8 – 5　游离腱索

1、2 – 游离小针刀顺时针一把,逆时针一把。专用腱索游离小针刀;

3 – 探针挂线小直刀

Figure 8 – 5　Dissociating muscle tendon

1,2. Dissociating acupuncture scalpel used especially to dissociate muscle tendon,

clockwise and counter-clockwise; 3. The small straight probing acupuncture scalpel with hanging thread

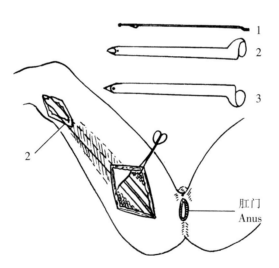

图 8 – 6　股薄肌游离小针刀

1 – 斜小针刀;2 – 顺时针专用游离小针刀;

3 – 逆时针专用游离小针刀,游离股薄肌后壁和两侧壁及前壁,

一般两刀操作后股薄肌,再用小针刀游离配合

Figure 8 – 6　Acupuncture scalpel used by dissociating the gracilis muscle

1. Inclined acupuncture scalpel; 2. Clockwise acupuncture scalpel used especially to dissociate;

3. Counter-clockwise acupuncture scalpel used especially to dissociate, acupuncture

scalpel combining to dissociate the posterior, two sides and anterior of gracilis muscular wall

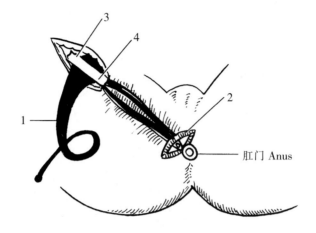

图8-7 建立隧道

1-股薄肌;2、3-隧道;4-隧道板

Figure 8-7 Setting the track

1. Gracilis muscle; 2,3. Track; 4. Board of track

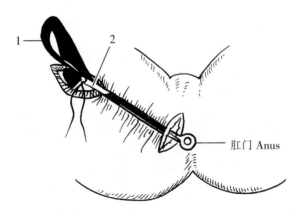

图8-8 插入引线用小针刀

1-股薄肌;2-引线用小针刀

Figure 8-8 Inserting the acupuncture scalpel with hanging thread

1. Gracilis muscle; 2. Acupuncture scalpel with hanging thread

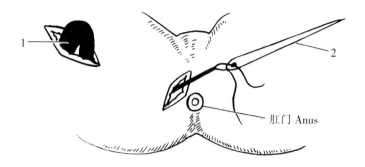

图 8 – 9 拔出引线用小针刀

1 – 股薄肌;2 – 引线用小针刀

Figure 8 – 9 Put out hanged thread with acupuncture scalpel

1. Gracilis muscle; 2. Hanged thread acupuncture scalpel

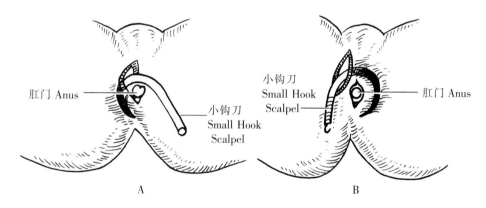

图 8 – 10 隧道探道小钩刀,顺时针,逆时针各一把,隧道探道小钩刀起探道和通开瘢痕的作用

Figure 8 – 10 Small hook style probing track acupuncture scalpels, clockwise and counter-clockwise, the small hook style probing track acupuncture scalpe takes part in probing track and opening the scar

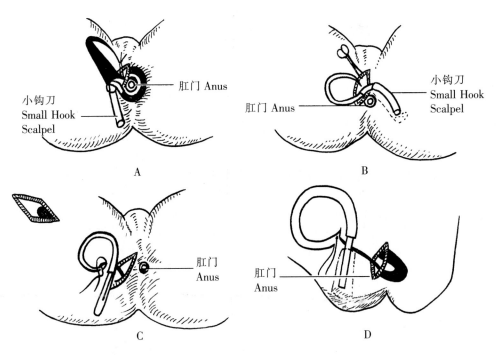

图8－11　小钩刀在建立隧道中的应用

A. 小钩刀通开隧道；

B. 拔出小钩刀；

C. 隧道器、小钩刀顺时针逆时针各一把，如用右大腿的股薄肌；

D. 逆时针隧道器小钩刀可顺利地把股薄肌引入肛门肛管周围

Figure 8－11　Carrying on small hook style acupuncture scalpel setting the track

A. Small hook style acupuncture scalpel opening the track；

B. Put out small hook style acupuncture scalpel；

C. Tunneler, clockwise and counter-clockwise acupuncture scalpels, right gracilis muscle；

D. Counter-clockwise acupuncture scalpels taking the gracilis muscle to anal canal region

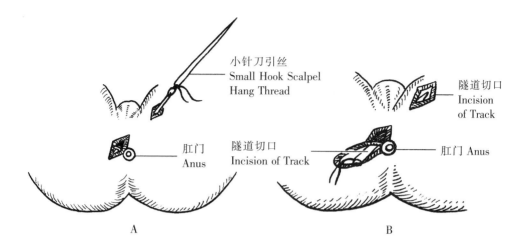

图 8 - 12 隧道器小针刀切口与隧道切口缝合固定

Figure 8 - 12 Tying and fixing incision of tunneler acupuncture scalpels and track

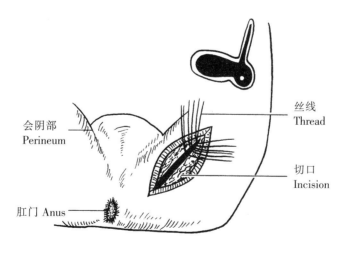

图 8 - 13 止腱固定缝合

Figure 8 - 13 Aponeurosis of insertion fixes and sutures

第 9 章　肛肠肿瘤

Chapter 9　Neoplasms of the Anus and Rectum

第一节　良性肿瘤

§ 1　Benign Tumor

一、直肠息肉

I. Rectal Polyps

息肉是肠道常见良性肿瘤,多发生于结肠和直肠,为球形或卵圆形肿物,由蒂与黏膜附着。可以有许多个集聚于一段或全部结膜或直肠(称为结肠息肉病),也可单发,或有数个分散于直肠内(称为直肠息肉)。大者直径可达数厘米,小者呈小结节样隆起于黏膜上。直肠息肉也有恶性变的可能,但远较结肠息肉病少见,以儿童多见。

Polyp is common in intestinal tract, colon and rectum mainly, ball or ovum shape, protrudes into the lumen of the gastrointestinal tract, there is a common stem adhering to mucosa. A broad spectrum of polyps occurs in the colon and rectum. There are also large numbers of tubular adenomas in the colon and rectum. They are characterized by polyposis coli. These small tiny mucosal excrescences are usually several milimeters in diameter. When multiple, there are usually only three or four polyps, the large polyp can arrive at several centimeters in diameter, but in rare instances the polyps may be so numerous that familial polyposis is simulated. This is now thought to represent an inherited polyposis syndrome.

【病因】

[Incidence]

发生原因目前还不太清楚,多发息肉病似与家族遗传有关;直肠息肉并无家族遗传因素。有人认为,可能由于胚胎发育异常,或因为慢性刺激所致。

The mode of inheritance is not clear, and multiple polypsmay have something to do with familial inheritance. Recal polyps have nothing to do with familial inheritance. Some persons think that the incidence of polyps has something to do with asyntaxia and chronic stimulation.

【临床表现】

[Clinical Manifestations]

最常见便后肛门出血,色鲜红,且与粪便不相混杂,或便后可见息肉脱出,其他无特别感觉。

The usual symptom of colorectal polyps is blood streaking of the stool. Rectal polyps may protude through the anus and be described as a small cherry by the patient. They are no special consequence.

【诊断】

[Diagnosis]

指检时可以摸到单个或数个质软而有弹力的小球状肿物(小者如豆,大者如核桃)。用窥肛器检查,可见到有蒂的卵圆形肿物吊挂在肠壁上,色红或紫赤,表面光滑,有光泽,质脆,易出血(图 9 – 1)。若便后能脱出肛外者,则更易诊断。

Diagnosis is by sigmoidoscopy, or by colonoscopy for polyps beyond the reach of the anoscope. Digital examination can feel single or some soft and elastic bodies. Polyps are nearly always pedunculated, from 3 to 10 mm in diameter, sometimes over 10 mm, even several centimeters, smooth, spherical, reddish brown, and often covered with mucus(Fig. 9 – 1).

但是,如果见到多发息肉,则应想到结肠息肉病的可能,应进一步确定发病部位和广泛程度。如在结肠息肉病患者的口腔黏膜及口旁皮肤处,可见到多数黑斑,或常有腹痛、腹泻症状,且大便多混有黏液。最好进行光导纤维结肠镜检查,以肯定诊断。因为息肉病的治疗和预后与直肠息肉不同,必须引起注意。

More commonly, however, rather marked symptoms develop consisting of frequent bouts of abdominal pain, passage of loose; multiple black spots oral mucosa and the skin beside the mouth show in multiple colonic polyposis. There are different therapies and prognosis between polyposis and rectal polyps, so it should be distinctly diagnosed. Fiberoptic colonoscopy can make clarity of diagnosis.

此外,直肠或乙状结肠另一种较少见息肉为乳头状或绒毛状瘤,多为单个且比较大(图 9 – 2),基底广阔,表面平滑,很易出血。

Villous adenoma, these polypoid lesions, also called papillary adenomas, are so named because of their characteristic frondlike projections. Grossly, villous tumors are poorly demarcated, bulky, broad-baoed lesions. They are smooth, soft and velvety, and therefore are difficult to be detected by palpation, and also easy to bleed(Fig. 9 – 2).

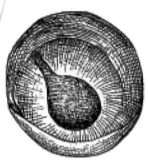

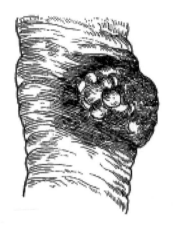

图9-1 带蒂直肠息肉

Figure 9-1 Rectal polyp with stem

图9-2 直肠广基良性息肉

Figure 9-2 Rectal polyp with broad-based

【治疗】

[Treatment]

1.**息肉套扎** 用弯头负压吸力套扎枪套扎小息肉。在胶圈套扎前注入亚甲蓝长效止痛剂,肛内挤入九华膏。

1. **Polyp Loop Ligation** To take angle head loop ligaturing gun with vacuum suction to ligate a small polyp. To inject and to squeeze cream into anus before loop ligature.

2.**结扎法或钝剥法** 对长蒂直肠息肉可用结扎法。方法是将息肉自根部单纯结扎,或以缝针贯穿结扎。术后于肛管内注入九华膏。一般3~5天息肉即可脱落。钝剥法是用手指自息肉根部钝性剥离,使息肉与蒂脱离(或捏断),不可用暴力扯掉,以防出血。

2. **Tying or Shaving Long** Long stem polyps can be treated by simple tying and sewing from the root of polyp. To squeeze the cream into anal canal in postoperative treatment. In 3~5 days the polyp drop out.

3.**小针刀切除** 息肉基底广阔者宜行小针刀手术切除。

3. **Cutting off by Acupuncture Scalpel** Broad-based polyps can be cut off by acupuncture scalpel.

二、肛门乳头状纤维组织瘤
II. Anal Papilloma

乳头状纤维组织瘤又称乳头瘤,是指肛门乳头肥大。

Papilloma also called hyperplastic polyps, results from hypertrophy of anal papilla.

【病因】
[Etiology]

多由于排便时创伤或肛门乳头附近组织炎症的影响而发炎,加之反复发作,日久逐渐肥大,在排便时可以脱出肛门外。

Since they arise as the result of localized minor imbalances between cell division and desquamation, the terms hyperplastic and metaplastic are appropriate. Taking hypertrophy with the time going, the papilloma can project out of anus.

【临床表现】
[Clinical Manifestations]

经常感觉肛门部瘙痒(似蚁走感),有时大便后乳头脱出肛门外,如有内痔脱出时更易将其带出。发炎时可有里急后重感。

Hyperplastic polyps cause no symptoms and of themselves are of no consequence. They are important only because they arise in the same location in the colorectum, greater normal. Patients often feel pruritus and pain in the anal area, and tenesmus if inflamed.

【诊断】
[Diagnosis]

根据特有症状,或便后脱出肛外时可看到如锥体形的小肿瘤,色淡,质稍硬,即可确诊。如不能脱出者,用窥肛器检查,可发现在齿线附近有灰白色肥大乳头(图9-3),指诊可摸到细长锥体形较硬的肿物。

According to its feature and a little small subuliform tumor with light color projecting out of anus after defecation, the diagnosis is clear. Anoscopy can check up the tumor without projecting out of anus, it locates near the dentate line, grey white hypertrophic papilla (Fig. 9-3), and digital examination can feel it.

【治疗】
[Treatment]

1. **结扎法** 用窥肛器扩开肛门,找到乳头瘤根部(在齿线上),用丝线从根部结

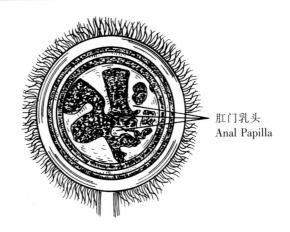

图 9 - 3　乳头瘤(窥肛器下观察可见肥大乳头)

Figure 9 - 3　Papilloma（hypertrophic papilla in anoscopy）

扎,以断绝血流。如有脱出肛门外者,可直接采用上法结扎(图 9 - 4)。

1. **Tying**　In anoscopy try to find out the root of papilloma（at dentate line）, tying it with silk thread（Fig. 9 - 4）.

2. **套扎枪治疗**　小乳头状纤维瘤合并有内痔者,分别用套扎枪套扎(图 9 - 4)。

2. **Loop Ligation Gun**　Loop ligation gun treats separately a small papilloma combined with internal hemorrhoids（Fig. 9 - 4）.

3. **小针刀切除**　乳头瘤基底宽者采用小针刀切除治疗,创面敷痔瘘散。

3. **Cutting off by Acupuncture Scalpel**　Broad-based papilloma can be cut off by acupuncture scalpel, then covered with gauzes on the wound.

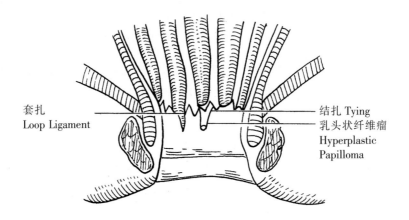

图 9 - 4　乳头状纤维瘤

Figure 9 - 4　Hyperplastic papilloma

第二节　肛门、直肠癌

§2　Anorectal Cancer

肛门、直肠癌在《外科大成》一书已有记载,如"锁肛痔、肛门内外如竹节锁紧,形如海蜇"。

Anorectal cancer has been recorded in <WaiKe DaCheng> (Surgery), for example, "it is a tumor in or out side of anus, liking jellyfish to close the anus."

一、肛　门　癌

I. Anal Cancer

肛门直肠癌之病因目前还不清楚。

Etiology of anorectal cancer is not clear at present.

肛门瘢痕、白斑、湿疹、痔瘘等均可能发生癌变,形成肛管癌(此多属于鳞状细胞癌)。

The cancer belong s mainly to squamous carcinoma in anus and anal canal.

【临床表现】

[Clinical Manifestations]

肛门或肛管癌,初起在肛门旁皮肤上出现硬的结节,逐渐长大,而表面出现破溃,形成特殊的边缘凸起,并向外翻、溃疡,常有血性分泌物,有疼痛感;如合并继发感染时,可出现红肿和剧烈疼痛;如侵犯到括约肌时,可有里急后重、大便失禁(严重者)或排便困难、粪便形状变细等症状。

Passage of bright red blood, and mucus are seen or on the stool. Dull, nagging, persistent pain even stab in anal area is frequent.

【诊断】

[Diagnosis]

根据上述病史和临床表现,应首先考虑到癌症的可能。因为这种癌瘤可以在肛门瘘管的基础上发生;也有由于癌的存在而继发感染形成肛瘘者,而两者在治疗和预后上则相差很远。因此,应早期做出诊断,遇有可疑时,最好做活检。

Patients with a histologic or clinical diagnosis of anal cancer who are not categorically inoperable because of far advanced disseminated metastatic disease. Biopsy can give a diagnosis clearly.

二、直 肠 癌

II. Rectal Cancer

【病因】

[Etiology]

直肠癌也有一部分是由息肉转变而来。另外,持久性肛瘘亦可能转变为癌(此多属腺癌)。

Rectal cancer develops in patients affected by familial polyposis villous tumors, and chronic inflammation, but these account for only a small minority of the total number. The extent of the contribution of adenomatous polyps is still speculative.

【临床表现】

[Clinical Manifestations]

直肠癌早期除直肠黏膜上触及较硬结节外,当出现症状时多已进入较晚期。其症状主要是由于癌体增大,大便中混有新鲜血液和黏液,并染有脓性物,出现粪便少而形状细扁。癌肿侵犯骶神经丛时,则在直肠内或骶部出现剧烈的持续性疼痛,且向腹、腰及下肢放射。如侵犯至膀胱及尿道时,则会出现排尿困难或尿频及尿痛感。晚期表现明显消瘦、食欲缺乏、贫血、水肿等。

Symptoms of anal cancer depend on several factors, including the anatomic location of the lesion, its size and extent, and the presence of complications such as obstruction, hemorrhage, etc. Dull, nagging persistent lower quadrant pain is frequent. These include pallor, easy fatigue, weakness, dizziness, dyspnea on exertion, and cardiac palpitation. Anorexia, indigestion, and weight loss are often presenting complaints. Severe symptoms such as excessive weight loss, cachexia, and hepatomegaly usually imply far advanced cancer. The caliber of the lumen is smaller and the fecal content more solid passage of bright red blood, and mucus are seen in or on the stool. Mild abdominal cramping may occur, but several rectal pain usually means extensive local disease, such as involving the urinary tract and bladder.

【诊断】

[Diagnosis]

1.**指检** 是十分重要的简易检查。在直肠黏膜上可以摸到有结节凸起,凹凸不平,质硬底宽,与下层组织粘连,固定不动。同时,周围黏膜糜烂,常有脓血黏于指套上。如多在癌的中央形成溃疡,边缘凸起不平。如位于肠壁周围,可触及环形狭窄。

1.**Digital Examination** The rectal carcinoma is usually easily diagnosed on the digital examination because of the hard, rough and irregular surface.

2. **窥肛器检查**　将窥肛器插入直肠后,可见癌的位置、形状、溃疡大小、有无脓血;可见底部宽广、边缘不整、色红紫、质脆、溃疡边缘凸起外翻、基底有坏死(图 9 - 5)。在插窥肛器前,须指诊了解肛门有无狭窄,无狭窄时才能用窥肛器徐徐插入,不得勉强插入,否则因肿瘤质脆,会引起大出血。

2. **Anoscopic Examination**　The surgeon can find by anoscopy the position, shape, ulcer, blood, the base, fringe, color, necrosis, anal narrow, etc(Fig. 9 - 5).

3. **活检**　可疑癌瘤均应做活检。方法是用窥肛器扩开肛门,于癌瘤边缘(不要选坏死组织和离癌远的组织)用刮匙小针刀旋切取一块组织,做病理检查。

3. **Biopsy**　The curette acupuncture scalpel shaves the tissue in endoscopy.

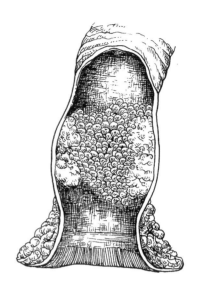

图 9 - 5　直肠癌

Figure 9 - 5　Rectal cancer

【治疗】

[Treatment]

肛门直肠癌目前较有效的治疗办法是争取早期做彻底切除,以达到根治。如晚期不能根治,只好采用中西医药物疗法,以减轻症状。

The rectum, for surgical purposes, is divided into unequal thirds. The proximal third extends from the junction with the sigmoid colon at the posterior peritoneal reflection. The middle third extends down to the lowest portion of the anterior peritoneal reflection, or pouch of Douglas. The distal third of the rectum, the entirely extraperitoneal portion, extends from the peritoneal reflection to the anal verge. Tumors with their lower margin can always be removed by low anterior resection and primary anastomosis. Since the anastomotic leak rate is somewhat higher than that in resections of the peritoneal colon, it is advisable to protect the anastomosis whenever possible by wrapping with a pedicle of great omentum. The uppermost component of the anal sphincter mechanism and thus the distal limit of sphincter operation is the puborectalis sling. The combined abdominoperineal resection, or Miles procedure, must be used. It is the standard by which all other procedures for rectal cancer must be measured.

1. **配合用双面小针刀手术**　在 Miles 手术基础上进行。将乙状结肠游离后提起,直视下剪开分离直肠上段的骶前筋膜和直肠固有筋膜之间的网状疏松结缔组织后进入该间隙。右手持小针刀仔细寻找前述延伸的间隙或薄弱处,边探边进,逐步扩大其孔隙。

用力点尽可能靠近肿瘤直肠壁一侧，切勿伤及骶前静脉，以免引起大出血。在左手示指辅导下从另一端拔出小针刀后，在小针刀柄孔系上丝线留挂在该间隙中。一旦发生大出血，则将该丝线立即结扎紧，可以起到止血作用。一般进展顺利则以线代刀，将丝线均匀地用力结扎（不打结），借其力勒割开该间隙。或小针刀将粘连在间隙中的癌肿块分别切开，或用线挂勒割开，或于相应的部位注射抗癌液以扩大其间隙，再从注射针眼处插入小针刀，分别用探切，再分别穿过丝线勒割该间隙。以点带面，逐渐扩大范围，逐步将直肠后壁癌肿从骶前筋膜间隙至尾骨尖完全分割切除。照此法从直肠两侧壁分离至肛提肌水平，男性从直肠前壁分离至前列腺的后方，勿伤精囊；对残留在骶前筋膜或输尿管上的癌肿，采用电刀烧灼和抗癌药物封闭给予配合治疗；勿再钝性分离或切除造成骶前大出血，之后酌情再做腹部人造瘘口或保留肛管，或行肛门重建术（图9-6）。

1. **Operation with Miles Combined Two-Edged Acupuncture Scalpel**　Lateral attachment of sigmoid colon is incised. The sigmoid colon is dissociated and held up. Peritoneal reflection between bladder and rectum is transected, and an anterior plane between these two organs is established. Posterior dissection is carried out in midline digitally. The finger establishes a plane just anterior to the anterior surface of the sacrum and continues the dissection as far caudad as possible. The lateral attachment of the rectum, including the middle hemorrhoidal vessels, is translated. These vessels are, at times, of sufficient size to require individual ligatures. Dissection carried down to coccyx and the posterior dissection is continued until it communicates with the space anterior to the sacrum which has been established previously transabdominally. The levator muscles are then transected on each side. Distal colon is brought down into the anal wound and dissection carried between it and the prostate or bladder (Fig. 9 - 6). The acupuncture scalpel operates as in the above space.

2. **小钩针配合螺旋管支架肠吻合术**　按 Miles 手术游离乙状结肠及直肠并松解结脾曲，采用 GF - Ⅰ 型（34mm）吻合器进行吻合。完成后用两叶肛门镜插入肛门内检查吻合口，如有钽钉脱落或吻合裂再给缝合。然后将螺旋塑料管于肛门口用小钩针置人吻合口及上端，起支撑吻合口，引流吻合口上端粪液作用。流出肛门外，防治吻合口漏。螺旋管下端再接肛管外引流瓶中（图9-7）。

2. **Anastomosis Combined Small Hook Style Acupuncture Scalpel**　In midrectal anastomosis with the GF-I (34mm) stapler, the proximal and distal purse-string sutures have been placed. The assembled instrument is passed up through the anus until the nose cone protrudes through the end of the rectal stump. The rectal purse-string has been tied. The nose cone containing the anvil portion of the cartridge is introduced into the proximal bowel and that purse-string securely tied. After the two ends of the cartridge are brought together approaching the purse-stringed ends of the proxima, and distal bowel, a squeeze of the instrument handle drives in a double staged circular row of staples and advances a circular knife just inside the ring of staples, cutting the double diaphragm made by the two apposed purse-stringed bowel ends (Fig. 9 - 7). To take catheter drainage by acupuncture scalpel.

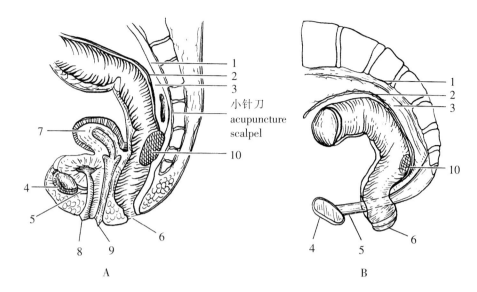

图 9 - 6　直肠后壁肿瘤双面小针刀配合手术
A. 直肠后壁处理;B. 骶前间隙处理
1 - 骶前筋膜;2 - 直肠固有筋膜;3 - 骶前间隙;4 - 耻骨联合;5 - 耻骨直肠肌;
6 - 肛门;7 - 子宫;8 - 尿道;9 - 阴道;10 - 肿瘤

Figure 9 - 6　Operation of tumor in posterior rectal wall combined double plane acupuncture scalpel
A. Postrectal wall management;　B. Postsacral space management
1. Presacral fascia;2. Rectal proper fascia;3. Presacral space;4. Pubic symphysis;
5. Puborectal muscle;6. Anus; 7. Uterus;8. Uretera;9. Vagina; 10. Tumor

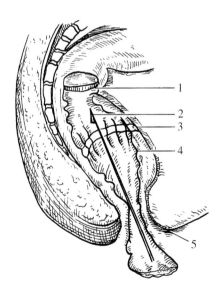

图 9 - 7　小钩针配合螺旋管支架肠吻合术
1 - 直肠上段;2 - 小钩针;3 - 吻合口;4 - 螺旋管;5 - 肛门

Figure 9 - 7　Anastomosis combined small hook style acupuncture scalpel
1. Proximal rectal lesion;2. Small hook style acupuncture scalpel;
3. Anastomosis stoma;4. Draining catheter;5. Anus

第 10 章　肛门直肠少见病

Chapter 10　Uncommon Diseases of the Anus and Rectum

一、肛门会阴坏死性筋膜炎

I. Necrotizing Fasciitis of Anal and Perineal Region

【病因】

［Etiology］

肛门会阴坏死性筋膜炎,可继发会阴部各种损伤肛周脓肿、肛门硬化剂注射治疗。肛门或会阴手术后,常合并有慢性消耗疾病,如糖尿病、肿瘤、肝硬化及长期使用免疫抑制药等。坏死性筋膜炎是一种少见的坏死性软组织感染,如不及时治疗,往往死于败血症和毒血症。

Anal and perineal necrotizing fasciitis is the secondary disease of perineal region such as perianal abscesses, commonly complicated with chronic wasting diseases such as diabetes, malignancy, liver cirrhosis, taking immunosuppressor for long time, etc. The necrotizing fasciitis is an uncommon necrotizing soft tissue inflammation. If untreated immediately the patient will die from septicemia and toxinemia.

致病菌多为溶血性链球菌、大肠杆菌,伴有厌氧菌感染多为混合感染。

The common bacteria are hemolysis streptococcus, colibacillus, etc. Anaerobic bacteria infection is usually a mixed infection.

【临床表现】

［Clinical Manifestations］

感染主要侵犯皮肤、皮下脂肪和浅筋膜,可出现广泛坏死,但不累及肌肉。表现主要为突然寒战高热,肛门会阴部皮肤开始红肿,类似蜂窝织炎或丹毒,进而引起浅筋膜广泛坏死。

The infection mainly involves skin, subcutaneous fat and fibro-areolar fascia, but not muscle. Main manifestations include sudden chill and high fever, the anal and perineal skin change red and swollen initially like cellulitis and erysipelas, leading to necrosis soon.

【治疗】

［Treatment］

硬膜外麻醉。肛门或会阴部胀肿可触及捻发感或波动感。在脓肿上下缘和内外缘分别用刮匙小针刀插入脓肿下缘,并在脓肿壁旋转切割多个圆洞,再在脓肿相对应的上缘与下缘各刺破并穿出脓肿壁,旋转切割成另 2 个圆洞,使脓肿上缘与下缘有两个对口。然后用粗丝线系在刮匙小针刀颈部,从脓肿下缘切口退出刮匙小针刀,使粗丝线留挂在脓腔作为引流丝线。照此方法,再将脓肿内缘与外缘做第 2 个对口挂线引流。再将脓肿中部做第 3 个对口挂线引流。将坏死的筋膜同时刮出脓腔。最后用过氧化氢冲洗脓腔,外敷中药消脓膏,黏膏固定(图 10 - 1)。

With extradural anesthesia, the doctor can feel the fluctuation in anal and perineal area, inserts the curette acupuncture scalpel to shave and cut the abscess wall from upper and two sides to bottom, goes through abscess out of the wall so that these courses form 2 holes style incision on the wall of abscess. To hold up thick silk thread on the neck of curette acupuncture scalpel, to return along the same way penetrating the abscess cavity from the inferior fringe, to put two thick silk thread out of the cavity from the two holes and to form arc circle and to take a part in open to open drainage. According to the method, to take the second hole to open seton drainage in inner and outer fringe of abscess, then the third in middle, meanwhile shave the necrotizing tissue out of the cavity of abscess, the last to wash the cavity by hydrogen peroxide, to apply gauze after the arrangement (Fig. 10 - 1).

二、肛门海绵状血管瘤

II. Anal Spongiform Vascular Tumor

病因不清。根据病史、大便有鲜血、坠胀感及肛门镜检查可确诊。

Etiology is not clear, according to medical history, blood with defecation, falling and distension in anal area, and anoscopy, the diagnosis can be made.

1. **小针刀疗法**　取侧卧位,消毒,局麻。术者先用左手示指插入肛管内约 1.5cm,确定括约肌间沟的上缘即为内括约肌,按压固定。右手持斜面小针刀从肛门外缘右侧点状局麻针眼插入。在肛管内左手示指引导下,隔着肛管左手示指尖摸到小针刀顶端,随着右手持斜面小针刀,两手指同时上下配合,纵行切开内括约肌 1.3 ~ 1.8cm。切忌横切,以免刺穿肛管腔。拔出小针刀,术毕(图 10 - 2)。

1. **Treatment with Acupuncture Scalpel**　Patient lies on side, being taken sterilizing and local anesthesia. The doctor's left index finger inserts into anal canal 1.5cm to define the position of

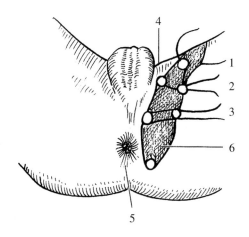

图 10 - 1 坏死性筋膜炎小针刀洞式对口挂线引流

1 - 上下缘口引流线;2 - 内外缘口引流线;3 - 中部口引流线;4 - 会阴;5 - 肛门;6 - 坏死筋膜

Figure 10 - 1 Necrotizing fasciitis is treated by acupuncture scalpel open to open hole style seton drainage

1. The thread of open to open drainage in upper and below fringe;

2. The thread of open to open drainage in inner and outer fringe;

3. The thread of drainage in middle incision;

4. Perineum; 5. Anus; 6. Necrotizing fascia

intersphincteric ditch, its upper fringe is the interna, sphincter, and to fix the iternal sphincter. His right hand handles the inclined plane acupuncture scalpel to insert into internal sphincter from local anesthetic points of right outside of anus, and in the guidance of his left index finger tip touching the top of acupuncture scalpel through anal canal, then his right hand handles the inclined plane acupuncture scalpel to insert into internal sphincter, two fingers coordinate each other, and cuts vertically internal sphincter 1.3 ~ 1.8cm, but don't cut horizontally. The acupuncture scalpel punctures anal canal, and then the doctor puts the acupuncture scalpel out (Fig. 10 - 2).

2. 套扎式和注射 在圆头缺口电池灯肛门镜下,使海绵状血管瘤凸入镜中,再用弯头负压吸引套扎枪扣入,使胶圈套扎在基底部,并于胶圈套扎后上端注入消痔灵 1ml 充盈,使呈水泡状。同法治疗另外血管瘤或内痔(图 10 - 2)。

2. Loop Ligation and Injection In optical anoscopy the doctor makes spongiform vascular tumor fall in anoscope, then ligates its base with rubber circle by angle head loop ligaturing gun with vacuum suction and then injects 1 ml XiaoZhiLing to enlarge and to form the rubber circle. According to the technique the other vascular tumor or internal hemorrhoids are separately ligated (Fig. 10 - 2).

三、大肠肛门放线菌病

III. Actinomycosis in Anus, Rectum and Colon

大肠肛门放线菌病多为慢性化脓性肉芽肿性炎症,有时伴脓肿和溃疡形成。

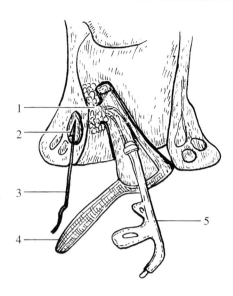

图 10 - 2　海绵状血管瘤套扎式注射,配合小针刀疗法
1 - 海绵状血管瘤;2 - 内括约肌;3 - 小针刀;4 - 肛门镜;5 - 套扎枪
Figure 10 - 2　The treatment of spongiform vascular tumor with loop ligation and injection by acupuncture scalpel
1. Spongiform vascular tumor;2. Internal sphincter;
3. Acupuncture scalpel;4. Anoscope;5. Loop ligating gun

肛周肿物没有明显的疼痛,只有坠胀感或坠痛,肿物质硬,一般 2cm 大小,没有波动感。

The large intestinal and anal actinomycosis is chronic suppurative granulomatous inflammation, sometimes accompanying with forming abscess and ulcer. There is no obvious pain except falling and distension. The tumor is hard, general, about 2 cm in size without fluctuation.

在超声波检查时也可用穿刺法吸出肿物内液体。如液体有臭味,呈硫黄色,内有颗粒,病检一般为放线菌。应与肛门脓肿、肿瘤、结核鉴别。鉴别依据为分泌物病检,也可用钩状小针刀,刺入肿物内钩取一些组织送病检确诊。

Ultrasonic examination or puncturing at the course of examination, if aspirating smell, yellow liquid with kernel from tumor, it may be actinomycosis. It should be differentiated from perianal abscess, cancer and tuberculosis. Biopsy of secretion is the help to differentiated diagnosis. The hook style acupuncture scalpel can also be used to insert into the tumor, and to hook some tissue for biopsy.

采用骶裂孔阻滞麻或局麻。手术前用亚甲蓝液划出肿物边界,用小针刀从肿物基底部刺入,连同皮肤、皮下整块,清除。如伤口有污染,可开放引流,外敷中药外痔贴;如伤口清洁,也可缝合。切除肿物,再送病理检查。

Methylene blue draws up the outline of tumor before taking operation with sacral hiatus block anesthesia or local anesthesia. Acupuncture scalpel punctures into the base of tumor, then puts the tumor with skin and subcutaneous tissue out. To open drainage and cover with herbs. The tissues being cut off should be taken for biopsy.

四、闭孔肌肥厚致肛门抽动痛
IV. Hypertrophy of Obturator Inducing Anal Witching Pain Syndrome

病因不清,病史间断,不明原因肛门内抽动痛。无肛门裂、肛窦炎,肛门外观无异常。肛门镜及盆腔 CT、B 超均无异常。肛指检查在肛管直肠两侧或一侧检查可触及约 2cm×4cm 大小,质软条索样肥厚闭孔内肌,上端入坐骨小孔,下端止于坐骨结节内侧。

It is a witching pain with unclear reason and intermittent spasm inside of anus, without anal fissure, anal sinusitis or abnormal anal exterior appearance. The examination results are normal such as anoscopy, CT and B ultrasonography of pelvic cavity. The digital examination can touch 2cm×4cm soft funicular hypertrophic obturator internus muscle in one side or two sides of anal canal and rectum, upwards till ischial tuberosity.

取截石位,消毒,局麻术者左手示指伸入肛管,隔着肛管壁触及索条状肥厚的闭孔内肌止于坐骨结节,其间隙为坐骨直肠窝。右手持斜面小针刀于肛门缘与坐骨结节、皮肤中点、经局麻针眼插入坐骨直肠窝。在肛管内的左手示指引导下隔着肛管,摸到小针刀顶端,随着右手持斜面小针刀两手指同时上下配合纵行切开索条状肥厚闭孔内肌 1.5~3cm,切忌横切,勿刺穿肛管腔,拔出小针刀,术毕(图 10-3,图 10-4)。对侧同法治疗。

Lithotomy position, sterilizing and local anesthesia, The doctor's left index finger inserts into anal canal to feel funicular hypertrophic obturator internus muscle resting on ischial tuberosity through anal canal, the space is ischiorectal fossa. His right hand handles the inclined plane acupuncture scalpel to insert into ischiorectal fossa from local anesthetic points in the middle between ischial tuberosity and anal fringe, and in the guidance of his left index finger tip touching the top of acupuncture scalpel through anal canal, then his right hand handles the inclined plane acupuncture scalpel, two fingers coordinate each other, to cut vertically funicular hypertrophic obturator internus muscle 1.5~3cm, but don't cut horizontally. The acupuncture scalpel punctures anal canal and then the doctor pulls the acupuncture scalpel out (Fig. 10-3, Fig. 10-4). The opposite side uses the same treatment.

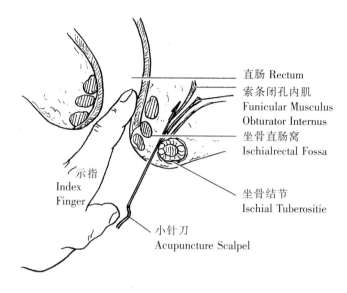

图 10 – 3 闭孔内肌纵切术

Figure 10 – 3 To cut vertically musculus obturator internus

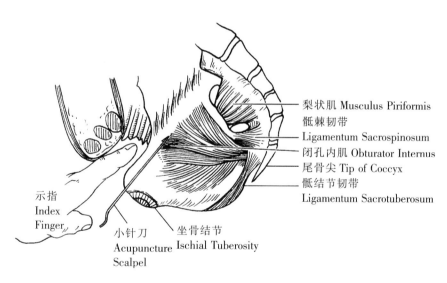

图 10 – 4 闭孔内肌肥厚纵切术

Figure 10 – 4 To cut vertically funicular hypertrophic musculus obturator internus

五、骶尾部脊索瘤疼痛

V. Chordoma of Sacrococcygeal Region

病因不清,排便后仍感排不尽,伴下腰骶臀部疼痛。尿频、排尿困难,无脓血便。腰骶 X 线未见异常,CT 和切除病检诊断"骶尾部脊索瘤"。肛门指检可扪及骶前肿块约 2cm×2cm,质硬、光滑移动差。指套无血染。

Etiology isn't clear, the feeling of incomplete evacuation in post-defecation, accompanying with pain in inferior lumbar and sacral parts and hips; frequency of urination and difficult urination without pus and blood. General X-way of lumbar and sacral portions doesn't discover abnormal graph, CT and postoperative biopsy confirms the diagnosis of chordoma of sacrococcygeal region. Digital examination can feel the 2cm × 2cm, hard, smooth, no moving tumor in anterior of sacrum, no blood on the glove.

取侧卧位,骶管阻滞麻醉,术者先用左手示指插入肛管内摸到尾骨尖,向上触及骶前肿块。右手持肛肠斜面小针刀,经尾骨尖前至肛门缘中点的点状局麻针眼插入。在肛管内的左手指引导下隔着肛管直肠左手指摸到小针刀顶端,随着右手持斜面小针刀,两手指同时上下配合纵行切割骶前肿块1圈,切忌横切,勿刺伤骶前静脉丛,以免出血。拔出小针刀,再用直血管钳插入针眼扩大间隙,将骶前肿物钳夹,拉出肛管外,针眼外敷创可贴(图10-5)。

Patient lies on side, being taken canalis sacralis block anesthesia. The doctor's left index finger inserts into anal canal to feel the tip of coccyx, its upper fringe is the tumor in the anterior of sacrum. His right hand handles the inclined plane acupuncture scalpel to insert into tumor from local anesthetic points of middle point between the tip of coccyx and anus, and in the guidance of his left index finger tip touching the top of acupuncture scalpel through anal canal while his right hand has handled the inclined plane acupuncture scalpel to insert into tumor, two fingers coordinate each other, and cut vertically the tumor one circle, doesn't cut horizontally to avoid injuring venous structures of anterior sacrum, and then the doctor puts the acupuncture scalpel out; then inserts straight blood-vessel forceps into the point to draw the tumor out of the anal canal. To cover with gauze on the point (Fig. 10-5).

六、肛门直肠子宫内膜异位症
VI. Anorectal Endometriosis

子宫内膜异位于小肠、大肠;好发于直肠;也可见于肛周或会阴皮下,引起周期性并与月经周期相关的便血。1860年,Roktansky首次发现子宫内膜异位症。Farinonam认为,结肠或直肠子宫内膜异位好发于育龄妇女,占15%~40%。

Endometriosis implies the occurrence of endometrial tissue at sites other than the lining of the corpus uteri. It was discovered by Roktansky. Farinonam thinks that it is found in 15% ~ 40% of women of child-bearing age.

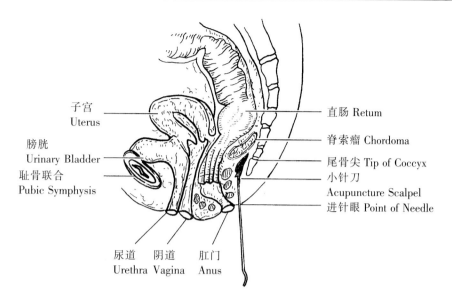

图 10 - 5　骶尾部脊索瘤切除术

Figure 10 - 5　Sacrococcygeal Chordomaectomy

【病因】

[Etiology]

子宫内膜种植。内膜异位为月经逆流所致,即子宫内膜碎片随月经倒流发生异位症,或与遗传基因、免疫因素等有关。

Endometrial ectopia is thought by most to result from influx of endometrial tissue through the fallopian tubes during menstruation. Lymphatic dissemination of endometrial emboli has also some adherents.

【病理】

[Pathology]

直肠子宫内膜异位症初期可见紫蓝色小点,并向阴道直肠隔发展,形成包块压迫直肠,向直肠壁浸润。肠道子宫内膜异位症,严重者可形成肿块导致肠梗阻。

The lesions of endometriosis, grossly and microscopically, essentially are identical to the normal uterine lining. Most frequently and most heavily involved are external surface of the uterus, broad ligaments, ovaries, cul-de-sac, rectosigmoid, rectovaginal septum, rectum, and sigmoid colon. Colonic lesions may be a single discrete implant in or on the wall, of the bowel, or involvement may be diffuse and extensive, and completely surrounding the bowel.

【临床表现】

[Clinical Manifestations]

有肠道症状与妇科子宫内膜异位的症状。如出现与月经有关的周期性腹泻、下腹痛、恶心、呕吐或肠梗阻,并有与月经有关的肛门出血,尤其是经期便血,严重者可出现贫血;伴有腹胀、周期性肠绞痛,可波及直肠,肛指检查可触及肿块或狭窄。

Symptoms may be present only at the time of menstruation or, if present throughout the cycle, are exacerbated at or just before the period. More common symptoms include gradually increasing dysmenorrhea, menstrual irregularities, rectal discomfort or pain on defecation, rectal tenesmus, lower abdominal cramps, constipation or diarrhea, abdominal distension, nausea, and dysuria. Less common is rectal bleeding and symptoms of intestinal obstruction, usually partial but occasionally complete. On digital rectal examination it may be felt anteriorly at the fingertip, representing cul-de-sac lesions.

【诊断】

[Diagnosis]

主要依靠病史、临床表现及相应的辅助检查。对周期性肛门便血,尤其与月经有关的便血,伴有腹痛或有不孕史、痛经史,均要进行妇科检查。肛门直肠检查发现有结节、肿块、狭窄的病灶,要进行活检,要与直肠癌或炎症疼痛便血鉴别。

Mainly relying on medical history, clinical manifestations and examinations. Pelvic and rectal examinations should be repeated at different phases of the menstrual cycle. Cyclic changes in the findings help to confirm the diagnosis.

【治疗】

[Treatment]

1. 药物

1. Medicine

(1)假孕法:应用孕激素造成类似人工闭经。甲孕酮(安宫黄体酮)加服乙炔雌二醇。

(1)Birth-control-pill:Provera and ethylidyne estradiol.

(2)假绝经法:应用药物诱导假绝经,以减少卵巢激素的分泌,使子宫内膜萎缩。口服达那唑。

(2)Suppression of menstruation:Danazol. Above two kinds of medicine on hormonal therapy can treat severe symptoms, suppression of menstruation with gradually increasing doses of a combination birth-control-pill, given continuously without cycling, usually causes regression of the lesions and relief of symptoms.

2. 激光小针刀治疗　在病灶部位进行激光,小针刀全切,汽化治疗。也可用高频小针刀电灼治疗。

2. Laser Acupuncture Scalpel Treatment　Laser acupuncture scalpel completely cut off and gasification the lesion, and also electrocauterize by high frequency acupuncture scalpel.

3. 手术治疗　切除卵巢内膜异位囊肿、肠道病灶(图 10 - 6)。

3. Operation　Solitary endometriomas that encroach on the lumen can be removed by anterior resection.

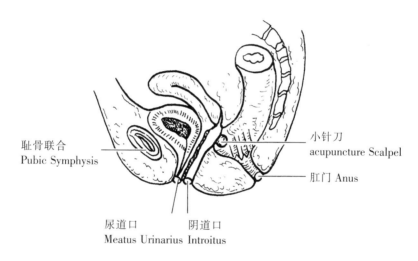

图 10 - 6　肛门直肠子宫内膜异位症小针刀疗法

Figure 10 - 6　Acupuncture scalpel treating anorectal endometriosis

本病预后良好。目前未见有肠道子宫内膜异位症癌变的报道。

This disease has good prognosis. There is no report on canceration of intestinal endometiosis.

七、肛尾肠囊肿
VI. Anal Hindgut Cyst

肛尾肠囊肿,即直肠发育期囊肿,主要是压迫直肠引起排粪便困难。常有排便困难、便秘、排便次数多或伴尿频、坐骨神经痛,女性患者伴会阴下坠。肛指检查可触及直肠前壁外肿块或囊肿,有波动者可以穿刺取液活检(图 10 - 7)。

An anal hindgut cyst is a cyst in rectal developmental phase, mainly pressing the rectum to cause serial symptoms such as common difficult defecation, constipation, or more times of defecation, frequency of micturition, sciatica, and feeling of perineal falling in female. A mass or cyst in the anterior rectal wall can be felt by digital examination, and the fluid in the cyst should be aspirated for biopsy (Fig. 10 – 7).

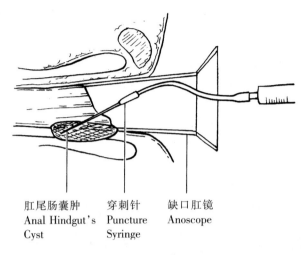

图 10 – 7　肛尾肠囊肿穿刺术

Figure 10 – 7　Puncture treating anal hindgut cyst

采用双面小针刀手术完整切除囊肿，并送病理检查（图 10 – 8）。身体衰弱不宜手术者，可以用刮匙小针刀行囊肿单纯引流术，以缓解压迫症状。

The doctor can carry on the double plane acupuncture scalpel to cut off completely the cyst, and takes biopsy (Fig. 10 – 8), meanwhile can also drain simply by the curette acupuncture scalpel.

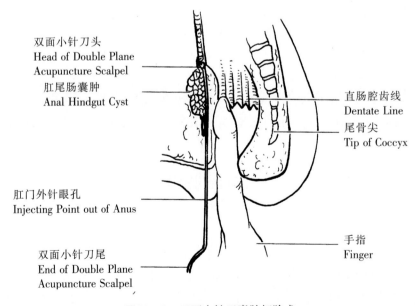

图 10 – 8　双面小针刀囊肿切除术

Figure 10 – 8　Double plane acupuncture scalpel cutting off cyst

八、肛旁藏毛窦

VIII. Perianal Pilonidal Sinus

肛旁藏毛窦是肛门旁皮肤上藏有毛发的窦道,多发生在肛门后方骶尾部。其发病常与肛旁皮肤损伤、感染等,致毛发侵入所致。局部检查常见肛门旁或骶尾部皮肤隆起、硬结、发炎或脓液,窦道内有毛发钻出。肛指、肛门镜检查均无异常。

Perianal pilonidal sinus is skinny sinus in which hair hides near the anus, mainly in posterior anus-sacrococcygeal region. It commonly results from the skinny trauma, infection, etc., to cause hair invading. Local examination usually shows skinny projecting, hard node, inflammation, pus hair drilling out of the sinus. Digital and anoscoopic examination can't discover abnormal condition.

化脓性藏毛窦用刮匙小针刀刮切窦道后引流,外敷消脓膏纱布条。硬结性藏毛窦用钩状小针刀完全切除后外敷痔瘘粉。

With the curette acupuncture scalpel the sinus can be curetted and pus drained for treating suppurative pilonidal sinus. With the hook style acupuncture scalpel the hard node like pilonidal sinus can be cut off completely.

附:典型病例
Classical Cases Report:

1. 肛门旁子宫内膜异位症
1. Perianal Endometriosis

例 1 因月经期间肛旁肿胀 1 年半,伴疼痛 4 个月,患者分娩时曾行会阴侧切,伤口愈合良好。于月经期出现肛旁坠胀,并可触及一鸽蛋大小肿块,月经过后坠胀缓解,肿块缩小。每逢月经来潮时肿块增大,伴剧烈疼痛,行走、坐位时更加明显。月经后肿块缩小,疼痛减轻。肛门检查:膝胸位肛门旁开处见 4cm×4cm 大小肿块,位于会阴切口处,拉之硬,有压痛。小针刀手术见肿物呈灰褐色,与皮下组织粘连,有多个囊腔,腔内有陈旧积血。病理检查示纤维组织中见子宫内膜组织、腺体及间质细胞,部分囊腔内见片状红细胞。诊断为子宫内膜异位症(附图 1)。

Case No. 1 In menses the patient suffered from perianal swelling 1 year and a half and pain for 4 months. Past medical history: She had ever been performed episiotomy, now the wound has healed well. In menses she felt pain of falling and distension around anus and caught a mass like a pigeon egg. Post-menses the feeling of falling and distension relieved, and the mass reduced. Every menses the mass increased in size gradually influencing sitting and walking, even more severe. On digital rectal examination, knee-chest position, the doctor may feel a mass 4cm×4cm near anus, located at the incision of episiotomy, hard and tender. The treatment with acupuncture scalpel and biopsy showed that the lesions also menstruate with the uterus, but since there was no cervix to drain off the effluvium, some glands and cysts filled with menstrual blood were found. Rupture of the cysts, with spillage of irritating contents, produced dense reactive fibrosis. Spillage of viable cells produced new implants and spread of the fibroplastic process. The lymphatic dissemination of endometrial emboli had some adherents. Diagnosis was endometriosis (Attached Fig. 1).

例 2 因月经期间肛旁肿痛 1 年多,近 2 个月加重。患者分娩时曾行会阴侧切,伤口愈合良好 03 年前发现肛门右前方有一肿块。月经来潮时增大,伴疼痛;月经过后肿块缩小,疼痛减轻,近 4 个月来症状加剧。肛门检查膝胸位旁开见 3cm × 3cm 大小隆起肿物,位于原会阴侧切口上,质硬,轻压痛。小针刀手术中见肿块呈灰褐色,与周围组织粘连,改用刮匙小针刀切除。病理检查报告:子宫内膜组织,诊断子宫内膜异位症(附图 1)。

Case No. 2 In menses the patient suffered from perianal pain over 1 year, severe pain near 2 months. Past medical history: She had ever been performed episiotomy, now the wound has healed well. In menses she felt increasing pain of falling and distension around anus and mass at anterior right side of anus. Post – menses the falling and distension reduced. On digital rectal examination the doctor felt the mass 3cm × 3cm near anus, located at the incision of episiotomy, hard and tender. The treatment with acupuncture scalpel and curette acupuncture scalpel was cutting the gray brown mass and adherent tissues, biopsy showed uterine endometrium tissues, diagnosis was endometriosis (Attached Fig. 1).

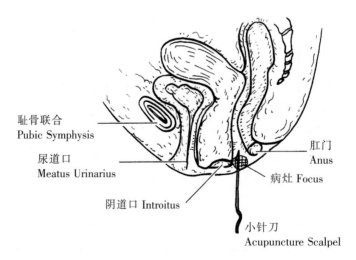

耻骨联合 Pubic Symphysis
尿道口 Meatus Urinarius
阴道口 Introitus
肛门 Anus
病灶 Focus
小针刀 Acupuncture Scalpel

附图 1 肛旁子宫内膜异位症小针刀疗法
Attached Fig. 1 Acupuncture scalpel treats perianal endometriosis

2.直肠异物

2. Foreign Body in the Rectum

例1　女,16 岁,学生。肛门坠胀,大便带血,指检直肠可触及金属异物。自述 3d 前将"发卡"吞入胃中。肛门镜下发现"发卡"嵌入齿线上 2cm 的直肠黏膜下,用钩状小针刀取出发卡,给予中药痔瘘粉外敷,治愈(附图 2)。

Case No. 1　A female student, 16yr of age, felt falling and distension in anus, and had blood on the stool. Digital examination showed a metal foreign body. She told that she swallowed a "hair clip" 3 days ago. Anoscopy discovered the "hair clip" inlaying in rectal submucosa 2cm above dentate line. With a hook style acupuncture scalpel the hair clip was taken out (Attached Fig 2).

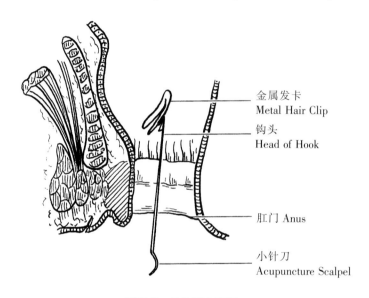

金属发卡
Metal Hair Clip

钩头
Head of Hook

肛门 Anus

小针刀
Acupuncture Scalpel

附图 2　异物嵌入直肠
Attached Fig. 2　Foreign body inlay the rectum

例2　男,58 岁,工人。肛门肿胀持续跳痛,大便带血伴发热,体温 39℃,指检直肠内可触及较硬异物。自述发病前 4 天不慎将"义齿"吞入胃中。肛门镜下发现"假牙"嵌顿在齿线上 2cm 黏膜下,隆起 3cm×3cm 脓肿,用钩状小针刀取出。有脓液流出,改换探针小弯刀,将齿线以下脓肿切开,齿线以上脓肿挂橡皮筋同步治疗。外敷痔瘘粉治愈。

Case No. 2　A male worker, 58yr of age, felt that anus was swollen, falling with persistent jumping pain. The body temperature was 39℃. On digital rectal examination the doctor felt a hard metal foreign body, and was told that the "false teeth" was swallowed 4 days ago. Anoscopy discovered the "false teeth" inlaying in rectal submucosa 2cm above dentate line to form a swelling of 3cm×3cm abscess. The hook style acupuncture scalpel took out the false teeth meanwhile draining pus. The doctor changed the small curving probing scalpel to incise the abscess below dentate line, and then to hang rubber loop treating the abscess above dentate line.

例 3 ，男，45 岁，工人。肛门剧痛，大便带血，指检直肠触及锐利异物，自述发病前暴食"猪排骨"。治疗经过：肛门镜下发现"骨片"卡在齿线以上黏膜层，用血管钳配合刮匙小针刀取出，给予中药痔瘘粉外敷治愈。

Case No. 3　A male worker, 45yr of age, felt sharp pain in anus, and had blood on the stool. On digital rectal examination the doctor felt sharp foreign body, and was told that the "pork chop" was gluttonized on the day before yesterday. Anoscopy discovered the "bone fragment" inlaying in rectal submucosa above dentate line. The doctor took vessel forceps cooperating with hook style acupuncture scalpel to take out the bone fragment.

例 4　男，62 岁。肛门针刺样痛，排便带血。指检触及类似"铁丝"样异物，自述发病前吃火锅暴饮史。肛门镜下发现铁丝嵌入直肠黏膜层内，血管钳、钩状小针刀取出。术后敷痔瘘粉治愈。

Case No. 4　A male, 62yr of age, felt pricking pain in anus, and had blood on the stool. On digital rectal examination the doctor felt that foreign body like "iron wire", and was told gluttonizing before the disease occured. Anoscopy discovered the iron wire inlaying in rectal submucosa. With the hook style acupuncture scalpel and vessel forceps the iron wire was taken out.

例 5　男，45 岁，农民。肛门持续跳痛，大便带血。指检直肠触及枣核异物，发病前有吞食大量"红枣"。肛门镜下发现一枚枣核尖部嵌入齿线上黏膜层，用刮匙小针刀取出，溃疡面敷中药痔瘘粉治愈。

Case No. 5　A farmer, 58yr of age, felt persistent jumping pain in anus, and had blood on the stool. On digital rectal examination the doctor felt foreign body like date pit, amd was told that he swallowed a lot of "red jujubes" before the disease occured. Anoscopy discovered the tip of date pit inlaying in rectal submuscosa above dentate line. With the curette acupuncture scalpel it was taken out.

3. 骶尾外伤后肌纤维粘连肛门直肠疼痛

3. Muscular Fibrous Adhesion Causing Anorectal Pain after Injuring Sacrococcygeal Region

例 1　患者，女，42 岁，肛周疼痛坠胀不适半年住院。经纤维结肠镜检查无异常，经追问病史有骶尾外伤史。X 线检查为尾骨陈旧骨折。肛指检查见肛门直肠后侧至尾骨尖有压痛，耻骨直肠肌紧张痉挛触痛。肛门直肠内示指和肛门外拇指双合诊检查尾骨尖成角屈曲，前后移位，疼痛加重。考虑陈旧尾骨骨折，至耻骨直肠肌粘连痉挛。入院诊断：骶尾外伤，肛门直肠疼痛综合征。

Case No. 1　A female patient, 42yr of age, was hospitalized because she felt falling and distension in anal region for half a year. Fiberopic colonoscopic examination didn't discover abnormalities. She had ever injured her sacrococcygeal region. X-ray showed old fracture of coccyx.

Digital rectal examination showed tenderness from posterior side of anus and rectum to tip of coccyx, spasm of puborectal muscle and tenderness. The index finger inside of anorectum and thumb outside of anus taking double fingers examination confirmed the tip of coccyx forming angle bend and anterior-posterior shift, with severe pain. So that old fracture of coccyx caused spasm and adhesion of puborectal muscle. The diagnosis is sacrococcygeal trauma, anorectal pain syndrome.

例 2　男 48 岁,肛门直肠疼痛 8 个月住院。经纤维直肠镜检查无异常,询问病史有骑车摔伤骶尾外伤史。X 线检查见尾骨向前错位。肛指检查肛门直肠内示指和肛门外拇指双合诊检查,尾骨尖前后移位,肛门直肠疼痛加重,考虑尾骨尖移位、粘连、痉挛。

Case No. 2　A male patient, 48yr of age, was hospitalized because he felt pain in anus and retum for 8 months. Fiberopic colonoscopic examination didn't discover abnormalities. Being asked his medical history, he had ever injured his sacrococcygeal region. X-ray showed shift of coccyx toward anterior. On digital rectal examination, the index finger inside of anorectum and thumb outside of anus taking double fingers examination confirmed the shift of tip of coccyx toward anterior-posterior, with severe pain. The diagnosis was shift of tip of coccyx, spasm and adhesion of muscles.

两例均取侧卧位,消毒,在肛门与尾骨尖之间的中点做点状局麻。术者先用左手指插入肛管直肠腔约 3cm,隔着肛管直肠后壁摸到尾骨尖上触及括约肌纤维粘连结节,按压固定。右手持钩状小针刀,从肛门外点状局麻的针眼插进。在直肠腔内左手指的引导下隔着直肠后壁,左手指尖先摸到钩状小针刀顶端导引,随着右手持钩状小针刀在两手指同时上下配合,纵行钩割开尾骨前的耻骨直肠肌纤维粘连结节。切忌横行钩割,勿刺穿直肠腔,拔除小针刀,术毕(附图 3)。两例全部治愈,无并发症。

The two persons were treated by hook style acupuncture scalpel. Coordinating with double fingers, the doctors' right hand handled the acupuncture scalpel to cut and hooked vertically spastic puborectal muscular adhesive node in front of coccyx. He didn't cut it horizontally lest puncturing to penetrate the rectal lumen. The doctor took out the acupuncture scalpel (Attached Fig. 3). The two cases were cured, with no complication.

4. 椎管内肿瘤　患者,男,37 岁。肛门下坠,排便困难,每天排便 3~5 次,每次排便伴有肛门下坠、疼痛、排便不尽感。有腰痛史,外院曾诊断为腰肌劳损,骨质增生。指诊:耻骨直肠肌痉挛,舒张障碍,触痛明显。直肠排便造影显示盆底失弛缓综合征。肌电图检查:耻骨直肠肌和肛门内括约肌均有静息压力反常收缩现象。腰椎 X 线片仅骨质增生。行小针刀闭合性耻骨直肠肌全束切开和内括约肌切开术,术后排便困难缓解,但仍有肛门下坠、疼痛和便不尽感,腰痛加重,再进行腰椎MRI 检查发现腰 4~5 椎管内占位性病变是椎管内肿瘤,转骨科手术。病检为椎管神经纤维瘤,术后腰痛缓解,排便困难缓解。肛门下坠,便不尽感均消失。

4. **Tumor in Vertebral Canal** A male patient, 37yr of age , felt falling in anus, difficult defecation every time, but 3 ~ 5 times every day with pain and uncompletely exhausted. He suffered from lumbar pain, and was diagnosed strain of lumbar muscles, hyperosteogeny. On digital rectal examination the doctor felt puborectal muscular spasm, difficult dilatation marked tenderness. Defecography showed nonrelaxing pelvic floor syndrome. Electromyogram showed that resting pressure of puborectal muscle and internal sphincter taking paradoxical contraction X-ray of lumbar showed only hyperosteogeny. To take closely puborectal musculotomy and internal sphincterotomy by acupuncture scalpel. Postoperatively the symptoms of difficult defecation improved, but falling in anus, pain and uncompletely exhausted defecation still existed, and more severe lumbar pain. Lumbar MRI showed a tumor in vertebral canal. So the patient was transfered to orthopaedic department. Biopsy confirmed the diagnosis being neurofibroma in the vertebral canal. The patient was cured after operation.

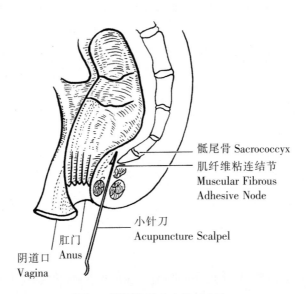

附图 3 骶尾肌粘连小针刀疗法

Attached Fig. 3 Acupuncture scalpel treats sacrococcygeal muscular adhesion

第11章　肛肠病治疗后并发症

Chapter 11　Postoperative Complications
of Anorectal Diseases

一、内痔注射并发症

I. Complications of Injection Therapy to Treat Internal Hemorrhoids

内痔注射是治疗内痔的方法之一。虽然操作简单,但操作不当,也会引起多种并发症,如感染、出血、疼痛、内痔脱出、前列腺炎和肛管狭窄、肠穿孔等。

Injection therapy is one of the methods to treat internal hemorrhoids. It is easy to induce some complications though the method is simple, such as infection, bleeding, pain projecting of internal hemorrhoids, prostatitis, inflammation and stricture of anal canal and perforation of rectum, etc.

(一)感染
(I) Infection

【临床表现】

[Clinical Manifestations]

局部感染多见,大多发生在注射后2~3天。表现肛门坠胀疼痛,有灼痛感、便血、黏液便、大便次数增多、便意不净感、肛门分泌物增多等。低热,周身不适。肛指检查触及注射区轻压痛、硬结、肿胀感,指套有脓血。肛门镜:痔注射后可见点或片状黏膜溃疡面积 $0.5 \sim 1cm^2$,中心有紫色血凝块,有少量渗血,周围黏膜水肿高起。继续发展可引起肛门脓肿,其肛门脓性分泌物,局部红肿、疼痛、畏寒、发热,甚至引起静脉炎、肝脓肿、患者往往伴有黄疸。B超检查可确诊。

Local infection is common, often takes place in 2 ~ 3 days after injection. The symptoms show in anus feeling distension and falling, hot and pain, bleeding or mucus defecation, more defecation and uncompletely exhausted, more secretion, with a low fever and uncomfortable status. On digital rectal examination, the doctor feels mild tenderness, hard node and swollen in injection area, blood and pus on the glove. On the anoscopic examination the doctor watches there are points or patched ulcers, $0.5 \sim 1cm^2$ area, purple blood clot and small oozing of blood in the centre, with surrounding edema and projective mucosa. If the disease is getting worse, it can form anal abscess so that the symptoms show pus secretion from anus, red and swelling locally, pain, shiver, fever, even liver abscess and jaundice. The diagnosis of liver abscess relies on B-us examination.

【防治措施】

[Prevention and Treatment]

(1)注射前选择病例:如有慢性肠炎或腹泻,尤其近期伴黏液血便,应先治疗肠炎,当症状好转,再选择注射疗法治疗内痔。注射前要排除直结肠炎或怀疑直肠癌,应做肛指检查,肛镜检查可以了解直肠内情况。注射前,伴发热、感冒、肺结核、肝炎活动期等,应等病情控制后再进行注射疗法。

(1)Choosing suitable cases:Patients suffering from chronic enteritis or diarrhea especially defecating pus and blood recently should first see the doctor for treating enteritis, wait for symptoms getting better, and then see the doctor for treating internal hemorrhoids by injection therapy; meanwhile the patients suffering from catching cold, phthisis, activity hepatitis should wait for symptoms having been controlled. Another problem which needs to get rid of the disease is rectal cancer. Anal digital and anoscopic examination are necessary for understanding the inner portion of rectum before injection.

(2)注射时要严格无菌、消毒措施;选择注射点尽量一次定针,不要反复多次、多针眼注射,以减少感染面。注射后,用无菌干棉或苯扎溴铵棉球压迫针眼,待数日再排便,排便后塞入痔疮栓,或九华膏。一旦出现脓肿,则配合小针刀挑割引流术。

(2)One must be strict, sterilizing as injection, should inject from one injected point, don't repeat injection for fear of infection. Once the abscess occurs, drainage should be done by acupuncture scalpel cutting.

(3)注射后口服甲硝唑(厌氧菌)、百炎净片(广谱杀菌药)预防,必要时用抗生素。

(3)After injection the patient should take medicine to prevent infection, such as antibiotics and herbs, etc.

(二)出血
(II) Bleeding

【临床表现】

[Clinical Manifestations]

多数为伴发感染后出现便血。主要是注射后,黏膜层创面渗血,量少。如溃疡糜烂面大、腐蚀到痔动脉则引起大出血。

Postoperative bleeding is related to either infective hemostasis at the time of operation or to heavy packing of the anal canal. The main symptom is a little amount of bleeding from mucous wound. If the ulcer area is large, and corrodes hemorrhoidal artery, then a large amount of bleeding will occur.

【防治措施】

［Prevention and Treatment］

（1）必须在麻醉下用细羊肠线，以出血点为中心进行置上海绵一同缝合。然后再用止血海绵蘸痔瘘粉或酌情用安全套气囊压迫止血。

（1）Direct suture of the bleeder is the treatment of choice to control postoperative hemorrhage. Thus, any patient who belongs to bleed postoperatively and doesn't respond to bed rest should be taken to the operating room, in which, under the proper anesthetic, the site of bleeding can be demonstrated and sutured.

（2）操作应轻柔准确，进针适当，药液不能外溢积留在痔核表面。

（2）The injection should be gentle and exact, the depth of injection should suit for the degree of disease, the liquid drug of using can't drip on the surface of the hemorrhoids.

（三）疼痛
（Ⅲ）Pain

【临床表现】

［Clinical Manifestations］

内痔注射后肛门轻度坠胀感，一般 6 小时消失。如操作不当，进针过深可损伤括约肌层，或波及齿线，药液弥散至齿线以下则引起肛门剧痛。继发感染也可伴疼痛加重。

Postoperative feeling of mild falling and distension around anus disappear generally in 6 hours, but unsuitable injection can induce severe pain in anal area, such as injecting in deeply, injuring sphincter, involving inferior of dentate line as drug spreading. If the pain is more, secondary infection is worse.

【防治措施】

［Prevention and Treatment］

进针勿过深，勿达肌肉（尤其是括约肌），只限黏膜层、黏膜下层。进针勿过低，应在齿线以上 0.5cm 处进针。注入药液勿过量，以痔黏膜下层变色、隆起为度。为了减轻注射疼痛及肛管水肿，降低肛门直肠角度压力，可配合小针刀闭合性切断内括约肌。

The tip of injector can't go in too deeply, can't arrive at muscular layer (sphincter especially). The injection should only locate in mucosa and submucosa. Meanwhile the position of injection should choose 0.5cm above dentate line, can't be too low. The drug of injection can't be of too large dose, the standard is that hemorrhoidal submucosa changes color and projects. The doctor can cut internal sphincter by acupuncture scalpel for reducing edema of anal canal and pressure of anorectal angle in order to decrease pain.

(四)内痔脱出
(Ⅳ)Prolapse of Internal Hemorrhoids

【临床表现】
[Clinical Manifestations]

多发生痔注射后 1 ~ 2 天。大便久蹲时,可见被注射的痔核完全或部分脱于肛门外。继发感染者肛管水肿、剧痛。

It occurs in the 1 ~ 2 days after injection as defecation, the hemorrhoid which has been injected prolapses outside of anus. It's very painful if infection occurs.

【防治措施】
[Prevention and Treatment]

切勿仅注射痔核,应在痔核上部,在黏膜下层一边注射,一边进行封闭各痔核,即对黏膜固有层注射,呈网状封闭。使之产生无菌粘连固定。对较大、较多的痔核应采用分次注射法。对注射后已脱出的痔核,应轻轻复位,外敷中药,外痔贴;送回肛门。严重者则配合小针刀,闭合切割外括约肌皮下部及内括约肌,以松解嵌顿环,利于脱出痔核送回肛管内。

Don't only inject into the hemorrhoid, one should inject into mucosa and submucosa above the hemorrhoid to form net style injection, and to produce adhesion and local fixing. Divide some times of injection for treating large and more hemorrhoids. The severe case should be treated with acupuncture scalpel to cut subcutaneous muscle of external sphincter and internal sphincter.

(五)前列腺炎或直肠阴道瘘
(Ⅴ)Inflammation of Prostate and the Fistula Between Rectum and Vagina

【临床表现】
[Clinical Manifestations]

多发生注射前位内痔。因进针穿进前列腺、膀胱、尿道,注射后表现尿痛、尿急、尿血、尿常规发现红细胞或脓细胞。发生尿潴留、前列腺炎。进针穿进阴道可引起直肠阴道瘘。

The injury mainly occurs in injection of anterior internal hemorrhoids, the injection mistakes to go into prostate, bladder and urinary tract. The manifestations are pain, rapid, bleeding as urination, routine urine examination shows red blood and pus cells. If the injection goes through vagina, then fistula between rectum and vagina will occur.

【防治措施】

[Prevention and Treatment]

注射前嘱患者先排尿、排大便;注射时勿过深,回抽无尿液。注射时必须直视下见痔核明显隆起。一旦发生隆起不明显,应回抽观察回吸液中有无尿液、前列腺液样浑浊物,一旦发生,则按泌尿系统感染或前列腺炎综合治疗。未婚女性可以配合肛管指检防止刺入阴道。

To telling the patient passing urine, and defecation if possible before injection. The injection should not go in too deep, or draw back urine. The doctor must observe obviously the hemorrhoids enlarging. If projection of hemorrhoids is not obvious, he should take care whether other muddy liquid was drawn back, such as urine, prostate fluid, etc. The women should be cared through anal digital examination with unmarried and vaginal digital with married lest the drug going into vagina.

二、直肠硬结症
II. Rectal Hard Node Syndrome

【病因】

[Etiology]

有内痔注射史,如注射消痔灵或其他硬化剂药量过多引起。内痔注射后引起内痔基底部肠壁广泛性变硬,弹性下降尤其注射过深,累及肠内壁肌肉层更易发生直肠硬结症。

The disease results from that the patient suffering from internal hemorrhoids was injected over doses XiaoZhiLing or other sclerosed drugs. Overdose injection make the wall of anal canal of internal hemorrhoidal base forming scar extensively, reducing elasticity, especially if injected too deeply it's easy to form hard nodes as involving intestinal muscular layer of inner wall.

【临床表现】

[Clinical Manifestations]

肛门直肠内有坠胀感,便意不尽,排便次数多,有异物堵塞感或大便变细。肛指检查触及直肠齿线附近孤立或盘曲、边缘清晰、表面光滑、质中度的硬结,移动差,无压痛和触痛。肛镜检查见隆起肿块,用刮匙小针刀旋转切除部分送病检为炎症。注意与直肠肿瘤鉴别。

The patients fill falling, distension, uncompletely exhausted defecation, multiple time defecation, foreign body blocking and thin stool. Anal digital examination shows hard nodes around rectal dentate line, curve, clearing fringe, smooth surface, little movement, no tenderness. Anoscopic examination shows projected masses, with curette acupuncture scalpel shaves them; pathological biopsy reveals inflammation. It should be differentiated from rectal tumors.

【治疗】

[Treatment]

1. 口服中药 行气活血,消肿散结。如散结汤,一煎口服,二煎保留灌肠。

1. Taking Herbs To take herbs of enhancing vitality and activating blood circulation and to remove swelling and nodes, such as decoction of SanJieTang, taking the decoction first and use the second boiled decoction for enema.

2. 刮匙小针刀治疗 排便后取侧卧位。用两叶肛门镜或斜缺口电池肛门镜,将其直肠硬结显露,亚甲蓝、利多卡因点状麻醉,用苯扎溴铵或碘伏消毒后,右手持刮匙小针刀,将硬结由底部从右向左旋转并切除,创面用敷有"痔瘘散中药粉"的棉球压迫。治疗后24小时再排便,以后每日肛内注入九华膏,疗程约3周。如没有痛苦,可照常饮食、排便活动(图11-1)。

2. Treating with Curette Acupuncture Scalpel Patient lies on side, with round head and notch mouth optic anoscope to show rectal hard nodes. Local anesthesia with lidocaine, sterilizing as usual, the doctor handles curette acupuncture scalpel to shave and cut the base of hard node from right to left. Cover and press with gauzes on the wound. Defecating after 24 hours, changing the gauzes everyday postoperatively, 3 weeks a therapeutic course (Fig. 11 -1).

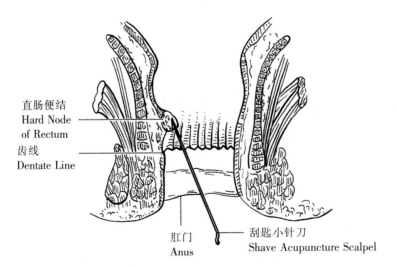

图11-1 直肠硬结症小针刀疗法

Figure 11 -1 Acupuncture scalpel treatment rectal for hard node syndrome

三、破　伤　风

III. Tetanus

破伤风在痔瘘的治疗合并症中虽然极为少见,但是由于病情严重,病死率高,处理比较困难,因此,应提高警惕。

Although tetanus is a rare complication in treating hemorrhoids and fistulas, it should be taken care because it is a very severe disease, difficultly treated and with high mortality.

【感染途径】

[Infection approach]

破伤风杆菌生存在动物及人的肠道中,随粪便排出体外,可形成芽胞,抵抗力较强,并能在土壤中长久生存,随灰尘飞散而沾染在衣物和皮肤上,因此,创伤总有被破伤风菌感染的可能。在治疗痔瘘的过程中,不论是"明矾压缩"、"简单开刀"、"枯痔法"等都会造成新鲜创口和溃疡,因而有发生破伤风的可能。另外,如在伤口内存有坏死组织及异物,组织因炎症引起氧化作用降低,或脓汁引流不畅及某些微生物同时存在等,均有利于破伤风杆菌的繁殖而发病。

Tetanus bacillus hide in the intestinal tract of human being and animals, excluded out of the body following the defecation. Tetanus bacillus form strong resistant gemma. The gemma can stay in the soil for long time meanwhile they can spread over with dust in the air, can infect the clothing and skin, so the wound may be infected. In the course of treating hemorrhoids and fistulas the fresh wound may be infected by tetanus whatever the methods are simple operation or injecting necrosis. In addition the tetanus bacillus can grow and breed in the focus such as necrotic tissues and foreign bodies in the wound, causing low oxygenization because of local inflammation, pus without being drained freely and other microorganisms existing here.

【临床表现】

[Clinical Manifestations]

前驱症状多表现四肢无力、多汗、头痛、腹肌疼痛、说话不便、吞咽困难或伤口处肌肉阵挛等。发病后最早出现最常见的症状是咀嚼肌痉挛,开口困难;以后便发生下颌痉挛、牙关紧闭,因表情肌痉挛而表现一种特有的"苦笑"面貌;当颈部及背部肌肉发生痉挛时会出现躯体向后屈曲,呈角弓反张。对外界任何刺激(如光、声、震动)均可诱发痉挛发作或加剧。

The symptoms of forerunner are feeble, multiple sweat, headache, abdominal pain, speech pause, difficult swallowing and the wounded muscular spasm, etc. The most initial symptoms show spasm of chew muscles and difficulty of opening mouth; the later are lower jaw spasm, teeth closeness, "bitter smile" expression because of facial muscular spasm; the body can bend toward posterior when the muscles of neck and back take place spasm, which is called opisthotonos. The every outside stimulation (light, sound, shake) can induce spasm or more severe spasm.

【诊断】

[Diagnosis]

当出现上述症状时,一般容易诊断,但对早期症状不显明容易误诊。如吞咽困难,开口不便,常被诊为咽峡炎、颈部淋巴结炎等;当出现神经系统症状时,有被误诊为脑膜炎者,应注意鉴别。因此,凡发现疑似破伤风症状者,均应仔细询问病史,注意近日来有无外伤或手术史等,严密观察,直至排除此病为止。当然,在伤口检出破伤风杆菌更有助于诊断。

The diagnosis is easy as occurring the above mentioned symptoms, however it is also easy to delay diagnosis when there is not obvious symptoms in the initial stage. For example, difficult swallowing and opening mouth usually mistaken to diagnose pharyngitis or inflammation of cervical lymph nodes. The nervous system symptoms sometimes were mistaken to diagnose cephalomeningitis, so we should pay attention to differentiation. All patients who are doubted of tetanus should be inquired carefully their medical histories, recent wounded histories, should be observed strictly till getting rid of the diagnosis of the disease. Of course, the most definite diagnosis is finding out the tetanus bacillus in the wound.

【治疗】

[Treatment]

目前由于采用中西医结合的综合疗法,疗效已大大提高。治疗方法主要是消灭感染病灶内的病原体,解除破伤风毒素的毒性,增加机体的抵抗力,预防及治疗并发症。

Recently because of carrying on the synthetical therapy of integrated traditional Chinese and western medicine, the curative effect have increased greatly. The method is mainly exterminating pathogeny, relieving toxin, improving resistance, preventing and treating complications.

1. **长期治疗**　进行系统全面的治疗,采取措施如下。

1. **Treatment Long Time**　Carrying on systematic and comprehensive treatment as follows.

(1)氯丙嗪 25mg,1 次/6 小时,肌内注射(或口服)。

(1)Chlorpromazine 25mg i. m. or oral taking, once/6h.

(2)水化氯醛合剂 10～20rnl,每天 3 次,口服或保留灌肠。

(2)Trichloraldehyde Hydrate 10～20mg, three times every day, taking orally or enema.

（3）混悬青霉素 40 万 U,每日 1 次,肌内注射(皮试阴性)。

（3）Penicillin 400 thousand units, once perday (after negative skin test).

（4）肾囊封闭,隔日 1 次,每次用 0.25% 普鲁卡因 60～100ml。

（4）Local block anesthesia at Kidney pouch, 0.25 % 60～100ml Procaine once per two days.

（5）玉真汤:每日 1 剂。

（5）Decoction of YuZhenTang:A dose per day.

（6）针刺:每日 1～2 次。常用穴位:人中、风府、大杼、合谷、少商、曲池、涌泉、哑门、百会、三阴交。

（6）Acupuncture:1～2 times per day, common points:RenZhong, FengFu, DaShu, HeGu, ShaoShang, QuChi, YongQuan, YaMen, BaiHui, SanYinJiao.

（7）饮食,给流质或半流质食物。

（7）Food:Liquid or semi-liquid.

（8）维生素 B、维生素 C:肌内注射。

（8）Vitamin B, Vitamin C:i. m.

2. 对症治疗

2. Treatment According to Symptoms

（1）为中和毒素,于入院后的第 1、2 天,每日用破伤风抗毒素 10 万 U,行肌内或静脉注射(以后可根据情况酌情应用)。

（1）Every day on first and second day after having been hospitalized for neutralizing toxin (the doctor can continue to carry on injection the medicine according to the disease development in later stage) with Tetanus Antitoxin 100 thousand units i. m. or i. v.

（2）痉挛严重时,用硫贲妥钠 0.5g,行一次肌内或静脉注射。

（2）Sodium pentothal 0.5g i. m. or i. v. once only for treating severe spasm.

（3）处理伤口,如适当扩创(并做细菌涂片及培养检查),并用过氧化氢冲洗或玉真散外敷。

（3）Local wound therapy, for example, the doctor can clear wound with washing aquae hydrogen dioxide or covering powder of traditional Chinese medicine (after taking bacterial culture examination for the infective wound).

3. 特别处理 如痰涎较多有窒息危险时,应以吸引器吸净。必要时宜及时做气管切开术。

3. Special Arrangement If the patient shows danger of asphyxia because of much saliva, sputum and water in the mouth, the doctor should remove secretions by suction, and perform tracheotomy in time.

重症患者在行针灸疗法时可诱发痉挛发作,但在行针后有全身肌肉松弛感。此法与制痉药配合使用,可加强治疗效果,故应在注射止痉药物后行针。

The method of acupuncture may induce spasm in the severe cases, but the whole body muscles can be relaxed after taking acupuncture, so the method should be used with medicine of relieving spasm to improve the curative effect. The doctor should give the acupuncture treatment after the patient having been injected with the medicine of relieving spasm.

【预防】
[Prevention]

除了在手术时注意无菌操作,应用器械、敷料也要求严格无菌外,对一些开放伤口(如肛瘘切开、外痔切除术后),应注意引流通畅,最好用痔瘘粉,以抑制破伤风杆菌。对有些伤口,如明矾压缩法、枯痔法、手术后留的伤口,深长的复杂瘘管配合高位挂线疗法者应及时换药。如多存有坏死组织或引流不畅者,除尽可能用痔瘘粉、消脓膏外敷,必要时可考虑给予破伤风抗毒血清(1500U)注射。

One must carry on aseptic manipulation strictly in operation, postoperative management and equipment maintenance. The opened wound should be drained free, changed gauzes in time for postoperative wound, such as hemorrhoids, deep and long complex fistula with hanging thread at high position, etc. To inject TAT (1500U) if necessary.

四、肛门疼痛
IV. Anal Pain

【病因】
[Etiology]

肛门周围神经末梢颇丰富,肛管直肠括约肌结构特殊。因肛门皮肤及括约肌受到刺激,加上括约肌痉挛性收缩,致术后剧痛。患者因怕痛而拒绝手术或治疗。有的因疼痛而排尿困难。因尿道与肛门属同一神经分支,相互影响,也可引起排便困难,并形成恶性循环。

There are very rich and sensitive nervous endings in anal area, meanwhile the sphincter structures of anal canal and rectum are special. Severe pain may come here postoperatively, because anal skin and sphincter are stimulated by contracting spasm. The patients are afraid of pain so as to refuse operation and other treatment. Some patients have difficult urination and defecation even vicious circle.

【治疗】

[Treatment]

1. **长效止痛药**　肛门术后应用。即在手术后注射于肛门术后的伤口,如封闭止痛药,疗效好,无不良反应。止痛药封闭后可缓解疼痛和括约肌痉挛,改善肛周血循环、淋巴回流及肛门缘水肿,促进伤口愈合。

1. **Long Effect Drugs for Stopping Pain**　Postoperatively the doctor injects the drugs into the wound to take part in local anesthesia for reducing sphincteric spasm, pain, and anal, fringe edema, and improving anal region blood circulation and lymph drainage, and promoting to wound healing.

2. 长效止痛剂组成

2. The Elements of Long Effect Drugs for Stopping Pain

(1)1 号液:0.25% 市比卡因 4ml,1% 亚甲蓝 1ml,肾上腺素 2 滴(高血压心脏病患者不用)。混合后伤口周围封闭。

(1)1# liquid; 0.25% bubicaine 4 ml, 1% methylene blue 1 ml, epinephrine 2drops (except for the patient with high blood pressure and heart diseases). The doctor combinds these drugs to inject into around wound.

(2)2 号液:0.5% 利多卡因 10ml,1% 亚甲蓝 1ml 混合加入肾上腺素 2 滴。混合后伤口周围封闭。

(2)2# liquid; 0.5% lidocaine 10 ml, 1% methylene blue 1 ml, epinephrine 2drops, compounding these drugs to inject into around wound.

(3)3 号液:1% 普鲁卡因 5ml,1% 亚甲蓝 1 支(2ml),肾上腺素 2 滴。混合后伤口周围封闭。

(3)3# liquid; 1% procaine 5ml, 1% methylene blue 2ml, epinephrine 2drops, compounding these drugs to inject into around wound.

(4)4 号液:复方利多卡因(曾用名,复方薄荷脑注射液)10ml,肾上腺素 2 滴。混合后伤口周围封闭。

(4)4# liquid; Compound lidocaine 10 ml, epinephrine 2drops, compounding these drugs to inject into around wound.

3. 长效止痛药穴位注射

3. Acupuncture Points Injection with Long Effect Analgesics

(1)适应证:肛门手术后患者,如肛瘘、肛裂、混合瘘、肛门乳头瘤、肛门脓肿术后。

（1）Indications：Every anal postoperative pain，such as anal fistulas，fissure，mixed hemorrhoids，papilloma，abscess.

（2）选用穴位：会阴穴、长强穴（图 11 – 2）。

（2）Points：HuiYin and ChangQiang （Fig. 11 – 2）.

（3）止痛药：1% 亚甲蓝 2ml，0.5% 利多卡因 10ml 混合。

（3）Analgesics：Mixed 1% methylene blue 2ml and 0.5% lidocaine 10 ml.

（4）操作方法：用 6 号针头，分别注入会阴、长强穴位，进针角度 45°，深 1.5 ～ 3.0cm。进针入穴位，回抽无回血无尿液，每个穴位注入 2 ～ 4ml 即可。

（4）Arrangement：The doctor takes 6# injected needle pin to inject 2 ～ 4ml analgesics，alter drawing back no-blood and no-urine，separately into points of HuiYin and ChangQiang 1.5 ～ 3cm from 45° angle.

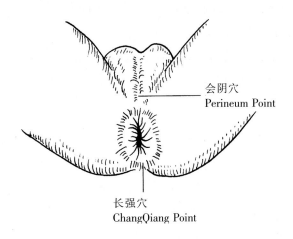

会阴穴
Perineum Point

长强穴
ChangQiang Point

图 11 – 2　长效止痛剂穴位注射

Figure 11 – 2　Acupuncture points injection with long effect analgesics

4. **效果**　会阴、长强两穴具有通络行气活血的作用，再加上长效止痛药的穴封，不但起到针灸的止痛作用，又有药理长效止痛的双重作用。不但止痛效果好，而且缓解了肛门括约肌痉挛，可治疗因膀胱会阴尿道内括约肌的痉挛并发的尿潴留。但应注意，会阴穴勿过深以免损伤尿道。

4. **Effect**　The points of HuiYin and ChangQiang take the part in dredging channels of acupuncture points，with the effect of invigorating vitality （Qi）and activating blood circulation meanwhile long effect analgesics cause the reaction of local anesthesia，so that acupuncture point injection with long effect analgesics own double effects for stopping pain. They not only stop pain，but also release spasm of sphincter so they can treat urinary retention resulting from spasm of internal sphincter of bladder，perineum and urinary tract. But it should be taken care that the point of HuiYin can't be injected too deep lest injuring the urinary tract.

五、肛门坠胀

V. The Feeling of Anal Falling and Distension

肛门手术后机械或炎症刺激,可引起肛门内坠胀不适感或胀满感,称坠胀。

The feeling of anal falling and distension results from the postoperative stimulation of machine and inflammation.

【病因】

[Etiology]

1.**机械刺激**　内痔结扎、直肠黏膜结扎、肛门瘘挂线等刺激均可以出现肛门坠胀感。

1. **Machinery Stimulation**　The feeling of anal falling and distension is due to ligation and seton, such as ligation of internal hemorrhoids and rectal mucosa, etc.

2.**换药刺激**　伤口换药、填塞、纱条引起坠胀。

2. **Changing Gauzes**　Covering and draining for wound cause the feeling of anal falling and distension.

3.**炎症刺激**　术后伤口充血、水肿、炎症刺激出现坠胀。内痔手术后因排便,内脱或外脱嵌顿引起坠胀。

3. **Inflammation**　Postoperative hyperemia, edema and infection stimulate to cause the feeling of anal falling and distension. .

【临床表现】

[Clinical Manifestations]

术后感觉肛门下坠、不适感或胀满感,往往引起便意或排便次数增多,也有欲便不解或是里急后重感,重者频频入厕,但便后坠胀感并不缓解,十分痛苦。

The postoperative feeling of anal falling and distension usually induces the sense of defecation and frequent defecation, feeling defecation but not to put feces out, uncompleted exhausted defecation and tenesmus. The patient feels very salary.

【治疗】

[Treatment]

1.**解除刺激病因**　消炎、消肿、治疗或重新换药。

1. **Relieving Stimulation Causes**　To remove inflammation and edema.

2. **药物治疗**　口服中药秦艽苍术丸。外洗药、祛毒汤、坐浴、肛门内注入九华膏中药。

2. **Medicine Treatment**　To take pill of QinJiuCangZhuWang, tub bath with herbs, and squeezing cream into anus.

3. **针灸封闭**　取气衡、长强、承山穴位。

3. **Acupuncture**　To puncture points QiHeng, ChangQiang, ChengShan.

4. **其他**　如合并肠炎应及时治疗。

4. **Others**　In case of complicated with enteritis, it should be treated in time.

六、肛肠术后尿潴留
VI. Postoperative Urinary Retention

尿潴留是肛肠术后常见并发症,以膀胱充盈,但排尿不行或不能排出为特征。确切机制尚不明确,但各种迹象表明,肛肠术后尿潴留与麻醉引起膀胱张力敏感性下降,或膀胱颈挛缩及尿道括约肌的痉挛有关。

The urinary retention is a frequent complication following anorectal operations. The urinary bladder is distended very much, but urine can't be put out. The mechanism has something to do with the decreasing sensibility of bladder tension, and with the spasm of bladder neck and sphincter of urinary tract.

【病因】
[Etiology]

(1)肛门局部水肿,压迫尿道。

(1)Local anal edema pressing the urinary tract.

(2)麻醉后膀胱功能失调。

(2)The function of bladder is maladjustment after anesthesia.

(3)有前列腺肥大病史或泌尿系感染。

(3)Existing medical histories of prostate hypertrophy and or urinary systemic infection.

(4)肛肠术后影响尿道或膀胱位置受牵连。

(4)Postoperatively the urinary tract or bladder position is involved.

(5)肛肠术中牵拉或损伤,尿道膀胱神经或因疼痛引起括约肌功能失调。

(5)In operation the nerves of the urinary tract or bladder are involved to cause malfunction of sphincter. The pain can also cause malfunction of sphincter.

（6）局部感染累及尿道。

（6）Local infection involved the urinary tract.

（7）填塞纱布过多压迫尿道。

（7）Too much gauzes covered wound pressing the urinary tract.

（8）年迈体弱膀胱无力。

（8）The weak and old person with deficiency of pressure in passing urine.

（9）精神过度紧张或肛肠术后伤口疼痛波及影响尿道或不习惯床上排尿。

（9）Nervousness very much or postoperative pain of wound involves passing urine.

【治疗】

[Treatment]

1. **针灸**　穴位：右侧足三里、三阴交、阴陵泉穴，进针深 1.5~2 寸，中强刺激，得气后留针 30 分钟，每 5 分钟行针 1 次。

1. **Acupuncture**　To puncture into points of right ZuSanLi, SanYinJiao, YinLingQuan, 1.5 ~2cm a unit of length（ = 1/3 decimetre）, middle strong stimulation, keeping acupuncture in the points 30 minutes after having effect of Qi, repeated puncturing once in every 5 minutes.

2. **穴位封闭**　关元、水道、气海、足三里穴位注射新斯的明封闭。

2. **Point Injection**　To inject neostigmine into acupuncture points, such as GuanYuan, ShuiDao, ZuSanLi.

3. **口服中药**　利尿汤：木通 30g，车前子 30g，通草 15g，黄连 20g，黄柏 20g。

3. **Taking Herbs**　Decoction of LiNiaoTang（helpful to pass urine）：Fiveleaf akebia 30g, Semen plantaginis 30g, Tetrapanacis medulla 15g, Rhizoma coptidis 20g.

4. **口服西药**　如硝苯地平片。

4. **Taking Western Medicine**　Nifedipine.

5. **导尿**　伴男性前列腺肥大者保留尿管。

5. **Urethral Catheterization**　Retention of catheter in case of prostate hypertrophy.

七、内痔术后出血

VII. Postoperative Hemorrhage of Hemorrhoidectomy

对早期内痔采用注射疗法，对较重的后期内痔或混合痔、脱肛，采用内痔结扎法,或贯穿缝扎法。并发手术后出血占 1% ~2% 。

Reappearance of bleeding following a hemorrhoidectomy is related to inadequate removal of redundant rectal mucosa or hemorrhoidal tissue. Postoperative bleeding occurred in 1% ~2% .

【病因】
[Etiology]

1. 感染
1. Infection

(1)内痔注射局部感染,导致痔蒂内动脉壁软化、分解、破裂出血,或引起肌层组织坏死脱落,血栓形成缓慢而出血。

(1)Injection therapy is easy to cause local infection, for hemorrhoidal arterial walls being softened, broken down and bleed; and easy to falling off from necrotic basic tissue.

(2)结扎的内痔脱掉后继发创面感染引起渗血。

(2)Secondary wound infection after internal hemorrhoids falling down induces bleeding.

2. 缝扎不适合
2. Unsuitable Ligation

(1)结扎不牢或仅结扎痔核下部,没有结扎在痔衬垫痔核的基底部。

(1)Untight or loose ligation.

(2)内痔缝合针贯穿过深,直接伤及痔上动脉。当痔核坏死脱落时,致深部创面血管出血。

(2)Too deep suture injuring anterior hemorrhoidal artery. The deep wound is easy to bleed as necrotic hemorrhoids falling.

(3)痔核过大,根部面积过大,单纯大块的一次结扎致痔核脱掉后引起创面过大引起出血。

(3)Too big hemorrhoid with wide base is tied only one time, the large wound area is easy to bleed after hemorrhoid falling down.

(4)花冠痔:结扎每个痔核后的间隙过小、过密,导致痔核脱掉后创面扩大而洛血。

(4)Crown style hemorrhoid: The space between tied hemorrhoids is too small and thick, wound area is easy to enlarge and bleed after hemorrhoid falling down.

(5)内痔缝合针贯穿过浅或血管钳钳夹痔核过浅或没钳夹于痔核的基底部伤及血管,痔核脱掉后引起出血。

(5) Too shallow suture by needle, or jaw by vessel forceps, the wound is easy to bleed after hemorrhoid falling down.

（6）结扎痔核后，剪除结扎线以上的痔核，组织过多，以致线滑脱引起出血。

(6) The doctor cuts more tied hemorrhoidal tissue below ligature thread so that ligature surged to bleed.

3. 大便干燥，排便过于用力　使痔核过早、过快脱掉，因坏死的痔核中血管闭锁不牢，凝血不牢而出血。

3. Dry Stool with Powerful Defecation　The tied hemorrhoid falls off sooner than do usually.

【治疗】

[Treatment]

1. 非手术治疗

1. Nonoperative Treatment

（1）轻度渗血：凡士林纱布条蘸痔瘘粉压迫即可。也可用 1% 明矾水 20ml，保留灌肠，以收敛出血，或 5%～10% 明矾水 50ml 保留直肠灌肠；或消痔灵 10ml，肛内注入保留肛管，直腔内。

(1) Slight oozing of blood: The gauzes press to cover the wound, or enema with pressure.

（2）中度出血：①用消痔灵，创面封闭注射，再于痔上动脉区封闭。②用橡胶肛管外包裹痔瘘粉插入肛门直肠腔中；注意要超过齿线以压迫创面。将橡胶肛管引出肛外，接盐水瓶，观察直肠腔有无再出血。③口服中药：凉血地黄汤＋黑地榆＋黑槐花＋紫珠草，水煎口服。④静脉输入止血定、安络血等。

(2) Middle bleeding: Local pressure, enema and taking medicine.

2. 重度出血安全套气囊治疗

2. Severe Bleeding

（1）安全套气囊疗法

(1) Ballonet

①安全套气囊制作：用 50ml 注射器将连接的粗针头插入细硬塑料管中，此后置入安全套中，将套口用丝线结扎紧。

①The making of ballonet: Inserting thick needle head of 50 ml syringe into thin and hard plastic pipe, to insert the plastic pipe into the ballonet, and then finally to tie the opening of ballonet tightly with silk thread.

②肛指检查并除去积血,将安全套气囊送入肛门,通过直肠环,放入直肠腔内。用 50ml 注射器吸人 150～250ml 空气并推入,使安全套气囊加大,然后用火柴将塑料管烧断封堵即可(图 11 - 3)。

②To take anal digital examination and put out hematocele, inserting the ballonet into rectum through anus and through rectal ring. The 50 ml syringe draws in air to insert into the ballonet, 150～250ml air enlarges the ballonet (Fig. 11 - 3).

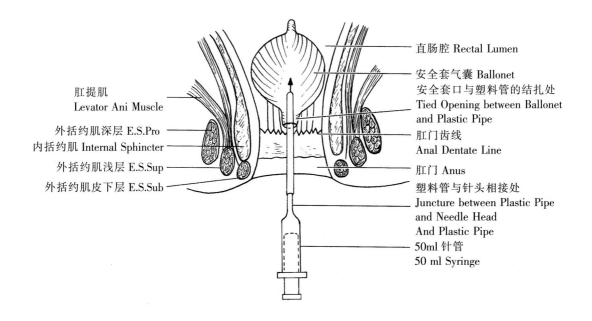

图 11 - 3　安全套气止血疗法

Figure 11 - 3　Stopping bleeding with ballonet

(2)手术治疗:结扎出血创面和痔上动脉手术关键是了解影响寻找出血点的因素,掌握寻找方法。

(2)Operation:Direct suture of the bleeder is the treatment of choice to control postoperative hemorrhage. Thus, any patient who begins to bleed postoperatively and doesn't respond to bed rest should be taken to the operating room to ligate the wound of bleeding and artery of anterior hemorrhoid. The key is to understand influential factors about looking for bleeding point and how to find out bleeding point.

①影响寻找出血点因素:a. 对肛肠术后、病情、手术方法应了解。不可慌张,不可盲目找出血点,应有的放矢,要心中有数,按步进行寻找。b. 正常肛管直径为 3cm,麻醉下扩张至 4.5cm。因管腔狭窄,影响视野,因此,光源要充足。c. 用肛门镜易刺激肛门括约肌,引起括约肌痉挛,反而压迫出血点而不易找到。有的肛门镜直接压迫出血点而不能发现出血点。d. 直肠腔内瘀血没清净时,出血点也不易

找到。

①Influential factors about looking for bleeding point:a. To understand the method of operation and postoperative recovering. Don't worry to look for aimlessly. b. The normal diameter of anal canal is 3cm, under anesthesia, it may be enlarged to 4.5 cm at the time the light must be abundant, c. The anoscope isn't suitable, it may stimulate sphincter spasm to looking for bleeding point meanwhile it may cover, the bleeding point to affect stopping bleeding, d. The bleeding point is not easy to find when the gore in rectum has not been put out cleanly.

②寻找出血点的方法:a. 麻醉要使肛管充分松弛。术前注入地西泮,消除紧张,利于术中配合;开通静脉输液,以利调正血压及血循环,以利显露出血点;用两叶肛门镜或电池灯圆头缺口肛门镜,先清除积血,并用纱布块堵塞直肠上腔,控制污物下流,使创面充分显露。b. 参照手术记录,从左至右,从上至下,依次对手术部位及创面逐一寻找出血点,重点是母痔区。c. 全面了解手术部位后,先从截石位12点钟位查起,从上至下观察内痔结扎线是否脱落,外痔延伸的切口有无渗血,缝合部位是否对合,有无出血。如结扎线已脱落,创面有无出血;是否还有残存的痔块。如没发现明显的出血点,应行全层贯穿缝合于痔块,使以前的结扎线在痔基底部。因组织脆弱,勿钳夹。也可于痔核块上敷止血海绵一块,并一同线扎。d. 由于麻醉或肛镜压迫,当发现创面只是渗血或充血,无明显出血点时,渗血点就是出血点。因出血的血管断端全部封闭,直视下未见出血,也不见渗血点创面上的充血点也应按出血点缝扎止血处理。e. 用肛镜观察创面,如无出血点、无渗血点或充血点,只寻见瘀血点,也应按出血点处理。全层缝合,深达肌肉层。f. 如查找不到出血点、渗血点、充血点和瘀血点时,观察到创面坏死组织、水肿糜烂或创面张裂,也应按出血点缝扎。如发现创面组织表面生长良好,伤口已修复,则应按新老创面的颜色、光泽进行比较,对已愈合与刚愈合的创面进行比较,尤其对创面黏膜鲜红而嫩的创面也应按出血点进行处理。g. 如按上述方法仍没找到出血点,出血已停止,也不可以结束检查。此时应取出肛门镜。输液中升血压观察30分钟后再次插入肛门镜查寻,如肛门镜下仍未发现出血点,但直肠上端有鲜血或血块流出,应改换纤维结肠镜检查,以了解直肠上部或乙状结肠其他病变有无诱发的出血点,例如溃疡、血管瘤、肿瘤等出血病灶。

②The method of looking for bleeding point:a. With proper anesthesia which makes anal canal being relaxed enough, the site of bleeding can be demonstrated and sutured, with evacuation of clots, and suture of the bleeding point. Keeping the venous drop to regulate blood circulation and to maintain blood pressure for showing the bleeding point; in bilobed anoscope or round head with notch mouth optic anoscope, the first putting out hematocele, then put gauzes to obstruct anterior rectum lumen to control excretion dripping down, to show wound. b. Looking for bleeding point from left to right, from upper to below. c. To observe whether the ligature thread node falls down, vestigital-hemorrhoid exists. The doctor should suture through the base even if the bleeding point has not been found out. Don't jaw because of frail tissue. May cover a Helistat on the wound then suture altogether, d. The oozing of blood should also be sutured while the bleeding point hasn't been found out. e. The point of gore should also be sutured while the point of bleeding, oozing and hyperemia haven't been found out under observing with anoscopy. f. The tissue with necrosis, edema, erosion should also be sutured while the point of bleeding, oozing, hyperemia and gore haven't been found out. The red fresh tender mucous wound should also be sutured while the wound tissue has healed. g. If the bleeding point still cannot be found according to the above method, don't stop examination easily. The doctor should continue to observe during transfusion, put out the anoscope to wait for 30 minutes, then insert the anoscope into anus again, if he finds out the fresh blood or blood clot draining from upper part of rectum he should take fiberoptic colonoscope examination instead of anoscopy to understand the damage in upper part of rectum and sigmoid colon, such as ulcer, hemangioma and tumor, etc.

E. S. Pro: Profundus Muscle of External Sphincter.

E. S. Sup: Superficial Muscle of External Sphincter.

E. S. Sub: Subcutaneous Muscle of External Sphincter.

（3）手术方法:腰俞麻醉。在两叶肛门镜下观察,先清除积血,寻找出血病灶。首先将痔创面上方的痔动脉用丝线贯穿缝扎一针。痔创面小的病灶,可用消痔灵于基底部封闭注射,大的痔创面有明显出血点时,置上海绵块用细肠线全层贯穿缝合。肛管留置,外裹中药痔瘘粉、云南白药。插入直肠腔内肛管引出肛门外,止血完成或再压迫止血。

（3）Operation therapy: Lumber anesthesia, in bilobed anoscope or round head with notch mouth optic anoscope, first putting out hematocele, then looking bleeding point. The doctor should suture a silk thread through the base above wound in which is similar to the position of upper hemorrhoidal artery, or cover a Helistat on the wound then suture altogether, then press gauzes on the wound.

【预防措施】

[Prevention]

1. 感染

1. Infection

（1）内痔注射后,应用苯扎溴铵棉球压堵注射针孔,24 小时后再排大便,口服甲硝唑(厌氧的细菌)。

（1）Strict sterilizing around operational course, taking metronidazole (anti-anaerobe), the best time of defecation is 24 hours.

（2）结扎内痔术后,肛门挤入中药九华膏或痔瘘粉。

（2）Strict hemostasis.

2. 注意缝扎技术

2. Ligature Techniques

（1）内痔结扎必须将痔核全部在基底部结扎牢。痔核基底部酌情注射消痔灵封闭。

（1）Suture must be in the base of internal hemorrhoid tightly and firmly.

（2）结扎的内痔不宜超过齿线上 1.5cm. 以免将痔上动脉也结扎在内。痔上动脉周围酌情注射消痔灵封闭。

（2）Ligated internal hemorrhoids should not beyond 1.5 cm above dentate line lest ligating the upper hemorrhoidal artery. The upper hemorrhoidal artery should be ligated separately.

（3）对多发痔或花冠痔,不要集团结扎,要逐个结扎;对较大痔核,可以分段单独结扎,以防痔核脱掉后创面过大。结扎痔蒂注入消痔灵。

（3）Multiple hemorrhoids or crown hemorrhoids can't be ligated together, should be ligated one by one. Large hemorrhoids should be ligated only singly in order to prevent a too large wound showing as hemorrhoid failing off.

（4）每个痔核之间留有黏膜桥（0.3~0.5cm）,防止痔核被结扎后间隙小,掉线后溶成大的创面而渗血。

（4）Leaving mucous bridge （0.3~0.5cm）between hemorrhoids in order to prevent a too large wound bleeding as hemorrhoids falling off.

（5）对较大的痔核,要单个痔核上先用手指触及按到痔上动脉搏动后,再在痔动脉下贯穿缝扎或配合消痔灵注射封闭。

（5）Large hemorrhoids should be ligated separately and gradually till or near the mucous roots, then sutured through inferior-hemorrhoidal artery.

3. 小针刀切断内括约肌,降低肛管内压力

因内痔形成与肛管内压力升高有关,尤其是肛管静息压增高,导致痔衬垫充血,痔核堵塞肛管出口,使排便时压力大增,造成排便费力,阻力加大,易引起痔术后出血。肛管内压力增加与内括约痉挛有关,也是导致被结扎痔核血管压力升高的原因。一旦结扎线脱掉,创面容易继发出血。因此,应用小针刀将痉挛的内括约肌切断,以降低肛管内压力。

3. Acupuncture Scalpel Cuts Internal Sphincter to Decrease the Inner Pressure of Anal Canal The formation of internal hemorrhoid is related to increasing inner pressure of anal canal, especially high resting pressure of anal canal to cause either hyperemia of hemorrhoidal cushion, or hemorrhoidal obstruction at the outlet of anal canal, so that during defecation the pressure and resistance increase highly, the energy wasting much, leading to postoperative bleeding. The increase pressure in anal canal one hand is related to the spasm of internal sphincter, the other hand is the reason of pressure increase of ligated vessels. Once the ligated thread falls off, the wound will be easy to bleed secondarily. Therefore the doctor carries on acupuncture scalpel to cut internal sphincter and to decrease the inner pressure of anal canal.

八、肛门直肠瘘术后复发
VIII. Postoperative Recurrence of Anorectal Fistulas

肛门直肠瘘是由于肛门直肠脓肿破溃而形成的。手术治疗后复发多为高位、低位的复杂肛瘘。

The fistula originates in an abscess, most patients present with previous history of anorectal abscess associated with intermittent drainage. Postoperative recurrence mainly results from completed high positional and low positional fistulas.

【病因】

1. 术前误诊　肛瘘虽然是局部病变,但与全身疾病有关系,故不能忽视全身情况。如伴有肺结核,应考虑是否为结核性肛瘘;如骶尾部囊肿或畸胎瘤,有破溃史引起的肛门直肠瘘;如肛门直肠癌引起肛瘘,以及直肠阴道瘘、会阴尿道瘘等误诊为肛门直肠瘘,治疗时只是按一般肛瘘手术或方法处理。

1. **Preoperative Misdiagnosis**　Anal fistula is related to systemic diseases, although it is a local damage, so we should not ignore the body state. For instance, accompanying with pulmonary tuberculosis, the anal fistula may be tubercular anal fistula; a cyst or teratoma in sacrococcygeal region may break up to form anorectal fistula; anorectal cancer may induce anal fistula; others may also be misdiagnosed to be anal fistulas, such as recto-vaginal fistula, perineal-urethral fistula, etc.

2. 术前分类不清　因术前未对肛瘘进行正确的分类,未确定瘘管的深度,内外口的部位与数量,以及病变范围与肛门直肠环的关系,如盲目手术可造成手术失败,因为未将瘘管全部切开或遗留瘘管。

2. **Preoperative Unclear Stages**　Anal fistulas haven't been divided stages exactly in preoperative period. Local damages are indistinct, such as fistulous depth, position and number of internal and external openings, extent and relationship with anaorectal ring. If the operation is performed aimlessly, it will be defeated, because the fistulous tracks are vestigital, they are not cut completely.

3. 未找到真正内口　肛瘘内口是肛瘘发生的主要病灶。手术中应准确找到内口的数量、部位,要防止因探查造成假道或假内口而致手术失败。如果未找到可信的内口而盲目手术,虽然肛瘘切开暂时会愈合,但肛瘘感染没有去除,仍难免复发。正确判定内口的位置是手术成败的关键,因此,寻找内口首先应仔细探查瘘管走行。除触诊外,应循瘘管弯曲度轻柔地探查,勿用力过猛。探针需多次弯成顺瘘管走行,探针能无阻力通过。肛指检查内口往往呈凹陷的硬结,这可能是内口部位,但探针往往需往上往前稍深入些,即从内口窝的顶上后端探出,勿在内口的中部或下部探出,以防遗留内口窝上部的死腔隙而复发。术前用肛门镜检查内口,可发现、了解齿线附近肛窦及其邻近区组织有无充血、水肿、隆突、起凹、陷窝、糜烂及溢脓的孔隙,配合肛瘘外口探针进入瘘管中,顺其弯度检查清楚。尤其是复杂肛瘘管道往往纵横交错,支管丛生,因此边探边切开前管壁,使探针顺肛瘘的后壁弯曲走行自然探查,较易找到真正内口。有时需用多根探针分别通过多个瘘管才能找到共同的内口。有的内口通向肛内,或为多发内口,或仅一个内口而为多发外口。因此探查弯曲瘘管须分别切开弯曲的肛瘘前管壁,才使探针顺利探行,不存留残余、盲端或腔隙。对敞切开的肛瘘支管壁仍需用刮匙、小针刀搔刮,发现有发黑的坏死点均要用探针再次探查,以防遗留下层支瘘管。对通过顺利的内口,也要将内口周围或感染的肛隐窝、肛门腺剪开、敞开瘘管,充分扩创、搔刮。切开、清除炎性腐败组织,以防遗留死腔。

3. **Exact Internal Opening not Found Out**　The principles of fistulotomy include unroofing all fistulas, eliminating the primary opening of infective source, and establishing adequate drainage. The tracks are unroofed from the primary source at the dentate line through the secondary opening or openings by excising all overlying tissue, including sphincter. Failure to unroof the entire track and divide the necessary amount of sphincter may lead to recurrence. The wound is allowed to heal by secondary intention. Fistulectomy in the excision of the entire fistulous track is rarely necessary. Occasionally, a patient may present with an acute perianal abscess associated with an obvious anal fistula. Incision and drainage of abscess and primary fistulotomy are indicated. If the fistula is high in relation to the anorectal ring, a two-stage procedure may be indicated. In the first stage, a seton of heavy black silk or a rubber band is placed loosely around the sphincter muscle as a marker. It stimulates fibrosis adjacent to the sphincter muscle so that when the second stage, which involves laying open the intersphincteric portion of the fistulous track, is completed, the sphincter will not gape. Bidigital palpation for locating the indurated fistulous track, using the index finger and thumb, delineates the indurated track to the primary opening. Probing the track from the external opening is successful, but care must be taken to avoid creating an artificial opening and seeding infected material into clean tissue, thus risking iatrogenic extensions above or beyond the original fistula. Latrogenic track created by injudicious probing of an anal fistula is easy to be misunderstood as internal opening. Probing fistulous tracks must cut their anterior walls respectively so that the probe can go freely, there would not be remaining spaces. Unroofed fistulous branches need still

take scoraping by curette and acupuncture scalpel. When doctor finds out a black necrotic point, he should check it up with probe lest remaining branch below layer. Although the internal opening probes freely, the doctor should also cut infective anal crypt and gland around the internal opening.

4. 瘘管清除不彻底　肛瘘支瘘管或窦道清除不彻底,尤其是复杂肛瘘,管道多弯曲,且伴有支瘘或死腔,一旦遗留必将会复发。因此,术中用多个探针均需一一切开,搔刮,利于通畅引流。不宜过多切除管壁,损伤肛管,以防术后肛门溢液,延长愈合时间。

4. Fistulous Tracks Haven't Been Eliminated Completely　The anal fistulous tracks or branches haven't been eliminated completely, especially complicated anal fistulas have curving tracks, branches and necrotic cavity, once they remain, then recurrence would be the case. So several probes need to be carried on in operation to cut and take scoraping one by one for free drainage. The wall of anal canal should be taken care lest rectal liquid going out postoperatively so as to prolong healing.

5. 肛瘘挂线位置不对　没有弄清内口位置与肛瘘走向的关系即挂线,使挂线不在内口的顶端或瘘管的上端,以致未真正切割开内口及肛瘘,造成病灶清除不彻底,引流不充分。

5. Use of Seton in Mistaken Position　Normally as use of seton in high fistula, the probe is in the fistulous track, and then a seton or suture is inserted into the fistulous track, the probe is put out, a seton or suture is tied loosely over the sphincter to create fibrosis. The fistulous track will be laid open in the second stage 6 ~ 8 weeks later. If the probe didn't find out clear internal opening, a seton has to be carried on, the seton is not in the top of internal opening or above fistulous track so as to cut them mistakenly. The fistula would still be there.

6. 引流不畅　虽然诊断明确,手术操作严谨,内口寻找正确,但忽视术后创口处理,如上皮组织内翻、内陷,造成对边粘连假愈合,也可引起肛瘘复发。因肛门直肠周围肌肉纵横交错,解剖复杂,术后创面清洁不彻底,引流不通畅。肉芽组织只有平行生长才能被上皮覆盖,过低或过高,如没有处理,上皮组织不能顺利生长也影响愈合。因此,换药时要剪修过高的肉芽组织,或引流低凹的肉芽伤口,使肉芽组织从伤口最底部往上生长,当肉芽组织与两边的皮肤平行时,两边的上皮组织才会生长,覆盖其上而愈合。术中要仔细检查瘘管与肛门直肠环和括约肌的关系,决定一期或二期手术,或是否用挂线疗法。特别注意不能切断肛管直肠环或耻骨直肠肌,以免发生肛门失禁。术后保持伤口引流,中药换药处理。伤口每隔数日须做直肠指检,扩张肛管,避免形成瘢痕性狭窄。

6. Little Free Drainage　Normally the probe is in the fistulous track, and then unroofing of the fistulous track over the probe must be done. Although the diagnosis is clear, operation is precise, and the internal opening is found out clearly, if postoperative wound is ignored to carry on then recurrence may occur, for instance epithelial tissue turns and sinks inwards to form pseudo-healing of side to side adhesion so as to cause recurrence. Granulation tissues need to be covered by skin only relying on their fiat growth, over high or low growth cause that the epithelial tissue can't crawl smoothly to influence healing. If the wound hasn't been carried on correctly the doctor should prune very high granulation tissues at the same time drain too low ones for making granulation tissues grow from the bottom in every dressing change. In operation the doctor should probe carefully the relationship between fistulous track and anorectal ring and sphincter to define performing the operation. Don't cut off anorectal ring or puborectal muscle lest anal incontinence would take place, so we must take care of these especially in the operation. Postoperatively the wound should keep drain smoothly and dressing change regularly, anal digital examination and enlarging for avoiding scarred stricture.

7. **正确处理内口及原发病灶**　肛腺感染是肛瘘形成的主要原因,因此,正确处理内口,彻底清除感染肛窦、肛门腺及其导管,是手术成败及防止复发的关键。借助钩针、小弯刀,必要时借助肛镜、指诊、染色和造影等,均可正确地寻找肛瘘内口。切开内口后,充分扩创、搔刮周围坏死组织,彻底清除感染的肛隐窝、肛门导管和肛门腺;彻底清除支管和死腔窦道内的感染物质,保证创口引流通畅和清洁。术后创口和支瘘管内滞留粪便等感染物质,如引流不畅,可剪开创口、支瘘管愈合延迟。在支瘘管或窦腔内挂人橡皮筋,应使橡皮筋松弛,才可持续发挥引流作用,使支管及窦腔彻底引流。换药时牵拉转动橡皮筋,并用过氧化氢液冲洗,促使创面及支管内清洁。主瘘管挂线须扎紧。伤口对拢粘连需全部剖开管道,应视病情而定。引流线不需扎紧,拆除时间视病情而定,一般当主瘘管伤口闭合可予拆除支瘘管引流线。

7. **Correct Management on Internal Opening and Primary Damage**　Anal fistula results mainly from infection of anal grands so that the keys of successful operation and preventing recurrence are to carry on internal opening correctly and eliminate anal crypt, gland and tract. When the doctor looks for the internal opening difficultly, he can get help from follows as small hook style head acupuncture, small curving probing scalpel, anoscope, digital, color and photography, etc.. After cutting off internal opening, to enlarge the wound enough, scoraping necrotic tissues around the wound, to eliminate infective anal crypt, tract and gland completely, to clear infective matters in branch, fistulous tracks and necrotic cavity, to keep free drainage and clean wound, otherwise prolonging the healing time. Hanging a rubber seton in branch or cavity to keep it loosely for developing its drainage reaction and making completed drainage from branch and fistulous cavity. To draw round rubber loop and wash with peroxide liquid as dressing change for improving clean in the wound. To put out the rubber seton according to state.

【治疗】

[Treatment]

综合上述 7 条,肛门直肠瘘术后复发虽然由多种因素引起,但只要术前正确诊断,术中按不同类型瘘管选择合适的手术,找到真正内口,敞开所有肛瘘管,注意术后换药,做到引流通畅,修整伤口,术后肛瘘复发是可以避免的。

In general above all, although postoperative recurrence of anorectal fistula results of several factors, only by relying on preoperative correct diagnosis, suitable choice of operation according to different kinds of anal fistulas, finding out true internal opening, roofing all fistulous tracks, to take care of dressing change postoperatively, free drainage, pruning wound, so to avoid postoperative recurrence.

九、术后肛缘水肿

IX. Postoperative Edema of Anal Fringe

【病因】

[Etiology]

1. **混合痔**　只治疗内痔或外痔,不是内外痔及时综合治疗。

1. **Mixed Hemorrhoids**　Only internal or external hemorrhoid is treated, but internal and external hemorrhoid is not given comprehensive treatment in time.

2. **内痔或直肠黏膜,结扎或套扎**　治疗后,因排粪便,被结扎的内痔或直肠黏膜组织外脱。

2. **Tied or Loop Ligated Internal Hemorrhoids or Rectal Mucosa**　Defecation causes mucosa prolapse

3. **嵌顿痔**　治疗后没再做肛缘减压术。

3. **Incarcerated Hemorrhoids**

4. **肛门手术牵拉、钳夹**　可损伤肛门缘皮肤。

4. **Traction and Jaw by Vessel Forceps in Anal Operation**　To injure the skin of anal fringe

5. **其他**

5. **Others**

(1)单纯结扎外痔,肛缘血液循环障碍。

(1) To ligate external hemorrhoids simply and singly to cause blood circulation obstruction in anal fringe.

（2）内痔注射或套扎内痔接近齿线以下。

（2）Injection or loop ligaturing of internal hemorrhoid below dentate line.

（3）肛门手术皮下止血不彻底，产生皮下血肿渗血。

（3）Uncompleted subcutaneous stanching in anal operation cause oozing of blood and hematoma in subcutaneous tissue.

（4）肛门病治疗后久蹲不起，排便用力过猛，使腹压、直肠腔内压升高，肛缘血流受阻。

（4）Mistaken position and power in defecation makes the pressure of abdomen and inner rectum increase to obstruct blood flowing in anal fringe.

【临床表现】

[Clinical Manifestations]

术后肛缘水肿，引起肛门疼痛、下坠、胀满感，排粪便受阻。

Postoperative edema of anal fringe induces anal pain, sense of falling and distension and difficult defecation.

【治疗】

[Treatment]

（1）口服中药通便，如润肠汤。

（1）To take herbs of moving intestine, decoction of YunChangTang.

（2）排粪便后，中药祛毒汤坐浴。

（2）Hip bath with herbs of XiaoDuTang (eliminate toxin)after defecation.

（3）外敷中药外痔贴。

（3）Cream covers wound.

（4）肛缘血肿、水肿，应用钩状小针刀治疗（见第 6 章第一节外痔局部治疗小针刀针孔法）。

（4）Carrying on acupuncture scalpel to treat edema and hematoma around anal fringe（see Chapter 6，§1 local treatment of external hemorrhoids with acupuncture scalpel point hole method）.

第 12 章　肛肠疾病伤口的治疗

Chapter 12　The Treatment of Wound in Coloproctology

第一节　肛肠术后换药

§ 1　Postoperative Dressing Change

1. 术后第 1 次换药　患者排便与否均要进行伤口检查和换药,以了解、处理、治疗术后伤口。例如,创面敷料血染程度,肛门缘水肿病灶脱出与否,切口皮瓣长合情况,长效麻药注射后组织情况等。对排便困难者口服液状石蜡 20～30ml,每晚饮用;排尿困难者可配合针灸治疗。伤口痛给 0.5% 丁卡因喷洒伤口;伤口渗血,便后滴血者可用痔瘘粉生皮膏纱布条用探针捅进肛门内与肛外伤口。换药时药纱布条要拉齐,理顺引出伤口外,勿扭曲或堵塞伤口,使中药纱布条起引流作用,发挥药效。肛门外水肿,包括脱出痔、脱出肛管,均可用中药熏洗后外敷中药外痔贴;肛门内一般挤入九华膏,可慢慢消肿恢复。

1. The First Postoperative Dressing Change　After undergoing operation, the patient needs to be changed dressing so that the doctor can look up if there is bleeding, infection, secretion of pus. The doctor should look for the state of wound, for example, the degree of bleeding on the gauze, edema in anal wound, skin of incision fringe, and the healing of wound. The patient with difficult defecation should take Whiteruss 20～30ml every night, combining with acupuncture to treat difficult urination. Use 0.5% Dincaine to spray the wound for pain; gauzes are inserted into anus and covered on outside as oozing of blood from the wound and dripping of blood after defecation. The gauzes should cover the wound regularly to facilitate drainage. The edema being outside of anus and hemorrhoids projecting outside of anal canal one can fume and wash with herbs, and can squeeze the cream into the anus for eliminating edema and improving recovery.

2. 内痔注射后换药　了解有无发热,如有黄疸应排除门静脉炎。排便后有无出血并观察痔核坏死脱落情况。适当给予止血药,如维生素 K、止血定。如便后有血块,给予生皮膏痔瘘粉纱布,用探针捅入到肛管内伤口处,可起到消炎、止血作用。

2. **Dressing Change After Injecting Internal Hemorrhoids**　To understand whether there is a fever. If the patient has jaundice, pylephlebitis should be differentiated. To look up whether there is bleeding after defecation and falling as hemorrhoidal necrosis. To give suitable stancher and adjuvant for preventing bleeding. In case of bleeding after defecation, to insert gauzes into anus by probe. In general, the aim is to eliminate inflammation and stop bleeding.

3. **肛周脓肿及肛瘘术后**　观察伤口引流是否通畅及肉芽生长情况,防止伤口两边缘粘连。肉芽过高应剪平。内陷纱布药条应置于伤口底部,超过上端伤口,往下引流超过下端伤口。生长肉芽可用中药生肌长皮膏纱布条平贴换药。肛周脓肿用消脓膏纱布引流换药,纱布条不可太紧、太严或过松,以平敞引流为适合。对挂线伤口,应于挂线的上前侧置 1 条,挂线伤口后下再置 1 条,将两条纱布条均引出、置平,并引出肛门外。

3. **Postoperative Dressing Change of Perianal Abscesses and Anal Fistulae**　To look for whether there is free drainage and granulation tissue growth and to prevent from adhesion of two sides of the wound. If the granulation is too high, it should be cut down. The gauzes are inserted deep to the upper wound and downward over the lower wound. Gauzes with herbal paste "Sheng-zhang Xiangpi Gao" can be used for granulation tissue. Gauzes with "Xiao Nong Gao" can be used for perianal abscess. For wounds with seton on probe, two gauzes should be put, one at the anterior upper part and the other at the posterior lower part of the seton, and both should be drained out of the anus.

4. **结核性伤口换药**　如伤口肉芽生长缓慢,引流物稀如米汤样,边缘高,中间凹陷,不规则,应考虑结核感染。可用抗结核药链霉素、雷米封治疗和换药,中药消脓膏、外痔贴效果较佳。

4. **Dressing Change for Tuberculosis Wound**　In case of slow granulation and porridge-like drainage in an irregular wound with a higher ridge and a deep center, tuberculosis infection should be diagnosed. Treatments with anti-TB drugs such as streptomycin and Rimifon, herbal paste "Xiao Nong Gao" or "Wai Zhi Tie" are preferable.

5. **尖锐湿疣换药**　应考虑抗感染、抗病毒,可用青霉素 80 万 U 肌内注射,口服病毒灵。局部可用氟尿嘧啶浸纱布条外敷创面,不要用膏剂油剂,保持伤口清洁干燥。

5. **Condyloma Acuminatum**　Anti-infection and ante-viral drugs should be considered, using Penicillin 800 000 units i. m. and "Bingdu Ling" p. o. Gauzes immersed with Fluril can be used for external application, but not oils and pastes. The wound must be kept clean and dry.

6. **注意肛门外观**　肛门变形,如肛门一侧移位,一侧凹陷,不规则,与手术不完善有关。如只注意治疗病灶,不重视肛门变形,可影响排便功能。因此,换药时应尽量矫正,如伤口一侧用粘膏布进行引拉性皮桥。但不要过早修剪,因为看似没生命的组织,可以起到一定的平衡和牵拉作用,可采取中药换药。可待恢复后,再进行处理。为防治肛门狭窄,在换药过程可扩肛,或配合小针刀治疗。

6. **Outlook of the Arms**　If the anus is deformed with irregular sides after improper surgery, defecation function may be interfered. So the disproportional anus should be regulated during dressing change. Traction with adhesive paste to one side of the anus can be done, but not early repairing by cutting. Extension of the anus can be done during dressing change or treated with acupunc-

ture scalpel.

7. 内扎痔核外脱或肛门水肿外翻 不要立即送回,可用外痔贴中药外敷治疗。因外脱痔送回易过早松动,且排便时仍会外脱,换药即可可以消肿回位。伤口粘连应分开,防止假道、窦道形成。酌情应用过氧化氢,但只限肛外伤口,勿滴入肛内,以利分泌清除。如合并感染的脓肿坏死组织出现窦道、凹陷,应用刮匙小针刀修整,以保证引流通畅。

7. Extrusion of Ligated Internal Hemorrhoid or anal edema The extruded hemorrhoid or anus may not be pushed in immediately, may be treated by herbal external application till the swelling being reduced. The wound adhesion should be separated to prevent from formation of false tracts or fistulae. Hydrogen peroxide can be used only on wounds out of the anus. Complicated necrotic tissue of abscess cavity can be treated with acupuncture scalpel to ensure free drainage.

8. 伤口感染 注意疾病和药剂对切口的影响,降低污染性手术切口与感染率的方法:

8. Wound Infection Methods to decrease incidence of wound infection:

(1)术前酌情用抗生素。

(1)Preoperative application of antibiotics.

(2)切口加垫,伤口平衡。

(2)Cotton pressing on the incision to give balance.

(3)橡皮条双片引流。

(3)Double plates rubber band.

(4)细菌培养和药敏试验后应用抗生素。

(4)Antibiotic application following bacteria culture and drug sensitivity tests.

(5)对污染性手术切口,应冲洗,以降低切口感染率。处理好切口感染的基本问题及术后感染因素,加速感染切口愈合。

(5)Washing infected wounds to accelerate wound healing.

(6)切口表浅感染的处理:如深及浅筋膜以外的皮肤感染或蜂窝织炎,应及早清创、搔刮。

(6)Early treatment for superficial infection by debridement and drainage.

(7)对深筋膜以下的严重切口感染,应及早扩创,如采用小针刀及时行切口引流减压,再用刮匙小针刀清除坏死组织,引流通畅,过氧化氢冲洗。

(7)Early treatment for deep infection by incision and drainage, with evacuation of necrotic tissue by a craping ladle acupuncture scalpel, followed by hydrogen peroxide washing.

（8）对大而浅的创面,如汗腺炎切除术后,应严格无菌操作、器械消毒,防止铜绿假单胞菌再感染,及时清除坏死组织。

（8）Strict aseptic technique is emphasized in resection of hidradenitis to prevent from pseudomonas infection. Prompt removal of necrotic tissue is necessary.

（9）如有窦道形成,应用刮匙小针刀,切口引流,同时清除管壁腐肉或增生的肉芽组织。

（9）Fistula can be treated by incision and drainage with craping ladle acupuncture scalpel.

（10）对少见的特异性感染切口可针对病因处理,扩创、清创要彻底,重视伤口的观察及处理。由于致病细菌和感染情况不同,脓液性质也不同,一般根据脓液的颜色、气味和稠度,可以鉴别细菌的种类,以利对伤口的处理和治疗。也要配合中药熏洗,应用痔瘘粉消脓膏、外痔贴等可消灭感染,提高愈合效果。

（10）For rarely seen specific infected wounds, full debridement is essential. Close observation on the color, viscosity, and swelling of the pus can be helpful to recognize the bacteria and to determine the wound treatment. Chinese herbal washing and powder or paste application are beneficial to wound healing.

第二节　肛肠术后伤口愈合延迟
§2　Delayed Healing of Anorectal Surgical Wounds

【病因】
［Etiology］

1. 伤口愈合分期
1. Staging

（1）凝血期:防止血液进一步流失,保证伤口处的机械强度。

（1）Coagulation stage:To prevent from further loss of blood and to protect wound mechanics.

（2）炎症反应期:使伤口与静脉回流分开,起到吞噬系统作用消灭异物、细菌,控制感染。

（2）Inflammation stage:To separate the wound from venous drainage, to form the action of phagocytosis, killing bacteria, removing foreign bodies and controlling infection.

（3）肉芽组织形成期:包括胶原纤维及细胞重新组合,提高机械强度。

（3）Granulation stage:Recombination of collagenous fibers and cells, to increase wound mechanics.

以上有其中一项受影响,均引起愈合迟缓。

Any factor under influence of the above will induce a delayed union.

2. 全身因素
2. Systemic Factors

(1)年龄:伤口愈合延缓多发生于老年人。

(1)Age:More delayed wound healing in the elderly.

(2)营养:蛋白缺乏可引起纤维增生和胶原合成不足,血浆胶体渗透压改变则可加重组织水肿,氨基酸和糖不足可以直接影响胶原和多糖合成,营养不良时对伤口愈合有多种作用的血浆纤维蛋白值下降。

(2)Nutrition:Protein deficiency may cause deficiency of fibrous proliferation and collagen synthesis; plasma collagen osmotic pressure change may cause edema; amino acid and sugar deficiency may affect collagen and sugar synthesis; thus decreasing plasma fibrin level which is essential in wound healing.

(3)维生素 C 对中性粒细胞产生过氧化物杀灭细菌,可促进胶原合成,影响巨噬细胞的游走和吞噬功能。

(3)Vitamin C can cause neutrophils to produce peroxide to kill bacteria and promote collagen synthesis, affecting wanderly and phagocytic functions of macrophages.

(4)维生素 A 可促进胶原聚合上皮再生,使受皮质类固醇抑制的创口恢复生长。

(4)Vitamin A can promote regeneration of collagen epithelial cells, leading to regeneration of wounds inhibited by corticoids.

(5)维生素 E 的抗氧化作用可保护伤口,不为中性粒细胞释出的氧自由基破坏。

(5)Vitamin E can protect wounds through antioxidation, not to be destroyed by oxygen free radicals.

(6)维生素 B_1 维持神经正常功能,促进糖类的代谢。

(6)Vitamin B_1 can maintain normal nervous function, promote sugar metabolism.

(7)微量元素:锌是多酶系统,包括 DNA 和 RNA 聚合酶的辅助因子,缺乏时可影响细胞增殖和蛋白的合成。

(7)Trace elements:Zn is in multienzyme, including adjuvant factors of DNA and RNA polymerase. Zn deficiency can affect cellular proliferation and protein synthesis.

（8）温度：过热或过冷能明显延迟愈合，因两者都能引起组织损伤和血管栓塞。

（8）Temperature：Too hot or too cold status may delay wound healing, due to tissue injury and vascular embolism.

（9）贫血：可伴发低血容量，出现组织缺氧，引起伤口愈合不良。

（9）Anemia or accompanied by low blood volume can cause tissue hypoxia, leading to mal-healing wound.

（10）糖尿病、高血糖可抑制中性粒细胞的功能，故减弱抗炎症作用。特别是对巨噬细胞的抑制，可影响成纤维细胞生长和胶原合成。糖尿病性动脉粥样硬化及小血管分布状态也可影响愈合。

（10）Diabetes：Hyperglycemia can inhibit neutrophilic function, thus reduce anti-inflammatory action, especially in inhibition of macrophages affecting fibrogen cell growth and collagen synthe-sis. Diabetic arterial atherosclerosis can also affect wound healing.

（11）恶性肿瘤扩散和转移及蛋白质缺乏，可影响伤口愈合。

（11）Malignant tumor metastasis with protein deficiency may affect wound healing.

（12）尿毒症：伤口低血容量和供氧减少，营养不良，均影响肉芽组织形成，延长伤口愈合。

（12）Uremia：Low blood volume and low oxygen support in wounds with malnutrition may af-fect granulation and delay wound healing.

（13）黄疸：影响维生素 K 吸收，使凝血因子减少，增加伤口血肿的发生，肝功能失调也妨碍蛋白代谢。

（13）Jaundice may affect Vitamin K absorption, reduce coagulation factors, and delay wound healing.

（14）药物：外源性皮质类固醇可影响炎症期伤口愈合，脲质素、阿霉素对伤口愈合也有明显抑制作用。

（14）Drug：Exogenic corticosteroids may affect healing of inflamed wounds. Some antibiotics may inhibit wound healing.

3. 局部因素
3. Local Factors

（1）感染：伤口感染则影响愈合，尤其是妨碍血供，不利于细胞生长，出现组织广泛坏死，异物、死腔、血管栓塞、低氧状态等均影响伤口愈合。

（1）Infection：Wound infection can affect healing by interfering with blood supply and cellular growth, causing extensive necrosis, foreign bodies, cavities, thrombosis and hypoxia.

（2）缺血：伤口局部压迫及血管本身病变，特别是动脉粥样硬化的影响。

（2）Ischemia：Due to local pressure and vascular disorders such as atherosclerosis.

（3）血肿：伤口血肿形成，压力加大，阻碍皮肤血液循环，甚至出现坏死、血肿，还可为细菌感染提供条件。

（3）Hematoma：Influence of blood circulation, causing necrosis, hematoma, providing conditions for bacterial infection.

（4）机械刺激：外科手术、换药、大便干燥等均影响伤口愈合；坏死组织清除不彻底、死腔、结扎、线头、异物残留也影响伤口；因肿瘤或伤口切除过多，组织缺损等也影响伤口愈合。

（4）Mechanical stimulation：Surgical procedures, dressing change, dry defecation, foreign bodies(silk threads)and cavities can influence wound healing.

（5）其他：合并有溃疡结肠炎、克罗恩病、肠瘘、滴虫、湿疹均影响伤口愈合。

（5）Other factors：Complicated with ulcerative colitis, Crohn's disease, colonic fistulae, trichomonads, and eczema.

【治疗】

[Treatment]

1. 全身治疗

1. Systemic Treatment

（1）抗感染：术前预防性应用抗生素。

（1）Anti-infection：Prophylactic use of antibiotics（preoperatively）.

（2）抗生素补充。

（2）Complement antibiotics.

（3）生物生长因子对伤口促进愈合。

（3）Biologic growth factors to promote wound healing.

（4）诱导单核细胞、吞噬细胞、上皮细胞合成纤维细胞的伤口运动，可促进吞噬系统清除细菌碎片净化伤口，促细胞生长活性。

（4）Wound movements.

（5）中医治疗：口服益气活血，增加机体免疫力。

（5）Chinese herbal treatment.

（6）支持疗法：补液注射丙种球蛋白、胎盘球蛋白。

（6）Supportive therapy：Gamma globulin，placental globulin.

2. 局部治疗

2. Local Therapy

（1）生长因子应用：外源透明质点状植皮。

（1）Growth factor application：skin graft.

（2）激光照射。

（2）Laser treatment.

（3）应用生物蛋白胶。

（3）Biologic protein glue.

（4）刮匙小针刀去除腐败组织。

（4）Necrotic tissue removal by acupuncture scalpel.

（5）斜面小针刀治疗致伤口引流通畅。

（5）Good wound drainage by acupuncture scalpel.

（6）采用中药膏换药，去腐生肌长皮。

（6）External application of herbal paste.

第 13 章　肛肠病的预防

Chapter 13　Prevention in Coloproctology

第一节　医源性肛肠病预防

§ 1　Prevention of Iatrogenic Diseases in Coloproctology

1.**肛指检查**　要综合考虑,尤其肛管与邻近组织器官的关系。如直肠前壁肿,此后会诊是子宫后倾直肠综合征。

1. **Digital Anal Examination**　The relationship between the anal canal and peripheral tissues and organs should be clearly considered. In case of swelling of the anterior wall of the rectum, that might be uterine retroversion-rectum syndrome.

2.**肛镜造成肛管撕裂伤**　肛镜插入肛管 2 ~ 3cm,即肛镜通过肛管直肠环,要拔出肛门镜内栓,再见腔进镜。

2. **Anal Canal Laceration Caused By Anoscopy**　When the anoscope is inserted into the anal canal 2 ~ 3 cm, it has passed the rectal ring of the canal. Then the plug should be pulled out to observe the canal prior to further getting the anoscope in.

3.**乙状结肠镜盲目插入造成肠穿孔**　要见腔进镜,尤其是直肠与乙状结肠交界狭窄处。

3. **Colon Perforation Caused By Blind Insertion of Sigmoidoscope**　The sigmoidoscope should be inserted slowly only with the view of the rectal canal, especially at the narrow point between the rectum and sigmoid colon.

(1)长期服用缓泻药:如服美鼠素皮药可引起结肠黑变病,直肠镜下见直肠黏膜黑色小斑点(蛇皮斑)。可酌情用中药,口服润肠汤治疗。

(1)Prolonged taking Caccagogues may cause blackening colon：This condition can be treated by herbal medicine："Ruanchang Tang"decoction.

(2)肠道菌群失调症:长期应用抗生素,应配合中药治疗。

(2)Intestinal bacterial disturbances induced by prolonged use of antibiotics：This condition can be treated by herbal medicine.

(3)外用药:引起瘀血、水疱,可改用外痔贴中药。

(3)External use of medicine causing hematemesis and bubbles：This condition can be treated with external use of herbs.

（4）普鲁卡因、布比卡因过敏：用药前试验，选用利多卡因。

（4）Allergy to Procaine or Bupivacaine：Select Lidamantle, to do sensitivity test before practice.

4. 肛管直肠溃疡　应用治疗机造成热灼伤，形成溃疡糜烂。应用中药消脓膏。

4. Anal Canal and Rectal Ulcer　Burning wound and ulcer caused by treatment machine can be treated by herbal "Xiao Nong Gao".

5. 污染肛门，尖锐湿疣　应用胸腺五肽皮下浸润封闭注射。

5. Contaminated Anus with Condyloma Acuminatum　Treated by subcutaneous infiltration injection with thymopeptide.

6. 肛周注射引起感染脓肿　刮匙小针刀治疗，外敷消脓膏中药。

6. Perianal Abscess Caused By Injection Infection　Treated by craping ladle acupuncture scalpel and external use of "Xiao Nong Gao".

7. 前列腺出血、血尿　因直肠前壁注射药液过深引起。输入等渗利尿液。

7. Prostate Hemorrhage Caused By Too Deep Injection　This is treated by infusion of isosmotic diuretic solution.

8. 肛管直肠硬化症　注射用药量过大或刺入过深引起肛管直肠硬化。口服中药治疗，刮匙小针刀治疗。

8. Anocanal and Rectal Sclerosis Caused By Too Deep Injection　This is treated by oral intake of herbal medicine and craping ladle acupuncture scalpel.

9. 人造假肛门瘘　探针误伤形成假道。应用探针小弯刀，可将检查切开挂线同步完成，可预防误伤。

9. Artificial Anal Fistula Caused By Traumatic Probing　Use craping ladle acupuncture scalpel together with incision and seton.

10. 肛管直肠狭窄　内外痔手术切除过多，形成瘢痕狭窄。应用弯头负压吸力式套扎枪治疗和探针小弯刀配合斜面小针刀。

10. Stricture of Anal Canal and Rectum Caused By Complicated Procedures for Internal and External Hemorrhoids　Treated by anal head loop ligating gun with acupuncture scalpel.

11. 肛门失禁　手术伤及肛门直肠环，给予直肠环修补。可采用挂线疗法，预防。

11. Anal Incontinence　Anorectal Ring Injury from Surgery, treated by seton on probe.

12. 肛管皮肤缺损 因肛门手术损伤造成直肠黏膜外脱,采用小针刀治疗皮条游离修补。弯头负压套扎枪治疗直肠黏膜外脱。

12. Skin Defect of the anal Canal with Extrusion of Rectal Mucosa Treated by acupuncture scalpel and angle head loop ligating gun, to repair the skin defect.

13. 肛管手术后大出血 给予安全套气囊压迫治疗。

13. Massive Hemorrhage after Anal Canal Surgery Treated by balloon pressure method.

第二节　肛肠病预防

§2　Prevention of Anorectal Diseases

早在 2000 年前《黄帝内经·四气调神大论》中就有记载:"是故圣人不治已病治未病,不治已乱治未乱。"从机体和外界环境统一的观点出发,预防疾病的原则应当是:既重视整体,也注意局部;要承认外因,更要考虑到内因。《黄帝内经·上古天真论》就提出"虚邪贼风,避之有时。"指预防外在致病因素的侵袭时,更强调人体的内在因素。又说:"恬憺虚无,真气从之,精神内守,病安从来。"说明疾病的发生,固然与外界刺激有着密切的关系,而发病的关键是由机体内在情况决定。因此,在肛肠病预防上,不仅要注意和防御一切与发病有关的诱因,而更重视如何保持精神愉快,通过锻炼保养正气,增强体质,提高抗病能力。只有内因与外因并防,整体与局部兼顾,使机体与变化着的环境经常处于平衡状态,才能达到有效地预防发病。主要预防措施如下。

As was mentioned in the famous literature < Huangdi Neijing > that a respectable doctor can treat the condition before the disease takes place, from the viewpoint of uniform idea of human body and environment. Therefore the principle of prevention is emphasized on both the body itself and the local portion, on both the external cause and the internal origin. So in the prevention of anorectal diseases, not only the predisposing causes of diseases should be noticed, but also the protection of spiritual happiness and strengthening the physical condition and disease-resistant energy must be emphasized.

一、保持精神愉快

1. Keeping Spiritual Happiness

人的精神状态与疾病的发生有密切关系。精神受到不良刺激,情绪发生波动,可影响正常生理活动,如刺激过大,或持续时间过久,就会引发疾病。《素问·阴阳应象大论》曾说:"喜伤心,怒伤肝,忧伤肺,思伤脾,恐伤肾";在《素问·疏五过论》

又说:"暴乐暴苦,始乐后苦,皆伤精气,精气竭绝,形体毁沮",都是中医学所说的七情内伤;如果有失节制,则可造成阴阳失调,气血虚损,引起疾病。因此说防止七情内伤,是可以增强防病能力的。纵然有外邪侵袭,可不引起发病。说明避免情绪过度波动、保持心情舒畅对预防疾病的重要性。

In the ancient medicine book ＜Su Wen＞ it was recorded:"Overjoy impairing heart, rage impairing liver, sorrow impairing lung, anxiety impairing spleen, and fright impairing kidney." Therefore, avoidance of too much excitement and keeping happiness are essential in prevention of diseases.

二、经常锻炼身体
2. Constant Physical Exercises

中医学很早就提倡锻炼身体,预防疾病。例如,早在公元 220 年以前,华佗创造了类似体操运动的"五禽戏"来锻炼身体,以调和内在平衡,促进气血周流,达到预防疾病的目的。久坐久站容易妨碍肛门直肠静脉血回流,使肠管运动迟缓,有诱发痔瘘的可能。因此,如经常锻炼身体,调和、促进血液循环,提高抗病能力,是非常必要的。坚持练太极拳和练习气功,除能治疗疾病外,对预防肛肠病也会发挥更积极的作用。

In traditional Chinese medicine, physical exercise is advocated for prevention of diseases. Early before 220 AD, Hua Tuo, a famous physician introduced a physical exercise movement "Five Birds Movement" for the people to regulate internal body balance, promote vital energy and blood circulation, thus prevent from diseases. Therefore, exercises of Taiji boxing and of Qigong can be beneficial in prevention of anal and rectal diseases.

三、注意节制饮食
3. Continence of Food and Drink

中医学在《素问·上古天真论》中就有"饮食有节,起居有常,不妄作劳。故能形与神俱,而尽终其天年,度百岁乃去"。说明生活、饮食节制对健康的重要作用。关于饮食不节与发病的关系,《疮疡经验全书》中更有具体的阐述:"……脏腑所发,多由饮食不节,醉饱无明,恣食肥腻,胡椒辛辣,炙煿酸酒,禽兽异物,任情醉饮……,遂致阴阳不和,关格壅塞,湿热下冲,乃生五痔。"

In ＜Su Wen＞ there was the advice:" continence of food and drink, regular daily life and avoidance of too much labor can be helpful to both spirit and body, leading to hundred years of age." Therefore, regular and proper food and drink and daily life are essential in prevention of diseases.

1. **每餐不要吃得过饱** 否则除会引起肠胃功能紊乱(消化不良等)外,还可增高腹腔内压力,影响痔静脉血回流,为痔形成创造有利的条件。

1. **Never Over Meal** Over meal can cause dysfunction of the gastrointestinal tract, increasing intraperitoneal pressure, interference of hemorrhoidal venous reflow, leading to formation of hemorrhoids.

2. **少吃或不吃刺激性食物** 如饮酒,过多地吃胡椒、芥末、辣椒等,以免刺激引起盆腔内充血导致便秘。

2. **Minimizing some irritating food and drink such as wines** Pepper, mustard which would cause pelvic congestion leading to constipation.

3. **其他** 如吞下鱼刺、碎骨片等异物,也可刺伤直肠,引起感染。

3. **Other Factors** Fish pin bones and pork bones, etc. causing injury and infection to rectum.

四、保持大便正常
4. Keep Normal Defecation

经常大便干结或泻痢既是肛肠病的结果,也可是肛肠病的重要原因。要保持大便正常除节制饮食外,更应养成定时排便的习惯,最好每天 1 次,排便时间以晨起或睡前为佳。这样可使胃肠蠕动正常,粪便水分不致被过多吸收而干硬。假如应该晨起排便而推迟到晚上或第 2 天,粪便水分就被过多吸收引起粪便干硬;干硬的粪便定会压迫直肠、阻碍血液回流,容易诱痔。用力排便易损伤肛门,形成肛裂,或损伤肛窦,甚至引起脓肿。如排便运动长期被有意识地控制、延长,则养成不良排便习惯,出现习惯性便秘。因此,如大便不正常时,必须及时调理,便干时可酌情服用缓泻药,如麻仁滋脾丸、槐角丸、脏连丸、液状石蜡等。或喝少许香油或蜂蜜,至大便恢复正常时为止。如患腹泻或痢疾时,应及时给适当治疗。

Constant dry stool or diarrhea is the result and also the cause of anorectal diseases. So keeping regular defecation habit preferably once a day, either in the morning or evening is essential. Water intake should be normal, not to make the stool too dry and hard, preventing injury of anus. Abnormal stool should be regulated or treated by laxatives such as "Maran Zipi Wan", "Huajao Wan", liquid paraffin, vegetable oil, honey, etc.

五、保持肛门周围清洁
5. Keep the Anus Clean

肛门部不洁可直接刺激局部引起发病,如妇女白带过多者常发生肛裂、感染或肛门直肠周围脓肿。因此,要经常保持肛门部清洁,尤其肛门或阴道分泌物较多者更应注意。如经常用温水洗肛门,不用不洁的便纸或土块、柴禾叶等擦肛门。应经常换衬裤。

Unclean anus may cause anal fissure or perianal abscess in women with vaginal secretions. So local cleaning is an essential habit. Warm water washing and frequent changing pants or undershorts are suggested.

六、孕期注意促进静脉血回流
6. Promote Venous Flow in Pregnancy

妊娠后,由于子宫逐渐膨大,压迫下腔静脉,使肛门直肠静脉的血液回流受到影响;尤其当胎位不正时,更容易造成明显压迫。因此,要及时矫正胎位,并应适当休息,更应注意避免便秘及久站久坐等。

During pregnancy the uterus is enlarging, pressing the inferior vena cava, thus the vascular flow of anal and rectal veins is influenced. So the fetal posture should be promptly corrected to decrease the pressure on the pelvic veins. Suitable rest, avoiding constipation and long lasting standing and sitting are essential.

总之,肛肠病的预防,除前面所说外,习惯性便秘、腹泻、痢疾、蛲虫病、白带过多等均可诱发肛肠病。因此,应注意及早适当治疗这些诱发病。如已发生痔、瘘、肛裂、湿疹等,也应该及时治疗,以免日久加重病情,给自己造成痛苦,增加治疗困难。

In general, prevention of anal and rectal diseases depends upon constant care of the anus and the rectal function. Prompt discovery or diagnosis and treatment of any disease if occurred should be one's proper habit.

第 14 章　肛肠科常用中药方剂

Chapter 14　Commonly Used Chinese Herbal Recipes

一、内服中药方剂

§1　Chinese Herbal Decoction

（一）痔瘘汤

1. Zhi Lou Decoction

【处方】　生地炭、赤芍、大黄、炒槐花、黄连、生槐角、防风各10g,当归、黄芩、地榆炭、红花、生栀子、升麻、金银花、枳壳、侧柏炭、芥穗、桃仁、麻仁、陈皮各9g,白芷、生阿胶各6g,乌梅5个,生白芍15g,甘草3g。

Prescription:Dried Rehmannia root carbon, Radix Paeoniae Rubra, Radix et Rhizoma Rhei, Flos Sophorae, Rhizoma Coptidis, Fructus Sophorae, Radix Saposhnikoviae,each 10g, Radix Angelicae Sinensis,Radix Scutellariae, Radix Sanguisorbae carbon, Flos Carthami, Cacumen Platycludi carbon, Semen Sinapi, Semen Persicae, Fructus Cannabis, Pericarpium Citri Reticulatae each 9g. Radix Angelicae Dahuricae, Colla Corii Asini each 6g,Fructus Mume×5, Radix Paeoniae Alba 15g,Radix Glycyrrhizae 3g.

【功能】　清热、除湿、止血、润便、消肿。

Function:Clearing heat, removing dampness, hemostasis, laxative, subsiding swelling.

【主治】　湿热型痔疮、肛瘘或肛门肿痛、大便出血,大便干燥。

Indications:Hemorrhoid of damp-heat type, anal fistula or anal pain, stool with blood, dry stool.

【用法及用量】　每天服1剂。

Application:1 dose per day.

（二）痔疮止血汤

2. Zhichuang Zixue Decoction

【处方】　大蓟、小蓟、侧柏叶、荷叶、茅根、茜草根、栀子、棕榈皮、槐花、麻仁各10g,陈皮、黄连、地榆、黄芩、荆芥穗、桃仁、生地各9g,大黄、牡丹皮各6g,甘草2g。

Prescription:Radix Cirsii Japanici, Herba Cephalanoploris, Cacumen Platycladi, Folium Nelumbinis, Radix Droserae Lunatae, Radix Rubiae, Fructus Gardeniae, Fibra Trachycarpi Vaginata, Flos Sophorae, Fructus Cammabis, each 10g, Herba Schizonepetae, Semen Persicae, Dried Rehmannia root each 9g, Radix et Rhizoma Rhei, Cortex Moutan Redicis each 6g, Radix Glycyr-rhizae 2g.

【制法】　将以上各药用 600ml 水煎至 200ml。

Production：Mixture of the above herbs ＋ water 600ml, boil to form 200ml.

【功能】　止血、祛瘀、生新、润便、消肿。

Function：Hemostasis, expelling stasis, laxative, subsiding swelling.

【主治】　便血(适用于内痔出血或手术后渗血)。

Indication：Hematochezia (bleeding internal hemorrhoid or postoperative oozing blood).

(三)润肠汤

3. Runchang Decoction

【处方】　生地、桃仁、火麻仁、郁李仁、杏仁、柏子仁、肉苁蓉(酒蒸)、广皮、熟军、当归、松子仁、枳实(麸炒)各 10g,生白芍 15g,厚朴(姜制)6g。

Prescription：Dried Rehmannia root, Semen Persicae, Fructus Commabis, Semen Pruni, Semen Armeniacae Amarum, Semen Platycladi, Herba Cistanches (alcohol steaming), Guangpi, Shujun, Radix Angelicae Sinensis, Simen Brassicae Chinensis, Fructus Aurantii Immaturus each 10g, Radix Paeoniae Alba 15g, Cortex Magnoliae Officinalis 6g.

【功能】　滋润大肠：健胃通便。

Function：Nourishing large intestine, strengthening stomach and purgation.

【主治】　肠热燥结、大便不通、腹胀胸满、产后及病后肠液不足的便秘。

Indications：Intestinal heat and dampness, constipation, full chest and abdomen, constipation following baby delivery or disease.

【用法及用量】　每晚服一剂。

Application：One dose every evening.

【禁忌】　孕妇忌服。

Contraindication：Pregnant women.

(四)通便粉

4. Tongbian Powder

【处方】　芦荟面 15g,大黄面 20g,朱砂面、芒硝面各 5g.

Prescription：Succus Aloes Folii Siccatus powder 15g, Radix et Rhizoma Rhei powder 20g,

Cinnabaris powder 5g, Natrii sulfas powder 5g.

【制法】 将以上四药研细合匀,以白酒泛为小丸 15 袋装,每袋 3g。

Production:Grind fine powder, add in white wine to make small pills, divided into 15 pockets, 3g per pocket.

【功能】 润肠、通便。

Function:Nourishing colon and purgation.

【主治】 习惯性便秘、大便燥结或数日大便不通而引起腹部胀痛、头晕胸闷。

Indications:Habitual constipation, dry stool with abdominal pain, dizziness, chest distress.

【用法及用量】每晚服一袋,米汤水送下。

Application:1 pocket of pills every evening, taken with rice soup.

【禁忌】 孕妇忌服。

Contraindication:Pregnant women.

(五)利湿止痒汤

5. Lishi Zhiyang Decoction

【处方】 苍术、蒿本、防风、黄柏、泽泻、紫花地丁、蒲公英各 9g,花粉、羌活、牛子、独活、苦参、川黄连各 6g。

Prescription:Rhizoma Atractylodis, Rhizoma Ligustici, Radix Saposhnikoviae, Cortex Phellodendri, Rhizoma Alismatis, Herba Violae, Herba Taraxaci, each 9g. Radix Trichosanthis, Rhizoma et Radix Notopterygii, Niuzj, Radix Angelicae Pubescentis, Radix Sophotae Flavescentis, Rhizoma Coptidis, each 6g.

【制法】 将以上各药用 600ml 水煎至 200ml。

Production :Mixture of the above herbs + water 600ml, boil to form 200ml.

【功能】 利湿、止痒、解毒。

Function:Eliminating dampness and relieving itching, detoxification.

【主治】 肛门周围湿疹及肛门瘙痒症;阴囊瘙痒等症。

Indications:Perianal eczema, anal pruritus, and scrotal pruritus.

【用法及用量】 早、晚各服 100ml。

Application:Take 100ml every morning and every evening.

(六)汤剂组方

6. Composed Decoctions

（1）**清热解毒汤**　太子参 6g,连翘、蒲公英、白头翁、红藤各 30g,白术、茯苓、当归、陈皮各 15g,白芷、皂角刺各 10g,生甘草 3g,炒白芍 20g,银花 60g,黄芪 5g,穿山甲（代）9g。

（1）**Qingre Jiedu Decoction**　Radix Pseudostellariae 6g, Fructus Forsythiae, Herba Taraxaci, Radix Pulsatillae, Caulis seu Radix Dalbergiae Hancei each 30g, Rhizoma Atractilodis Macrocephalae, Poria, Radix Angelicae Sinensis, Pericardium Citri Reticulatae each 15g, Radix Angelicae Dahuricae, Spina Gleditsiae each 10g, Radix Glycyrrhizae 3g, Radix Paeoniae Alba 20g, Fructus Lonicerae 60g, Radix Astragali 5g, Squama Manitis 9g.

（2）**升举汤**　白术、当归各 15g,柴胡、桔梗各 5g,陈皮、枳壳各 10g,延胡索 9g,甘草 3g,知母 9g,炙黄芪 50g,党参 25g,升麻 20g。

（2）**Sheng Ju Decoction**　Rhizoma Astractylodis Macrocephalae, Radix Angelicae Dahuricae each 15g, Radix Bupleuri, Radix Pladicodi each 5g, Pericardium Citri Peticulatae, Rhizoma Anemarrhenae 9g, Radix Astragali 50g, Radix Codonopsis 25g, Rhizoma Cimcifugae 20g.

1）气阴虚加生地 30g,玄参 15g,山药 10g,扁豆、莲子肉各 6g,大枣 5 个,谷芽 9g。

1）In case of asthenia of Qi（Vitality deficiency）, add：Radix Remanniae 30g, Radix Scrophulariae 15g, Rhizoma Dioscoreae 10g, Semen Dolicoris 6g, Semen Nelumbinis 6g, Fructus Jujubae ×5, Fruxtus Oryzae Germinatus 9g.

2）脾肾阳虚加陈皮、吴茱萸各 9g,白芍 15g,防风、川芎、补骨脂各 6g。四神丸：肉豆蔻、五味子各 3g。

2）In case of asthenis of splenorenal Yang, add：Pericardium Citri Reticulatae 9g, Fructus Evodiae 9g, Radix Paeoniae Alba 15g, Radix Saposhnikoviae 6g, Rhizoma Chuanxiong 6g, Fructus Psoraleae 6g, 'Four Shen Pills', Semen Myristicae 3g, Fructus Schisandrae 3g.

（3）**清热解毒汤**　健脾清热汤　白头翁 20g,黄连 6g,秦皮、黄柏各 10g,赤芍、银花各 15g,当归、枳壳、川芎、茯苓各 9g。

（3）**Jianpi Qingre Decoction**　Radix Pulsatillae 20g, Radix Coptidis 6g, Cortex Fraxini 10g, Cortex Phellodendri 10g, Radix Paeoniae Rubra 15g, Fructus Lonicerae 15g, Radix Angelicae Sinensis 9g, Fructus Aurantii 9g, Rhizoma Chuanxiong 9g, Poria 9g.

（4）**健脾疏肝汤**　白术、陈皮各 9g,白芍 15g,防风、升麻、黄芪、川芎各 6g,乌梅 5 个,五倍子 2g。

（4）**Jianpi Shugan Decoction**　Rhizoma Atractilodis Macrocephalae 9g, Pericardium Citri Reticulalae 9g, Radix Paeoniae Alba 15g, Radix Saposhnikoviae 6g, rhizome Cimcifugae 6g, Radix Astragali 6g, Rhizoma Chuanxiong 6g, Fructus Mume ×5, Galla Chinensis 2g.

（5）**健脾和胃汤**　党参、茯苓、炒白术、山药、扁豆、莲子肉、黄芪、升麻各 9g，太子参、谷芽各 6g，炙甘草 3g，大枣 5 个，诃子肉、肉豆蔻各 2g。

（5）**Jianpi Hewei Decoction**　Radix Codonopsis , Poria, Rhizoma Atractyladis Macrocephalae, Rhizoma Dioscoreae, Semen Dolicoris, Semen Nelumbinis, Radix Astragali, Rhizoma Cimcifugae each 9g, Radix Pseudostellariae 6g, Fructus Oryzae Germinatus 6g, Radix Glycyrrhizae 3g, Fructus Jujubae ×5, Fructus Kopsiae Officinalis, Semen Myristicae each 2g.

（6）**健脾补肾汤**　补骨脂、肉豆蔻各 3g，陈皮、党参、白术、川芎各 9g，五味子 2g，吴茱萸 6g，大枣 5 个，生姜三片。

（6）**Jianpi Bushen Decoction**　Fructus Psoraleae 3g, Semen Myristicae 3g, Pericardium Citrii Reticulatae, Radix Codonopsis, Rhizoma Astractylodis Macrocephalae, Rhizoma Chuanxiong each 9g, Fructus Schisandrae 2g, Fructus Evodiae 6g, Fructus Jujubae ×5, Rhizoma Zingiberis Recens 3 slices.

（7）**健脾化瘀汤**　当归、香附、枳壳、乌药、五灵脂、木香、桃仁、没药、丹皮、红花、川芎、甘草、延胡索各 6g，茯苓 9g。

（7）**Jianpi Huayu Decoction**　Radix Angelicae Sinensis, Rizhoma Cyperi, Fructus Auranti, Radix Linderae, Faeces Trogopterori, Radix Auklandiae, Semen Persicae, Myrrha, Cortex Moutan Radicis, Flos Carthami, Rhizoma Chuanxiong, Rhizoma Corydalis each 6g, Poria 9g.

（8）**散结汤**　木香、桃仁、红花、秦艽、秦皮、川楝子各 9g，延胡索、防风、柴胡、炙大黄各 6g，当归、夏枯草、乌药各 10g，白芍 15g。

（8）**Sanjie Decoction**　Radix Auklandiae, Semen Percicae, Flos Carthami, Radix Gentianae Macrophilae, Cortex Fraxini, Fructus Toosendan , each 9g, Rhizoma Colydalis, Radix Saposhnikoviae, Radix Bupleuri, Radix et Rhizoma Rhei, each 6g, Radix Angelica Sinensis, Spica Prunellae, Radix Linderae each 10g.

（9）**玉真汤**　天南星、白附子、防风、白芷、羌活各 9g，明天麻 6g。

（9）**Yu Zhen Decoction**　Rhizoma Arisaematis, Rhizoma Typhonii, Radix Saposhnikoviae, Radix Angeliocae Dahuricae, Rhizoma et Radix Notopterygii, each 9g, Rhizoma Gastrodiae 6g.

1）若病在半表半里者，在原方基础上加大黄、柴胡、细辛、僵蚕、蝉蜕、朱砂、钩藤、甘草等。

1) In case the disease is in semi-exterior and semi-interior situation, add：Radix et Rhizoma Rhei, Radix Bupleuri, Herba Asari, Bombyx Batriticatus, Periostracum Cicadae, Cinnabaris, Radix Cryptolepic Buchanani, Radix Glycerrhyzae.

2）病情重而入里者，在原方基础上加大黄、钩藤、僵蚕、全蝎、蝉蜕、蜈蚣、橘红、橘络、苏梗、生石膏、粉草、羚羊粉(冲服)。

2) In case the disease is severe and get into interior, add: Radix et Rhizoma Rhei, Radix Cryptoleptic Buchananii, Bombyx Batriticatus, Scorpio, Periostracum Cicadae, Scolopendra, Exocarpium CitriTangerinae, Vascular Aurantii Citrii Tangerinae, Lignum Sappan, Gypsum Fibrosum, Fan Cao, Cornu Saigae Tartaricae powder, drink with warm water.

3) 病情急重危者,在病情重而入里之处方基础上去石膏、大黄、羚羊粉;加川乌、草乌、雄黄、干姜。

3) In case the disease is very severe, from the prescription of 2), delete: Gypsum Fibrosum, Radix et Rhizoma Rhei, Cornu Saigae Tartaricae powder, but add: Radix Aconiti, Radix Aconiti Kusnezoffii, Realgar, Rhizoma Zingiberis.

4) 煎法:用水 600ml 煎成 300ml。

4) Production : Boil with 600ml of water to form 300ml.

5) 服法:每日 1 剂,3 次分服,病人清醒能吞咽者口服,不能口服者采用保留灌肠法。

5) Application:1 dose a day for 3 times, take p. o. or by retention enema.

(10) **通便汤**　火麻仁、柏子仁、肉苁蓉各 20g,起润肠通便作用;枳壳 10g 消积止痛;大黄 6～15g 较坚攻下,增强胃肠蠕动而促使排便;玄参、煅牡蛎各 9g,滋阴生津,潜阳补阴软坚散结,止血收口;黄芪、白术各 10g,补中益气健脾和胃;甘草 4g 调和诸药。全方组合,共奏润肠通便、行气活血、通络止血、健脾和胃、驱风散热之功效。

(10) **Tong Bian Decoction**　Semen Canabis, Semen Platycladi, Herba Cistanches, each 20g, for moistening intestines to relieve constipation, Fructus Auranti 19g for removingfood retention and relieving pain, Radix Rhizoma Rhei 6～15g for softening hardness to purgate and increase G-I tract peristalsis, Radix Scrofulariae , Charring Ostrea each 9g for nourishing Yin to produce fluid, softening hardness to dissipate mass and hemostasis, Radix Astragali, Rhizoma Astractylodis each 10g for strengthening middle energizer to nourish Qi and invigorating spleen and regulating stomach, Radix Glycyrrhizae 4g to harmonize all herbs, giving a best effect of purgation.

二、外敷中药制剂
§2　Herbal Medicine for External Application

(一)痔瘘粉
1. Zhi Lou Powder

【处方】　冰片、狗胆、乳香、没药、血竭、儿茶、鹿茸各 5g,驴皮、海巴、龙骨、猫骨、赤石脂各 10g,炉甘石、石膏、海螵蛸、花蕊石各 15g,珠子 3g,三七 7g。

Prescription：Borneolum Syntheticum, Dog's gall, Olibanum, Myrrha, Resina Draconis, Catechu, Cornu Cervi Pantotrichum, each 5g, Donkey skin, Hai Ba, Os Dragonis, Os Sepiae, Ophicalcitum, each 15g, Pearl 3g, Radix Notoginseng 7g.

【制法】 先将珠子、海巴、花蕊石、石膏、猫骨煅制,驴皮(炙)、乳香、没药(去油),然后把上述各药共研细末,越细越好。(本药敷在新鲜伤口处微有刺痛感,因药内有腐蚀及杀菌药物。)一般经过 7~10 分钟就可消失。如在此药内加 10% 的苯唑卡因或普鲁卡因,疼痛即可减轻或消失。

Production：First forge pearls, Hai Ba, Ophicalcitum, Gypsum Fibrosum and Cat bone, remove oil from Donkey skin, Olibanum and MYrrha, then grind the herbs to form fine powder.

【功能】 止血、消炎、杀菌、去腐、生肌、收口。

Function：Hemostasis, anti-inflammation, killing bacteria, removing necrotic tissue and promoting granulation, and helping healing.

【用法】 于肛瘘、肛裂、外痔等手术后,敷于伤口。

Application：Apply on wounds after surgeries for anal fistulae, fissures and external hemorrhoids. There may be painful for fresh wounds due to the presence of corrosive and antiseptic medicine, but pain will be disappeared after 7~10minutes. Addition of 10% Benzocaine or Procaine to the above medicine would be beneficial to reducing pain.

(二)外痔贴
2. Wai Zhi Tie

【处方】 珍珠、红粉各 3g,冰片、生乳香、海螵蛸(去壳)、官粉各 5g,生白石脂、煅海巴、煅龙骨、煅炉甘石各 30g,儿茶 4g,炉甘石 10g,煅石膏 17g。

Prescription：Pearl, Hydragyri Oxydum Rubrum, each 3g, Borneolum Syntheticum, Olibanum, Os Sepiae (shell removed), Guan Fen, each 5g, Sheng Bai Shizhi, Duan Hai Ba, Os Dragonis, Forged Calamina , each 30g, Catechu 4g, Calamina 10g, Forged Gypsum Fibrosum 17g.

【制法】 将以上各药研成细粉,混合调匀即可。取散 30g,凡士林 70g,成 30% 的外痔贴(冬天或较浓时,可加些液状石蜡或麻油)。

Production：Grind all the above herbs to form fine powder and mix them together. A 30% paste can be made by 30g of the powder and 70g Vaseline, Liquid Paraffin or Oleum Sesami can be added in winter.

【功能】 消肿、止痛、生肌、收口。

Function：Reducing swelling, stopping pain, invigorating granulation and helping wound healing.

【用法】 用于各型痔瘘感染发炎、肿胀、疼痛等,敷之有卓效,可立即止痛、消肿。

Application：Local application on any inflammation, swelling and painful parts.

（三）消脓膏
3. Xiao Nong Gao

【处方】 当归、白脂各 60g,甘草、麻油各 30g,白芷、血竭各 5g,紫草 3g。

Prescription：Radix Angelica Sinensis, Semen Sesami, each 60g, Radix Glycyrrhizae, Oleum Sesami, each 30g , Radix Angelicae Dahuricae, Resina Draconis, each 5g, Radix Arnebiae seu Lithospermi 3g.

【功能】 用于一切感染之伤口。

Function：To be used for all infected wounds.

（四）痔裂膏
4. Zhi Lie Gao

【处方】 氧化锌 60g,凡士林 30g,硼酸、驴皮各 10g,冰片、银朱各 5g,乳香、没药各 9g。

Prescription：Zinc oxide 60g, Vaseline 30g, Boric acid and Donkey skin, each 10g, Borneolum Syntheticum and Hydragyrum Sulphuratum, each 5g, Olibaman and Myrrha, each 9g.

【制法】 将各药研成细粉,用凡士林调匀成软膏,冬天可加些麻油。

Production：Grind the herbs to form fine powder, making paste with Vaseline. Oleum Sesami can be added in winter.

【功能】 去腐、生肌、收口、止痛。

 Function：Removing necrotic tissue and promoting granulation, helping wound healing and stopping pain.

【用法】 用于初期单纯或复杂性肛裂,将此膏注入肛内可治愈;对肛门湿疹及瘙痒症涂敷此膏也很有效。

Application：Insert the paste into the anus to treat simple or complicated anal fissure, anal eczema and pruritus.

（五）生皮散
5. Sheng Pi San

【处方】 熟石膏、炉甘石、赤石脂各 30g,驴皮（炙）5g。

Prescription：Gypsum Fibrosum, Calamina, Halloysittum, each 30g, Donkey skin 5g.

【制法】 将以上各药研成细粉,混合调匀即可。

Production:Grind the herbs to form fine powder and mix together.

【功能】 生皮、收口、去湿。

Function:Skin regeneration, wound healing, removing dampness.

【用法】 用于一切将愈合的伤口,敷之可促进增长上皮,提早愈合。

Application:Apply the mixed powder for healing wound.

附:生皮膏取生皮散30g,凡士林70g,混合调匀即为30%的生成膏。敷用于一切将愈之伤口,其功能与生皮散相同。

Note:Mix 30g of ShengPi San with 70g of Vaseline to form 30% Sheng Pi Gao(Paste).

(六)收湿散
6. Shou Shi San

【处方】 枯矾30g,樟丹、炉甘石、白芷、冰片、驴皮、乳香、没药、儿茶各2g。

Prescription:Withered alumina cement 30g, Cortes Cinamami Camphorae , Calamina, Radix Dahulicae, Borneolum Syntheticum, Donkey skin,Olibamum, Myrrha, Catechu, each 2g.

【制法】 将以上各药研细,混合调匀即可。

Production:Grind the herbs and mix together.

【功能】 去湿、止痒、消肿、生皮、杀菌。

Function:Removing dampness, stopping itching, reducing swelling, skin regeneration, killing bacteria.

【用法】 用于肛门周围湿疹、肛门瘙痒症及伤口分泌物过多等症,敷之颇效。

Application:Apply the powder on the lesion to treat perianal eczema and pruritus, and wound secretion.

附:收湿膏 取收湿散30g,凡士林70g,混合调匀即可。

Note: Mix 30g of Shou Shi San with 70g of Vaseline to form Shou Shi Gap (Plate).

三、熏洗中药

§ 3　Fumigating and Washing Herbs

（一）祛毒汤

1. Qu Du Decoction

【处方】　瓦松、马齿苋、川文蛤、苍术、防风、枳壳、侧柏叶各 15g,朴硝 30g,甘草、川椒、葱白各 5g。

Prescription：Herba Orostachydis, Herba Portulacae, concha Meretricis, Atractylodis, Radix Saposhnikoviae,Fructus Auranti, Cacumen Platycladi, each 15g Natrii sulfas 30g, Rhdix Glycyr-rhizae, Fructus Copsici Frutescentis, Bulbus Allil Fistulosi, each 5g.

【制法】　每剂可用水 1000ml,煮沸后放于坐盆内。

Production：1 dose ＋ water 1000ml, put in a large basin after boiling.

【功能】　消肿、解毒、止痛。

Function：Reducing swelling, anti-toxicity, stopping pain.

【用法】　用于发炎感染之痔瘘,患者先坐于盆上,借热气熏之,待水温后再洗。用后将药放于阴凉处,可于次日加热再用,每剂可用 1～2 天。

Application：Use for treating hemorrhoids and fistulae. The patient sits on the large basin to receive the hot vapor from the basin, later washes his anus portion with the warm liquid. After washing, the liquid can be put in a cool place and be used again on the next day.

（二）止痒汤

2. Zhi Yang Decoction

【处方】皮胶 120g,白矾(研末)、硫黄、蛤蟆草各 30g。

Prescription：Skin Glue 120g, Alumen powder, sulfur, Herba Woodfrog, each 30g.

【制法】　将以上各药放入沙锅内,加水 1000ml(5 茶碗)在火上煮沸后,放入熏洗盆内即可。

Production：Boil the above drugs in 1000 ml of water, then put in a large basin.

【功能】　止痒、收敛、消毒、杀菌。

Function：Stopping itching, astriction, aseptic, killing bacteria.

【用法】　用于肛门瘙痒症或肛门周围湿疹。要先熏后洗,至凉时用净布蘸药汤擦洗,每日 1～2 次,每次 20～30 分钟。

Application: Use for treating pructus and perianal eczema. Use the vapor first and wash with warm liquid once or twice daily, 20 ~ 30 minutes each time.

(三)去肿汤
3. Qu Zhong Decoction

【处方】 川乌、草乌、马齿苋、蛤蟆革各 15g,葱白 2 根。

Prescription: Radix Aconiti, Radix Aconiti Kusnezoffii, Herba Portulacae, Herba Woodfrog, each 15g, Bulbus Allii Fistulosi ×2.

【制法】 将以上各药放在沙锅内,加水 1000ml(约 5 茶碗),煎半小时将汤滤出,放在洗盆内即可。

Production: Boil the above drugs in 1000ml of water for 0.5 h. Put in a large basin.

【功能】消肿、止痒、止痛。

Function: Reducing swelling, stopping itching and pain.

【用法】用于一切感染发炎时期之内外痔及肛门瘘等;对肛门瘙痒也有效。每日熏洗 1 ~ 2 次,每次半小时。

Application: Used for treating infected internal and external hemorrhoids and fistulae, and anal pruritus. Use the vapor first, then wash with the warm liquid, once or twice a day, 0.5 h each time.

第 15 章　肛肠科器械及发明专利证书

Chapter 15　Otoproctologlc Instruments and Patent Certificates

一、肛肠科器械

I. Otoproctologic Instruments

（一）探针小弯刀

1. Small Curving Probing Scalpel

【适应证】　肛门瘘、肛门直肠狭窄、肛门脓肿一期手术等。

Indication：Anal fistula, ano-rectal stricture, anal abscess primary operation.

【操作方法】　先用探针小弯刀前端的探针(图 15－1)。插入肛门瘘外口。肛指触及内口，探针从内口探出。内口在直肠环以下(齿线为界)，则将探针弯叠扣出肛门外，并顺弯刀将肛门瘘管割切开；如内口在直肠环以上，则需用探针头部挂线于肛门直肠环部，以防损伤括约肌。但直肠环以下部分的肛瘘则应用弯刀切割开。

Procedure：Insert the probe needle at the front part of the small curving probing scalpel (Fig. 15－1)into the external orifice of the anal fistula. When the finger in digital examination touches the internal orifice, let the probe get out of the internal orifice. If the internal orifice is below the rectal ring (dentate line), then bend the probe to let it getting out of the anus, and incise the fistula canal with the curving scalpel. If the internal orifice is above the rectal ring, then hold up thick silk thread at the rectal ring to avoid injuring the sphincter. The part of the fistula lower than the rectal ring should be incised with the curving scalpel.

【功能】　探针小弯刀可将术中的探查、切开、挂线同步完成。

Function：With the small curving probing scalpel one can furnish the procedures of examination, incision, and seton drainage in one operation.

（二）钩状小针刀

2. Hook Style Acupuncture Scalpel

【适应证】　肛窦炎、肛门裂、痉挛耻骨直肠肌、外括约肌皮下部。

Indication：anal sinusitis, anal fissure, spasm of puborectalis muscle, subcutaneous part of external sphincter.

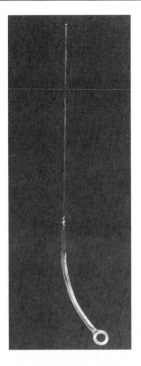

图 15 - 1 探针小弯刀
Figure 15 - 1 Small curving probing scalpel

【操作方法】

Procedure:

1. **肛窦炎** 在肛门镜下,用钩状小针刀(图 15 - 2),从肛窦上缘往下钩开肛,因肛窦敞开引流,故解除炎症。

(1) **Anal Sinusitis** Using the hook style scalpel (Fig. 15 - 2) under anoscopy, incise and drain the anal sinus valve to eliminate the infection.

2. **肛门裂** 将肛窦肛裂溃面及哨兵痔从上内至下外纵行钩割开。

(2) **Anal Fissure** Incise the ulcer portion of the sinus fissure and sentinel pile longitudinally from the upper internal part to the lower external part.

3. **痉挛耻骨直肠肌** 用示指先伸入肛管内,触及到痉挛耻骨直肠肌后缘(搁板征)。右手持钩状小针刀从肛门缘与尾骨尖之中间的皮肤插入并潜行纵深伸入,在肛管内手指导引下,将其痉挛耻骨直肌后缘往下钩割开,达松解仍原路退出钩状小针刀完成治疗。

(3) **Spasm of Puborectal Muscle** The doctor's index finger inserts into the anal canal, touching the posterior margin of spasmotic puborectal muscle. Then his right hand takes the curving probing scalpel to insert deeply from the skin at the midpoint between anal margin and coccyx tip, with the guidance of the finger in anal canal, incise the posterior margin of puborectal muscle downward till the feeling of release.

【功能】　钩状小针刀尖顶为探针头,侧面为钩刀,因此可将探查、钩割、切开同步完成。

Function：With a probing tip and curving knife, the curving probing scalpel can furnish the procedures of examination, curving cutting incision in one operation.

（三）斜面小针刀

3. Inclined Plane Acupuncture Scalpel

【适应证】　闭合切断内括约肌、切开肛门内脓肿、切开肛门内瘘、肛门瘙痒症。

Indication：To close cut internal sphincter, to incise anal abscess, to incise internal anal fistula, anal pruritus.

【操作方法】

Procedure：

1. **切断内括约肌**　先用斜面小针刀(图 15 - 3)的前端的探针头,插入尾骨尖与肛门缘连线的中点(即点状局麻的针眼)在肛指的导引下,将内括约肌纵行闭合切开、松解,即可从原路退出。

（1）**To Cut Internal Sphincter**　Insert the probe tip of curving probing scalpel to the midpoint between the coccyx tip and the anal margin（i. e. the needle point of anesthesia injection）, then with the guidance of the finger in anal canal, close cut longitudinally the internal sphincter till the feeling of release.

2. **切开肛门内脓肿**　在肛门镜下将脓肿纵行由下往上切开引流。

（2）**To Incise Internal Abscess**　With the anoscope to incise longitudinally from lower to upper part of the abscess and drain.

3. **切开肛门内瘘**　在肛门镜下,将内瘘用斜面小针刀由瘘口插入、切开即可。

（3）**To Incise Internal Anal Fistula**　During anoscopy to incise the fistula with the inclined plane acupuncture scalpel.

4. **肛门瘙痒症**　将斜面小针刀插入皮下组织,割断神经末梢,用斜面小针刀呈扇形扫切。

（4）**To Treat Pruritus Ani**　To insert the inclined plane acupuncture scalpel into subcutaneous tissue to cut nervous endings.

【功能】　斜面小针刀可将探查与切开同步完成。

Function：With an inclined plane acupuncture scalpel the examination and incision can be furnished in one operation.

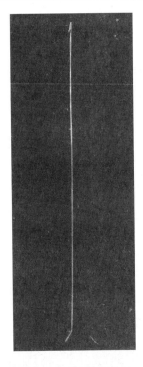
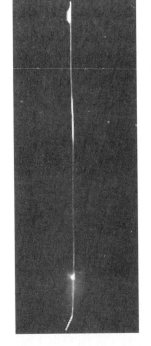

图 15 − 2　钩状小针刀　　　　　　　　图 15 − 3　斜面小针刀

Figure 15 − 2　Hook style acupuncture scalpel　　　Figure **15 − 3**　Inclined plane acupuncture scalpel

（四）刮匙小针刀
4. **Curette Acupuncture Scalpel**

【适应证】　肛门周围脓肿、肛门直肠硬结症和直肠内活检。

Indication:Perianal abscess, anorectal nodes, and intrarectal biopsy.

【操作方法】

Procedure:

1. **肛门脓肿**　先用刮匙小针刀(图 15 − 4)由脓肿下缘垂直插入,旋转一圈,使切口呈圆洞形,继之在深插后在脓肿上缘穿出再旋转一圈,完成第 2 个洞形开口。将粗线系在刮匙小针刀颈部,并由原路退出刮匙小针刀,剪断系在刮匙小针刀颈部粗线,并打成线圈,起(两个洞或切口)挂线、引流作用。

（1）**Perianal Abscess**　Insert the curette acupuncture scalpel (Fig. 15 − 4) vertically at the lower margin of abscess and turn around to make a circular hole, then insert deeper to reach the upper margin and turn around again to make a second hole. Tie the scalpel neck with a silk thread and make a thread ring to drain the pus.

2. **硬结症**　在肛门镜下,由刮匙小针刀顺时针旋转,直接切割直肠硬结症。

（2）**Anorectal Nodes**　With the aid of anoscopy insert the curette acupuncture scalpel and turn clockwise to cut the node.

3. **直肠内活检**　在肛门镜下将需活检组织先用刮匙小针刀前端探针头部插入,随之顺时针旋转切入刮匙中活检组织。退出肛门,倒入甲醛液中,送病理。

（3）**Intrarectal Biopsy**　With the aid of anoscopy insert the curette acupuncture scalpel and turn clockwise to cut off the tissue for biopsy.

【功能】　洞式切口、挂线引流、取病检同步完成。

Function:Hole-like incision, threading drainage and biopsy can be done in one operation.

（五）探针双面小针刀
5. **Probing Double-Edged Acupuncture Scalpel**

【适应证】　直肠后壁癌和肛门外多发窦道硬皮。

Indication:Cancer at posterior wall of rectum and extraanal multiple sinuses hard skin.

【操作方法】

Procedure:

1. **直肠后壁癌**　先将探针头(图 15 – 5)插入骶前筋膜与直肠固有筋膜间隙,双面刀深切,扩大间隙。探针头部从肿瘤下缘探出,在上探头针眼系上粗线,然后双面小针刀从原路退出,粗线留置间隙中打滑结扣,顺粗线下滑勒割肿瘤自骶前筋膜并分离开,而不要损伤骶前静脉丛。

（1）**Cancer at Posterior Wall of Rectum**　Insert the probe（Fig. 15 – 5）into the space between presacral fascia and rectal proper fascia and cut deeply with the double-edged scalpel to enlarge the space. Tie the scalpel tip with a silk thread making knot, and pull out the tumor without injuring the presacral venous plexus.

2. **肛门外多发窦道**　先用探针从窦道或硬皮下缘探人,即用双面刀切开。

（2）**Extraanal Multiple Sinuses**　Insert the probing Scalpel from the sinus or lower margin of hard skin and cut with the double-edged acupuncture scalpel.

【功能】　将探查、切开、挂线与分离同步完成。

Function:Examination, incision, threading and separation can be done in one operation.

（六）挑穴小针刀
6. **Pricking Acupuncture Scalpel**

【适应证】　内外痔和肛瘘。

Indication:Internal and External hemorrhoids, anal fistulae.

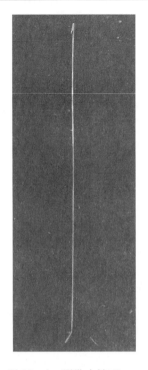

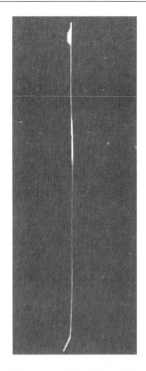

图 15 - 4　刮匙小针刀　　　　　　　图 15 - 5　探针双面小针刀

Figure 15 - 4　Curette acupuncture scalpel　　　Figure 15 - 5　Probing double-edged acupuncture scalpel

适用于内痔、外痔、肛瘘等。挑治腰背部穴位(图 15 - 6)。只是对症治疗便血、疼痛等。

Procedure：Picking acupuncture points at the dorsal and lumbar regions (Fig. 15 - 6), indicated for bloody defecation and pain over anal region.

(七)钩头小针
7. Small Hook Tip Acupuncture

【适应证】　肛门松弛症和肛门术后溢液。

Indication：Loosing anus, effusion of anus postoperatively.

【操作方法】　于尾骨尖与肛门中点距肛门缘约 1.5cm 处先点状局麻,将钩头小针(图 15 - 7)从点状局麻针眼插入肛门缘皮肤,从肛门外括约肌皮下环钩挑出肛门外。用羊肠线对拢结扎,缩小肛门环。再原针眼送回,外敷创口贴。

Procedure：Local point anesthesia at 1.5cm away from the midpoint between the coccyx tip and center of anus. Insert the small hook tip acupuncture (Fig. 15 - 7) from the anesthesia point into subcutaneous tissue near the anus and hook out of the anus from the subcutaneous ring of external anal sphincter.

【功能】　针眼微创,可将肛门口缩紧。

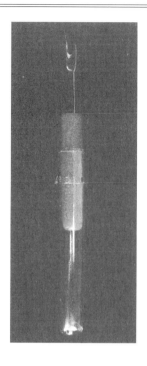

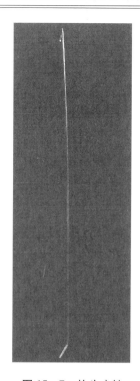

图 15 − 6　挑穴小针刀

Figure 15 − 6　Pricking Acupuncture Scalpel

图 15 − 7　钩头小针

Figure 15 − 7 Small hook tip acupuncture

Function：Constriction of the anus by the minimal wound. Thread embedding by small hook tip acupuncture.

（八）钩针埋线

8. **Hook Style Head Acupuncture with Hanging Thread**

【适应证】　结肠炎、肛门病等。

Indication：Colitis and other diseases of anus.

【操作方法】　将结肠炎或肛门病相对应的体表穴位消毒、涂搽，丁卡因表皮麻醉。用钩针(图15−8)从穴位一端插入，再由另一端穿出，用羊肠线结扎钩针头部，然后原路退回钩针，羊肠线留置穴位内。

Procedure：Local acupuncture points for colitis and other diseases giving superficial anesthesia with Dicaine. Insert the thread embedding hook tip scalpel from one end of acupuncture point to the other end getting out, leave a catgut in the point(Fig. 15−8).

【功能】　通过针眼，埋入羊肠线治疗结肠炎、肛门病。

Function：Leaving catgut to treat colitis and other anal diseases.

（九）双挂线探针

9. Double Threading Probe

用于肛肠病,尤其肛瘘探查挂双线。将探针(图 15 – 9)插入肛门瘘或肛门脓肿腔内,探查或引流,探针头与探针尾端可各挂线引流。

Indication：Anorectal diseases. Procedure：Insert the probe（Fig. 15 – 9）into the anal fistula or abscess. Double threading can be set at both ends of the probe. Function：Examination and drainage can be done.

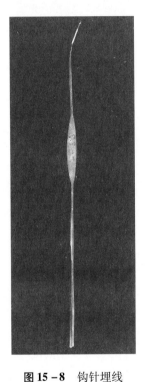

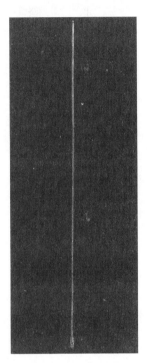

图 15 – 8　钩针埋线

Figure 15 – 8　Hooking and threading

图 15 – 9　双挂线探针

Figure 15 – 9　Double threading probe

（十）弯头负压吸力式套扎枪[（专利号第 469197 号）]见图 15 – 10

10. Curve Tip Negative Pressure Absorption Lasso Pistol [（Patent No. 469197）]（Fig. 15 – 10）

（1）使用前后,枪头用乙醇碘伏棉球消毒,用 50ml 注射器吸入消毒液,自枪尾胶管人端将消毒液由枪口推出。一则消毒,二则通畅。

（1）Asepsis of pistol tip with iodine alcohol cotton ball. Using a 50ml syringe, absorb aseptic solution at the back of pistol and push the solution through the plastic tube to get out of the pistol at the front orifice.

（2）检查枪口凹处与"顶针"应纠正或检查。在同一纵沟中,胶圈应置枪口凹,顶针前侧,可同时套入 2 个胶圈。没创伤、安全、有效。

（2）To examine the concave portion of pistol orifice and "roof needle". In the same longitudinal sulcus the rubber ring should be put in the concave portion. Two rubber rings can be put at the front of roof needle.

（3）在肛门镜下,将被套入的内痔、息肉、乳头瘤,或直肠黏膜脱垂。一定要将弯枪头口稍加压扣入基底层(肛垫)组织。勿只扣一半,因不完全扣入易可引起术后出血或复发。当完全扣入枪口中,助手再用 50ml 注射器一次性"外吸",并固定枪头。再扣动一扳机,胶圈即套扎入基底部。如发出"喳喳"的声音,则说明漏气,勿再套扎。应检查枪尾管紧否,应纠正枪口是否往下,加压使完全扣入。

（3）Under anoscopy relax the lassoed internal hemorrhoid, polyp, papilloma or rectal mucosal prolapse. The curve pistol tip should be gently pressed to join completely in the basal tissue（anal base）. Then the assistant does absorption once again with the syringe and fix the pistol tip. When the trigger is pushed, the rubber ring will be pushed to the bottom to encircle the lesion mass.

（4）治疗可以重复进行,1 个月内最好分 3~4 次完成多个痔核的治疗。套扎后,组织 5~7 天干枯,脱掉自行随粪便排出。

（4）The lassoed hemorrhoid mass will be withered and dried-up in 5~7 days and be expelled out with the stool. Repeated treatment can be done 3 or 4 times in a month.

（5）用枪套扎"内痔"后,再往套扎住的内痔上端,注入消痔灵液(用蓝心针管,消痔灵加入 1% 利多卡因,共计 1ml)使痔核隆起。一则套扎胶圈更紧;二则痔核产生无菌纤维化粘连,可防止术后出血和感染。

（5）"Xiao Zhi Ling" solution and 1% Lidocaine in total 1ml can be injected into the lassoed hemorrhoid.

（十一）圆头缺口电池灯肛门镜
11. Anoscope with Battery Light and Notch Round Opening

使用说明如下(图 15-11)。

Procedure（Fig. 15-11）.

（1）将肛门镜芯的横针拔出,插头部固定。

（1）Pull out the central part of anoscope, fix the plug.

（2）圆头缺口肛门镜头部对准需治疗内痔的一侧,以利痔核突人肛门镜缺口处和暴露。

（2）Turn the notch opening to expose the hemorrhoidal mass to be treated.

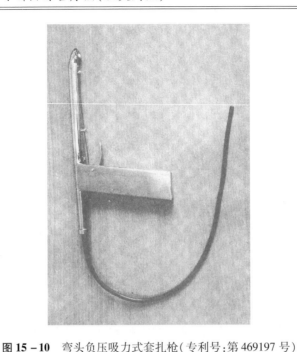

图 15 – 10 弯头负压吸力式套扎枪(专利号:第 469197 号)

Figure 15 – 10 Curve tip negative pressure absorption lasso pistol (Patent No. 469197)

(3)往后按肛门镜电池灯的红色开关。

(3) Switch on the battery light and perform the planned procedure.

(4)使用后,肛门镜常规消毒,但电池灯把先顺时针往后、往下,朝前扣出卡片框。灯泡头顺其自然一同退出。勿用手拨动灯泡头,以防扭断电线。再行消毒。

(4) After the operation, sterilize the anoscope routinely. The battery light should be turned clockwise backward and downward, the card frame being taken forward out together with the light bulb.

(5)往上拔电灯泡头的基底部金属盖,更换新的电池灯泡。

(5) Exchanging batteries and bulbs can be done by pulling out the metallic cover.

(6)电池灯把上盖上拔,更换电池。

(6) The battery light should be sterilized by iodine alcohol gauge rubbing or by steaming heat of Realgar.

(7)电池灯把用碘伏擦抹,或雄黄蒸熏消毒。

(7) The battery light handle should be wiped with iodophor, or sterilized by realgar fumigation.

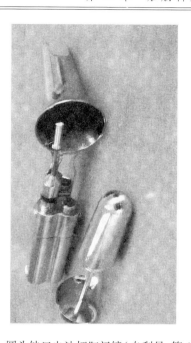

图 15 – 11　圆头缺口电池灯肛门镜(专利号:第 468052 号)

Figure 15 – 11　Anoscope with battery light and notch round opening (Patent No. 468052)

（十二）肛肠多功能检查手术床

12. **Multifunctional Anorectal Examination and Operation Table**

使用说明如下:用于肛肠手术或换药,也可用于妇科或外科手术。取半坐位下躺,骶尾部板可以手摇顶起,利于肛肠病变术中显露,此后下降为凹陷,便于冲洗。手术器械盘可置于床下,医师坐凳操作,可自选合适位置,方便快捷。腿架可自由外展,并可加大外旋角度,利于显露肛门疾患(图 15 – 12,图 15 – 13)。

Procedure:For anorectal operations or dressing change, or gynecologic or surgical operations, patient at semireclining position, the sacrococcygeal plate of the table can be elevated to fascilitate exposure of anorectal lesions, and lowering the plate may favor the irrigation. Surgical instrument plate can be put under the table. The surgeon can work upon sitting. The leg frames may be extended laterally to give better exposure(Fig. 15 – 12, Fig. 15 – 13).

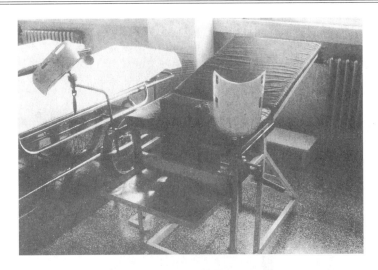

图 15 - 12　肛肠多功能检查手术床(1)

Figure 15 - 12　Multiple function anorectal examination and operation table（1）

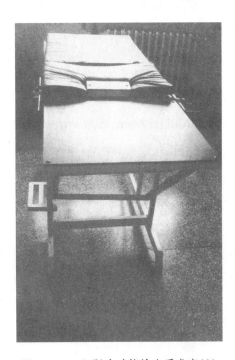

图 15 - 13　肛肠多功能检查手术床(2)

Figure 15 - 13　Multiple function anorectal examination and operation table（2）

二、专利证书

II. Patent Certificates

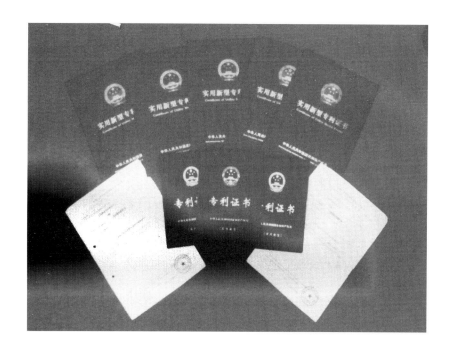

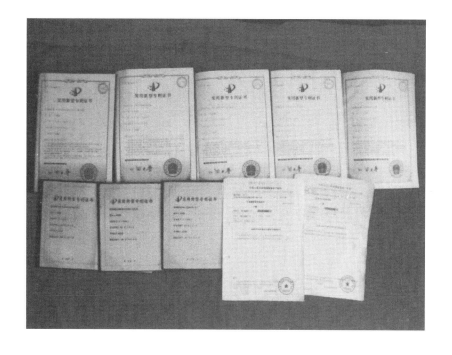

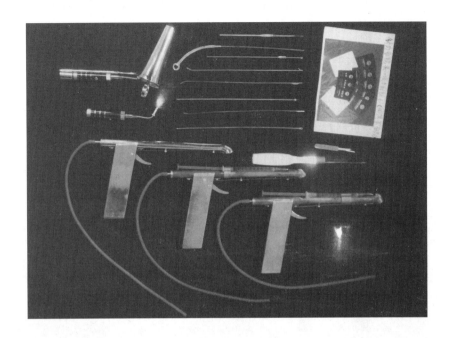

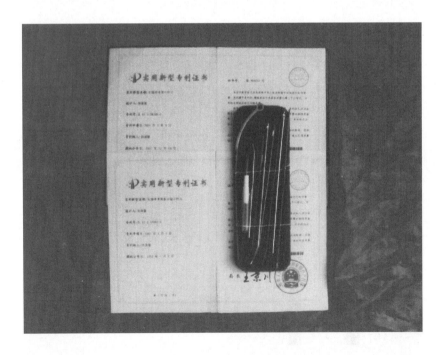

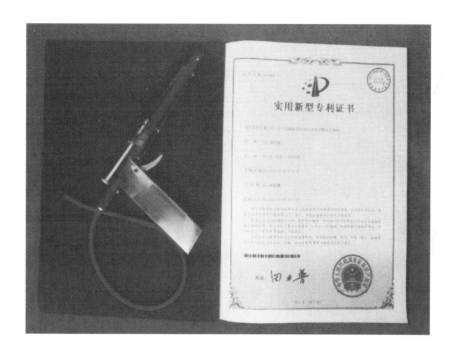

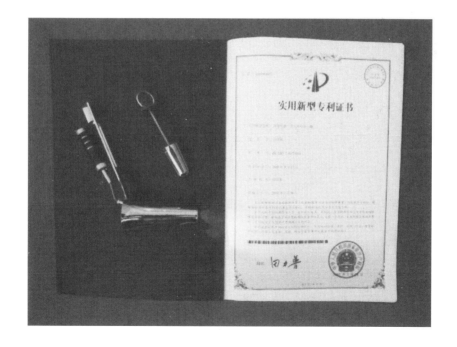

实用新型专利证书

实用新型名称: 弯头负压吸压力式套扎枪

设计人: 田淇第

专利号: ZL 01 2 08298.8

专利申请日: 2001 年 3 月 9 日

专利权人: 田淇第

授权公告日: 2001 年 12 月 19 日

第 1 页(共 1 页)

证书号　　第 469197 号

　　本实用新型经过本局依照中华人民共和国专利法进行初步审查,决定授予专利权,颁发本证书并在专利登记簿上予以登记.专利权自授权公告之日起生效.

　　本专利的专利权期限为十年,自申请日起算.专利权人应当依照专利法及其实施细则规定缴纳年费.缴纳本专利年费的期限是每年 3 月 9 日 前一个月内.未按照规定缴纳年费的,专利权自应当缴纳年费期满之日起终止.

　　专利证书记载专利权登记时的法律状况.专利权的转移、质押、无效、终止、恢复和专利权人的姓名或名称、国籍、地址变更等事项记载在专利登记簿上.

专利号 ‖‖‖‖‖‖‖‖‖‖‖‖‖‖‖‖‖‖

局长 王景川

二○○一年十二月十九日

实用新型专利证书

实用新型名称: 肛肠手术用小针刀

设计人: 田淇第

专利号: ZL 01 2 08300.3

专利申请日: 2001 年 3 月 9 日

专利权人: 田淇第

授权公告日: 2001 年 12 月 19 日

第 1 页(共 1 页)

证书号　　第 468052 号

　　本实用新型经过本局依照中华人民共和国专利法进行初步审查,决定授予专利权,颁发本证书并在专利登记簿上予以登记.专利权自授权公告之日起生效.

　　本专利的专利权期限为十年,自申请日起算.专利权人应当依照专利法及其实施细则规定缴纳年费.缴纳本专利年费的期限是每年 3 月 9 日 前一个月内.未按照规定缴纳年费的,专利权自应当缴纳年费期满之日起终止.

　　专利证书记载专利权登记时的法律状况.专利权的转移、质押、无效、终止、恢复和专利权人的姓名或名称、国籍、地址变更等事项记载在专利登记簿上.

专利号 ‖‖‖‖‖‖‖‖‖‖‖‖‖‖‖‖‖‖

局长 王景川

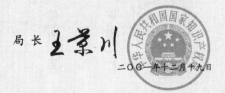

二○○一年十二月十九日

中华人民共和国国家知识产权局

地址：北京市海淀区蓟门桥西土城路6号　　国家知识产权局专利局受理处　　邮政编码：100088

邮政编码：300192 天津市南开区科研西路2号（科技园区）金辉大厦5楼　　2G **天津市专利事务所** **卢枫** 申请号：　01109666.7	发文日期： 2001年7月27日

申请号：　01109666.7	申请人：　田淇第

发明创造名称：外痔贴

发明专利申请初步审查合格通知书

1. 上述专利申请经初步审查，符合专利法及其实施细则的规定。

2. 根据专利法第三十四条规定，上述专利申请自申请日起满十八个月即行公布。

提示：

　　发明专利申请人可以自申请日起三年内提出实审请求，并同时缴纳审查费，申请人逾期不请求实质审查的或逾期不缴纳审查费的，该申请即被视为撤回。

审查员：	审查部门： 初审及流程管理部

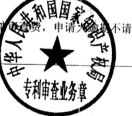

2123 — 1

实用新型专利证书

实用新型名称: 肛肠手术用多功能小针刀

设计人: 田淇第

专利号: ZL 01 2 07802.6

专利申请日: 2001 年 3 月 9 日

专利权人: 田淇第

授权公告日: 2002 年 1 月 2 日

第 1 页（共 1 页）

证书号　　第 471228 号

　　本实用新型经过本局依照中华人民共和国专利法进行初步审查，决定授予专利权，颁发本证书并在专利登记簿上予以登记、专利权自授权公告之日起生效.

　　本专利的专利权期限为十年，自申请日起算，专利权人应当依照专利法及其实施细则规定缴纳年费。缴纳本专利年费的期限是每年 3 月 9 日前一个月内。未按照规定缴纳年费的，专利权自应当缴纳年费期满之日起终止.

　　专利证书记载专利权登记时的法律状况，专利权的转移、质押、无效、终止、恢复和专利权人的姓名或名称、国籍、地址变更等事项记载在专利登记簿上.

专利号 ||||||||||||||||||||||

局长 王景川

二〇〇二年一月二日

中华人民共和国国家知识产权局

地址：北京市海淀区蓟门桥西土城路6号　　国家知识产权局专利局受理处　　邮政编码：100088

邮政编码：300192 天津市南开区科研西路金辉大厦611室 **天津德赛律师事务所** **卢枫**		2G	发文日期： 2002年12月27日
申请号：02148657.3			

申请号： 02148657.3	申请人： 田洪第
发明创造名称：肛肠激光小针刀	

发明专利申请初步审查合格通知书

1. 上述专利申请经初步审查，符合专利法及其实施细则的规定。

2. 根据专利法第三十四条规定，上述专利申请自申请日起满十八个月即行公布。

提示：

　　发明专利申请人可以自申请日起三年内提出实审请求，并同时缴纳实审费，申请人逾期不请求实质审查的或逾期不缴纳审查费的，该申请即被视为撤回。

审查员：	审查部门： 　　初审及流程管理部	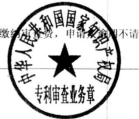

2123 — 1

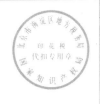

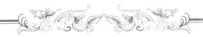

实用新型专利证书

实用新型名称：多功能检查手术治疗床

设　计　人：田淇第

专　利　号：ZL 2005 2 0027317.0

专利申请日：2005 年 9 月 12 日

专利权人：田淇第

授权公告日：2007 年 1 月 24 日

　　本实用新型经过本局依照中华人民共和国专利法进行初步审查，决定授予专利权，颁发本证书并在专利登记簿上予以登记。专利权自授权公告之日起生效。

　　本专利的专利权期限为十年，自申请日起算。专利权人应当依照专利法及其实施细则规定缴纳年费。缴纳本专利年费的期限是每年 9 月 12 日前一个月内。未按照规定缴纳年费的，专利权自应当缴纳年费期满之日起终止。

　　专利证书记载专利权登记时的法律状况。专利权的转移、质押、无效、终止、恢复和专利权人的姓名或名称、国籍、地址变更等事项记载在专利登记簿上。

局长　田力普

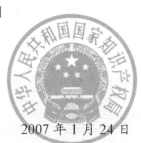

2007 年 1 月 24 日

第 1 页（共 1 页）

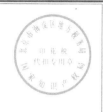

证书号 第884840号

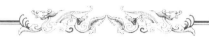

实用新型专利证书

实用新型名称：自带电源一体式组合肛门镜

设　计　人：田淇第

专　利　号：ZL 2005 2 0027316.6

专利申请日：2005 年 9 月 12 日

专利权人：田淇第

授权公告日：2007 年 3 月 28 日

　　本实用新型经过本局依照中华人民共和国专利法进行初步审查，决定授予专利权、颁发本证书并在专利登记簿上予以登记。专利权自授权公告之日起生效。

　　本专利的专利权期限为十年，自申请日起算。专利权人应当依照专利法及其实施细则规定缴纳年费。缴纳本专利年费的期限是每年9月12日前一个月内。未按照规定缴纳年费的，专利权自应当缴纳年费期满之日起终止。

　　专利证书记载专利权登记时的法律状况。专利权的转移、质押、无效、终止、恢复和专利权人的姓名或名称、国籍、地址变更等事项记载在专利登记簿上。

局长 田力普

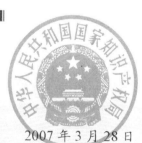

2007 年 3 月 28 日

第 1 页（共 1 页）

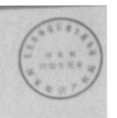

证书号第1586451号

实用新型专利证书

实用新型名称:自带冷光源的肛肠腔内多功能小针刀

发　明　人:田淇第

专　利　号:ZL 2010 2 0139503.4

专利申请日:2010 年 03 月 24 日

专利权人:田淇第

授权公告日:2010 年 11 月 17

　　本实用新型经过本局依照中华人民共和国专利法进行初步审查,决定授予专利权,颁发本证书并在专利登记簿上予以登记。专利权自授权公告之日起生效。

　　本专利的专利权期限为十年,自申请日起算。专利权人应当依照专利法及其实施细则规定缴纳年费。本专利年费应当在每年 03 月 24 日前缴纳。未按照规定缴纳年费的,专利权自应当缴纳年费期满之日起终止。

　　专利证书记载专利权登记时的法律状况。专利权的转移、质押、无效、终止、恢复和专利权人的姓名或名称、国籍、地址变更等事项记载在专利登记簿上。

局长　田力普

2010 年 11 月 17 日

第 1 页 (共 1 页)

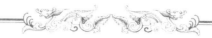

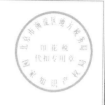

证书号第 1586449 号

实用新型专利证书

实用新型名称：卡带冷光源的腔内注射器

发　明　人：田淇第

专　利　号：ZL 2010 2 0139501.5

专利申请日：2010 年 03 月 24 日

专利权人：田淇第

授权公告日：2010 年 11 月 17 日

　　本实用新型经过本局依照中华人民共和国专利法进行初步审查，决定授予专利权，颁发本证书并在专利登记簿上予以登记。专利权自授权公告之日起生效。

　　本专利的专利权期限为十年，自申请日起算。专利权人应当依照专利法及其实施细则规定缴纳年费。本专利的年费应当在每年 03 月 24 日前缴纳。未按照规定缴纳年费的，专利权自应当缴纳年费期满之日起终止。

　　专利证书记载专利权登记时的法律状况。专利权的转移、质押、无效、终止、恢复和专利权人的姓名或名称、国籍、地址变更等事项记载在专利登记簿上。

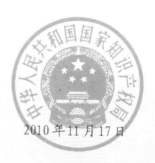

局长　田力普

2010 年 11 月 17 日

证书号 第1859429号

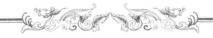

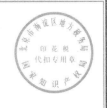

实用新型专利证书

实用新型名称：用于治疗肛肠疾患的弯头式负压吸扎注射枪

发　明　人：田淇第

专　利　号：ZL 2010 2 0642350.5

专利申请日：2010 年 12 月 03 日

专利权人：田淇第

授权公告日：2011 年 07 月 13 日

　　本实用新型经过本局依照中华人民共和国专利法进行初步审查，决定授予专利权，颁发本证书并在专利登记簿上予以登记。专利权自授权公告之日起生效。

　　本专利的专利权期限为十年，自申请日起算。专利权人应当依照专利法及其实施细则规定缴纳年费。本专利的年费应当在每年 12 月 03 日前缴纳。未按照规定缴纳年费的，专利权自应当缴纳年费期满之日起终止。

　　专利证书记载专利权登记时的法律状况。专利权的转移、质押、无效、终止、恢复和专利权人的姓名或名称、国籍、地址变更等事项记载在专利登记簿上。

局长　田力普

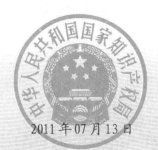

2011 年 07 月 13 日